Key Questions in
CARDIAC SURGERY

Narain Moorjani

Nicola Viola

Sunil K. Ohri

Foreword by And

tfm Publishing Limited, Castle Hill Barns, Harley, Nr Shrewsbury, SY5 6LX, UK. Tel: +44 (0)1952 510061; Fax: +44 (0)1952 510192
E-mail: nikki@tfmpublishing.com; Web site: www.tfmpublishing.com

Design & Typesetting:	Nikki Bramhill BSc Hons Dip Law
First Edition:	© March 2011
Reprinted:	December 2011

ISBN: 978 1 903378 69 4

Printed by Gutenberg Press Ltd., Gudja Road, Tarxien, PLA 19, Malta. Tel: +356 21897037; Fax: +356 21800069.

Contents

iv

Preface

Cardiac surgery is a continually expanding field with the development of novel techniques and operations as well as the refinement of well-established surgical procedures. These developments fuel the demand for knowledge regarding cardiac surgical disease processes and the optimal therapeutic strategies currently available. Although several large volume texts exist, there are very few which aim to deliver this knowledge base in one concise book. *Key Questions in Cardiac Surgery* systematically covers all the main topics involved in the contemporary practice of an adult cardiac surgeon using numerous illustrations to enhance the reader's understanding.

In keeping with modern practice, the data and body of knowledge presented is strictly evidence-based. The book incorporates the current guidelines for practice from the American Heart Association and European Society of Cardiology, with up-to-date information based on current scientific literature. Each chapter contains important references for further reading and greater in-depth study. All the chapters have been written by a cardiac surgeon who has recently undertaken cardiothoracic examinations and reviewed by a cardiothoracic surgery examiner. Uniquely, the images have been drawn by a cardiac surgeon from an operative perspective.

This book is relevant to all cardiac surgical trainees and residents, at any stage of their training programme, as it provides them with the necessary knowledge base to carry out their daily duties. Adult cardiologists, cardiothoracic intensive care unit specialists, nursing staff, physiotherapists and other allied professionals working with adult cardiac patients, either pre-operatively or postoperatively, will also find this book key to facilitating their understanding of the principles surrounding adult cardiac surgical disease management. Importantly, the book is also an ideal revision aid for trainees and residents undertaking their cardiothoracic surgery board examinations around the world. Its concise yet complete coverage of the important topics make it the perfect guide to answer the

Key Questions in Cardiac Surgery that are often asked within the confines of an examination. The style and content of the book allow the reader to obtain information in an easily accessible format.

Narain Moorjani MB ChB, MRCS, MD, FRCS (C-Th)
Department of Cardiothoracic Surgery
Hahnemann University Hospital
Drexel University College of Medicine
Philadelphia, USA
Nicola Viola MD
The Hospital for Sick Children
University of Toronto
Toronto, Ontario
Canada
Sunil K. Ohri MD, FRCS (Eng, Ed & CTh), FESC
Department of Cardiothoracic Surgery
Wessex Cardiothoracic Centre
Southampton University Hospital
Southampton, UK

Foreword

There are many ways to learn a subject. A traditional method is to read and review a large body of visual material and, having performed that exercise, to be subjected to testing to see what has been learned. Unfortunately, when the body of knowledge is large, it is sometimes unclear as to the relevance of individual items as they are perused. The consequence may be inordinate amounts of time spent on inconsequential bits of knowledge at the expense of the most critical components of the subject matter.

In his textbook, *Key Questions in Cardiac Surgery*, Narain Moorjani, writing from the vantage point of one who has recently undertaken specialty exams following completion of his cardiac surgery training, provides a most interesting alternative. Specifically, the work of determining the most critical aspects of the body of knowledge has been thoroughly reviewed and questions are asked as a teaching tool without the antecedent didactics. In this system, there is no uncertainty as to the elements that are regarded as important for the student. The text in this book is accompanied by very useful illustrations and photographs. Once again these visual tools are pointedly related to the question surrounding the anatomic or disease process. I have found this a rather fun way to test my own knowledge, even though I have been practicing cardiac surgery for thirty-five years and teaching residents during most of that time. The danger of a question and answer approach to learning or knowledge testing is the presence of ambiguity in either the questions or the answers. Reassuringly, such instances are remarkably rare in this book and it is clear that important forethought was given to the formulation of the test items. Moreover, there is a strong didactic component to the text because the answers to the question are brief, to the point and authoritative.

The strength of this book lies in one of the important words in the title, that being 'key': it focuses on the essential information that every cardiac surgeon should have at their fingertips. For this reason, I believe the book is particularly appropriate for those in the late stages of their training or the early stages of their practicing career.

Andrew S. Wechsler, M.D.
Stanley K. Brockman Professor and Chairman
Department of Cardiothoracic Surgery
Hahnemann University Hospital
Drexel University College of Medicine
Philadelphia, USA
Editor Emeritus, *The Journal of Thoracic and Cardiovascular Surgery*

Acknowledgements

We would like to thank and acknowledge the consultant surgeons at Southampton General Hospital, Southampton, UK (Mr Steven Livesey, Mr Marcus Haw, Mr Geoffrey Tsang and Mr Clifford Barlow) and the attending surgeons at Hahnemann University Hospital, Drexel College of Medicine, Philadelphia, USA (Professor Andrew Wechsler, Dr John Entwistle, Dr Percy Boateng) for imparting the knowledge described in this book and also for the opportunity to take the operative photographs.

As regards some of the individual chapters, we are grateful to Professor John Morgan, Dr Alison Calver, Dr Steven Harden, Dr Ivan Brown, Dr Arthur Yue, Dr Michael Rubens and Dr James Shambrook for their images. In particular, we would like to thank Dr Tom Pierce for access to his collection of electrocardiograms. We are grateful to Edwards Lifesciences and Eurosets Medical Devices for permission to reprint their copyrighted images.

Finally, we are deeply indebted to Nikki Bramhill of TFM Publishing, whose enthusiasm, endless patience and hard work has resulted in the production of this cardiac text.

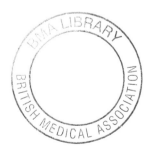

Abbreviations

AC	assist control
ACC	American College of Cardiology
ACEI	angiotensin-converting enzyme inhibitor
ACS	acute coronary syndrome
ACT	activated clotting time
ADH	anti-diuretic hormone
ADP	adenosine diphosphate
AF	atrial fibrillation
AHA	American Heart Association
AL	anterior leaflet of the tricuspid valve
ALT	alanine transaminase
AMVL	anterior mitral valve leaflet
ANP	atrial natriuretic peptide
AoV	aortic valve
AP	anteroposterior
APTTR	activated partial thromboplastin time ratio
AR	aortic regurgitation
ARB	angiotensin II receptor blocker
ARDS	adult respiratory distress syndrome
ART	Arterial Revascularisation Trial
ARTS	Arterial Revascularisation Therapies Study
AS	aortic stenosis
ASA	American Society of Anesthesiologists
ASH	asymmetrical septal hypertrophy
AST	aspartate aminotransferase
AT	acceleration time
ATG	anti-thymocyte globulin
ATLS®	Advanced Trauma Life Support
ATP	adenosine triphosphate
AVA	aortic valve area
AVN	atrioventricular node
AVR	aortic valve replacement
BARI	Bypass Angioplasty Revascularisation Investigation
BNP	brain natriuretic peptide
BP	blood pressure
BSA	body surface area
Ca	calcium
CABG	coronary artery bypass grafting

cAMP	cyclic adenosine monophosphate
CAPRIE	Clopidogrel versus Aspirin in Patients at Risk of Ischaemic Events
CASS	Coronary Artery Surgery Study
CBF	coronary blood flow
CHARM	Candesartan in Heart Failure Assessment of Reduction in Mortality and Morbidity
CI	cardiac index
Cl	chloride
CK	creatinine kinase
CK-MB	creatinine kinase MB isoenzyme
CMV	cytomegalovirus
CO	cardiac output
CO_2	carbon dioxide
COCPIT	Comparative Outcome and Clinical Profiles in Transplantation
CONSENSUS	Cooperative North Scandinavian Enalapril Survival Study
COPD	chronic obstructive pulmonary disease
COPERNICUS	Carvedilol Prospective Randomised Cumulative Survival
CP	constrictive pericarditis
CPAP	continuous positive airway pressure
CPB	cardiopulmonary bypass
Cr	creatinine
CS	coronary sinus
CSA	cross-sectional area
C-SMART	Cardiomyoplasty-Skeletal Muscle Assist Randomised Trial
CT	computed tomography
CURE	Clopidogrel in Unstable Angina to Prevent Recurrent Events
CVA	cerebrovascular accident
CVP	central venous pressure
Cx	circumflex artery
CXR	chest X-ray
DBP	diastolic blood pressure
DC	direct current
DES	drug-eluting stent
DFP	diastolic filling period
DHCA	deep hypothermic circulatory arrest
ECG	electrocardiogram
ECSS	European Coronary Surgery Study
EEG	electroencephalogram
EF	ejection fraction
EOAI	effective orifice area index

EROA	effective regurgitant orifice area
ESC	European Society of Cardiology
$ETCO_2$	end-tidal carbon dioxide
ETT	exercise tolerance test
FDG	fluorodeoxyglucose
FEV_1	forced expiratory volume in 1 second
FFP	fresh frozen plasma
FFR	fractional flow reserve
FiO_2	inspired oxygen concentration
FRISC	Fragmin in Unstable Coronary Artery Disease Study
FS	fractional shortening
GTN	glyceryl trinitrate
Hb	haemoglobin
Hct	haematocrit
HFSS	heart failure survival score
HLA	human leucocyte antigen
HMG	3-hydroxy-3-methylglutaryl
HOCM	hypertrophic obstructive cardiomyopathy
HR	heart rate
HS	heart sound
HU	Houndsfield units
IABP	intra-aortic balloon pump
I:E	inspiration: expiration ratio
IL	interleukin
IMAGE	International Multicenter Aprotinin Graft Patency Experience
IMV	intermittent mandatory ventilation
INR	international normalized ratio
ISHLT	International Society for Heart and Lung Transplantation
ITU	intensive therapy unit
IV	intravenous
IVC	inferior vena cava
IVS	interventricular septum
IVUS	intravascular ultrasound
JVP	jugular venous pulse; jugular venous pressure
K	potassium
LA	left atrium
LAA	left atrial appendage
LAD	left anterior descending (coronary artery)
LAHB	left anterior hemiblock
LAO	left anterior oblique
LAP	left atrial pressure
LBBB	left bundle branch block

LCC	left coronary cusp of the aortic valve
LCCA	left common carotid artery
LCS	left coronary sinus
LED	light emitting diode
LGL	Lown-Ganong-Levine
LICA	left internal carotid artery
LiDCO	lithium indicator dilution cardiac output
LIMA	left internal mammary artery
LIMV	left internal mammary vein
LIPV	left inferior pulmonary vein
LMCA	left main coronary artery
LMS	left main stem
LMWH	low-molecular-weight heparin
LPHB	left posterior hemiblock
LSPV	left superior pulmonary vein
LV	left ventricle
LVAD	left ventricular assist device
LVEDP	left ventricular end-diastolic pressure
LVEDV	left ventricular end-diastolic volume
LVEF	left ventricular ejection fraction
LVESV	left ventricular end-systolic volume
LVH	left ventricular hypertrophy
LVIDd	left ventricular internal diameter in diastole
LVIDs	left ventricular internal diameter in systole
LVM	left ventricular mass
LVMI	left ventricular mass index
LVOT	left ventricular outflow tract
LVOTO	left ventricular outflow tract obstruction
LVPW	left ventricular posterior wall
MACS	maximal aortic cusp separation
MADIT	Multicenter Automatic Defibrillator Implantation Trial
MAGIC	Myoblast Autologous Grafting in Ischaemic Cardiomyopathy
MAP	mean arterial pressure
MECC	minimal extracorporeal circulation
MI	myocardial infarction
MMF	mycophenolate mofetil
MPAP	mean pulmonary artery pressure
MR	mitral regurgitation
MRI	magnetic resonance imaging
MRSA	methicillin-resistant *Staphylococcus aureus*
MS	mitral stenosis
MUGA	multi-gated acquisition
MUSTIC	Multisite Stimulation in Cardiomyopathies
MV	mitral valve

MVA	mitral valve area
MVR	mitral valve replacement
Na	sodium
NCC	non-coronary cusp of the aortic valve
NICE	National Institute for Health and Clinical Excellence
NSTEMI	non-ST elevation myocardial infarction
NYHA	New York Heart Association
O_2	oxygen
OM	obtuse marginal artery
OPCAB	off-pump coronary artery bypass grafting
PA	pulmonary artery; posteroanterior
$PaCO_2$	partial pressure of carbon dioxide
PADP	pulmonary artery diastolic pressure
PaO_2	partial pressure of oxygen
PAP	pulmonary artery pressure
PASP	pulmonary artery systolic pressure
PAU	penetrating aortic ulcer
PAWP	pulmonary artery wedge pressure
PCI	percutaneous coronary intervention
PCV	pressure controlled ventilation
PDA	posterior descending (coronary) artery
PEA	pulseless electrical activity
PEEP	positive end expiratory pressure
PET	positron emission tomography
PHT	pressure half-time
PISA	proximal isovelocity surface area
PL	posterior leaflet of the tricuspid valve
PLSVC	persistent left superior vena cava
PMBV	percutaneous mitral balloon valvuloplasty
PMVL	posterior mitral valve leaflet
PPM	patient prosthesis mismatch
PS	pressure support (ventilation)
PTCA	percutaneous transluminal coronary (balloon) angioplasty
PV	pulmonary vein; pulmonary valve
PVC	polyvinyl chloride
PVR	pulmonary vascular resistance
PVRI	pulmonary vascular resistance index
PWT	posterior wall thickness
RA	right atrium
RAA	right atrial appendage
RALES	Randomized Aldactone Evaluation Study
RAO	right anterior oblique
RAP	right atrial pressure
RAPCO	Radial Artery Patency and Clinical Outcome

RBBB	right bundle branch block
RCA	right coronary artery
RCC	right coronary cusp of the aortic valve
RCCA	right common carotid artery
RCM	restrictive cardiomyopathy
RCS	right coronary sinus
RECA	right external carotid artery
REMATCH	Randomised Evaluation of Mechanical Assistance for the Treatment of Congestive Heart Failure
RESTORE	Reconstructive Endoventricular Surgery Returning Torsion Original Radius Elliptical Shape to the Left Ventricle
RICA	right internal carotid artery
RIMA	right internal mammary artery
RIPV	right inferior pulmonary vein
RITA	Randomised Intervention Treatment of Angina trial
ROOBY	Randomized On/Off Bypass Study
RPA	right pulmonary artery
RPV	right pulmonary vein
RR	respiratory rate
RSCA	right subclavian artery
RSPV	right superior pulmonary vein
RV	right ventricle
RVOT	right ventricular outflow tract
RVSP	right ventricular systolic pressure
SAM	systolic anterior motion (of the mitral valve)
SAN	sino-atrial node
SaO_2	arterial oxygen saturation
SAVER	Surgical Anterior Ventricular Endocardial Restoration
SBP	systolic blood pressure
SEP	systolic ejection period
SIADH	syndrome of inappropriate anti-diuretic hormone
SIMV	synchronised intermittent mandatory ventilation
SIRS	systemic inflammatory response syndrome
SL	septal leaflet of the tricuspid valve
SNP	sodium nitroprusside
SOLVD	Studies of Left Ventricular Dysfunction
SoS	Stent or Surgery
SPECT	single photon emission computed tomography
SR	sinus rhythm
STEMI	ST elevation myocardial infarction
STICH	Surgical Treatment for Ischaemic Heart Failure
SV	stroke volume
SVC	superior vena cava
SVD	structural valve deterioration

SVG	saphenous vein graft
SvO_2	mixed venous saturation
SVR	systemic vascular resistance; surgical ventricular restoration
SVRI	systemic vascular resistance index
SYNTAX	Synergy between PCI with TAXUS and Cardiac Surgery
SZA	solitary zone of apposition
TEG	thrombo-elastogram
TIMI	Thrombolysis in Myocardial Infarction
TM	tropomyosin
TMR	transmyocardial revascularisation
TOE	transoesophageal echocardiography
Tp	troponin
TR	tricuspid regurgitation
TS	tricuspid stenosis
TTE	transthoracic echocardiography
TV	tricuspid valve; tidal volume
TVA	tricuspid valve area
UA	unstable angina
UNOS	United Network for Organ Sharing
VA	Veterans Administration
VAC	vacuum-assisted closure
Val-HeFT	Valsartan in Heart Failure Trial
VSR	ventricular septal rupture
VTI	velocity time integral
WL	window level
WPW	Wolff-Parkinson-White
WW	window width
YAG	yttrium aluminium garnet

Recommendations and evidence

The classification of recommendations and the levels of evidence used in this book are taken from the American Heart Association guidelines:

Class I:	Conditions for which there is evidence or general agreement that a given procedure or treatment is beneficial, useful, and effective.
Class II:	Conditions for which there is conflicting evidence or a divergence of opinion about the usefulness/ efficacy of a procedure or treatment.
Class IIa:	Weight of evidence/opinion is in favour of usefulness/efficacy.
Class IIb:	Usefulness/efficacy is less well established by evidence/opinion.
Class III:	Conditions for which there is evidence or general agreement that a procedure/treatment is not useful/ effective and in some cases may be harmful.
Level of Evidence A:	Data derived from multiple randomised clinical trials or meta-analyses.
Level of Evidence B:	Data derived from a single randomised trial or non-randomised studies.
Level of Evidence C:	Only consensus opinion of experts, case studies, or standard-of-care.

Chapter 1

Cardiac anatomy

1 **Describe the anatomy of the coronary artery system (Figure 1)**

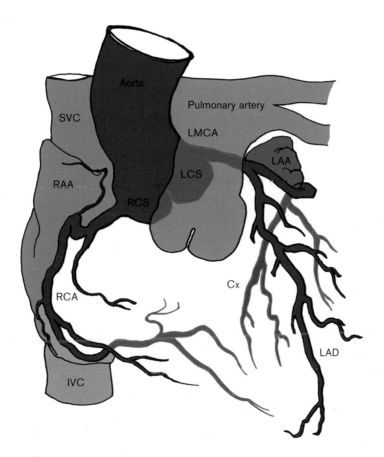

Figure 1. Coronary artery system. SVC = superior vena cava; RAA = right atrial appendage; IVC = inferior vena cava; RCS = right coronary sinus; RCA = right coronary artery; LCS = left coronary sinus; LMCA = left main coronary artery; LAA = left atrial appendage; Cx = circumflex artery; LAD = left anterior descending artery.

- The coronary artery system originates from the aortic root and consists of the left and right coronary arteries and their individual branches.
- The left coronary artery originates from the left coronary ostium as the left main stem and divides early into the left anterior descending artery (also known as the anterior interventricular artery) and circumflex artery (see below).
- The right coronary artery originates from the right coronary ostium and eventually terminates as the posterior descending artery (also known as the posterior interventricular artery) and posterior left ventricular artery (see below).

2 Describe the anatomy of the left main coronary artery (Figure 2)

- The left main coronary artery (left main stem) courses from the left coronary sinus of the aorta in an anterior and inferior direction between the pulmonary trunk and the left atrial appendage.
- It then divides into two major arteries of nearly equal diameter, the left anterior descending artery and the circumflex artery. Typically, no branches are seen before this bifurcation.

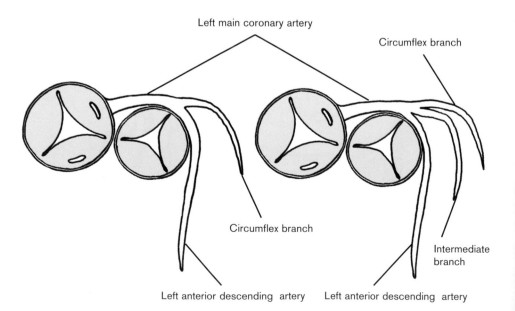

Figure 2. Bifurcation and trifurcation of the left main coronary artery.

- In some patients, the left main coronary artery trifurcates into the intermediate coronary artery (ramus intermedius), left anterior descending artery and circumflex artery.
- The left main coronary artery is typically 10-40mm in length but may be absent in patients with separate circumflex and left anterior descending coronary ostia.

3 **Describe the anatomy of the left anterior descending (LAD) artery (Figure 3)**
- The LAD artery courses anteriorly and inferiorly in the anterior inter-ventricular groove towards the apex of the heart.

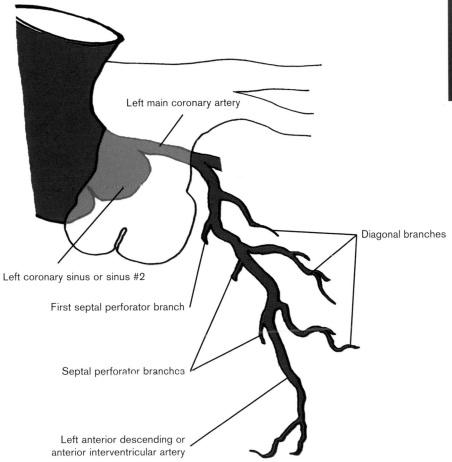

Left main coronary artery

Diagonal branches

Left coronary sinus or sinus #2

First septal perforator branch

Septal perforator branches

Left anterior descending or anterior interventricular artery

Figure 3. Left anterior descending (LAD) artery and its branches.

- Occasionally, the LAD continues around the apex to supply part of the posterior interventricular groove and rarely even replaces the posterior descending artery.
- In 4% of patients, the LAD bifurcates proximally and continues as two equal sized parallel vessels down the anterior interventricular groove.
- The main branches of the LAD include:

    a) diagonal arteries (usually 2-6 in number) which course along and supply the anterolateral wall of the left ventricle;

    b) septal perforator arteries (usually 3-5 in number) which branch perpendicularly into and supply the anterior two thirds of the ventricular septum. The first septal artery is the largest and runs perpendicularly towards the medial papillary muscle of the tricuspid valve. It is at risk during the Ross procedure as it lies immediately beneath the right ventricular outflow tract and pulmonary valve;

    c) right ventricular branches, which supply blood to the anterior surface of the right ventricle but are not always present.

4

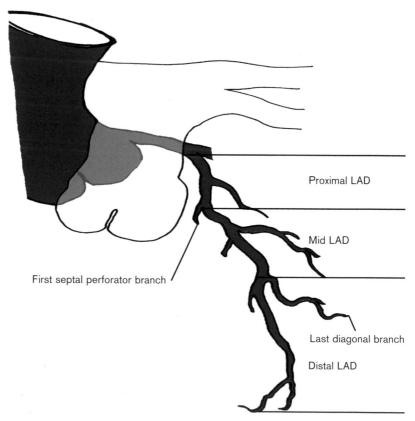

Proximal LAD

Mid LAD

First septal perforator branch

Last diagonal branch

Distal LAD

Figure 4. Segments of the left anterior descending (LAD) artery.

- The LAD is divided into (Figure 4):

    a)   a proximal third, which runs from the origin of the LAD to the origin of the first septal artery;
    b)   a middle third, which runs from the first septal artery to the origin of the last diagonal artery;
    c)   a distal third, which runs from the last diagonal artery to the termination of the LAD.

4   Describe the course of the circumflex coronary artery (Figure 5)

- The circumflex coronary artery courses along the left atrioventricular groove and in 85-90% of patients terminates before reaching the posterior interventricular groove. In 10-15% of patients, the circumflex coronary artery continues as the posterior descending artery.

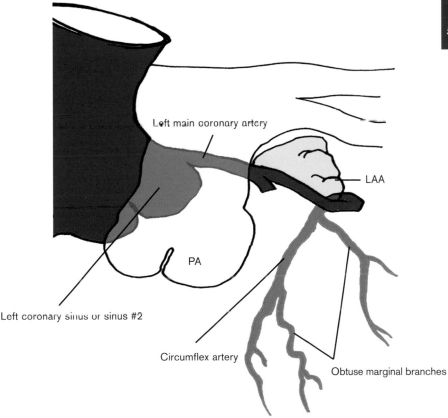

Left main coronary artery

LAA

PA

Left coronary sinus or sinus #2

Circumflex artery

Obtuse marginal branches

Figure 5. Circumflex artery and its branches. LAA = left atrial appendage; PA = pulmonary artery.

- The main branches of the circumflex coronary artery include:

    a)   obtuse marginal arteries that supply the lateral aspect of the left ventricular wall, including the anterolateral papillary muscle of the mitral valve;
    b)   left atrial branches;
    c)   sino-atrial nodal artery (in 45% of patients);
    d)   atrioventricular nodal artery (in 10-15% of patients);
    e)   posterior descending artery (in 10-15% of patients).

5   Describe the anatomy of the right coronary artery (RCA)(Figure 6)

- The RCA courses anteriorly and laterally from its origin at the right coronary ostium, descending into the right atrioventricular groove and inferiorly towards the acute margin of the right ventricle.
- It courses around to the inferior surface of the heart and after giving off the posterior descending artery, it continues as the posterior left ventricular artery.

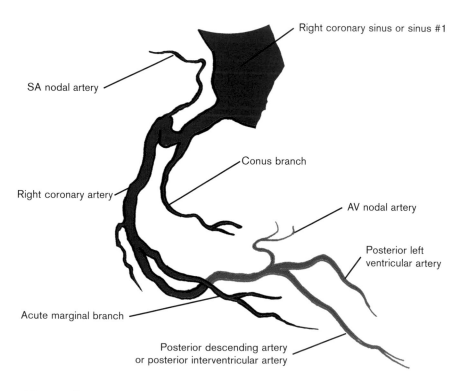

Figure 6. Right coronary artery (RCA) and its branches. SA = sino-atrial; AV = atrioventricular.

- The main branches of the RCA include:

  a)   sino-atrial nodal artery (in 55% of patients) (see below);
  b)   infundibular (or conus) branch that courses anteriorly over the right ventricular infundibulum;
  c)   acute marginal branch that courses over the acute margin of the right ventricle;
  d)   anterior right ventricular branches that supply the anterior free wall of the right ventricle;
  e)   atrioventricular nodal artery (in 85-90% of patients) (see below);
  f)   posterior descending artery (in 85-90% of patients), which runs in the posterior interventricular groove and gives off septal perforator arteries which branch perpendicularly into and supply the posterior one third of the ventricular septum;
  g)   posterior left ventricular artery that supplies the posterior surface of the left ventricle.

7

6   How is dominance of the coronary artery system determined?

- Dominance refers to the artery from which the posterior descending artery originates and not the vessel which supplies the greater absolute myocardial muscle mass.
- A right dominant system occurs in 80-85% of patients, with a left dominant system in 10-15% and a codominant system in approximately 5% of patients.
- Left dominance occurs slightly more frequently in males and in patients with a bicuspid aortic valve.

7   Describe the coronary venous drainage system

- The majority of coronary veins (see below) drain via the coronary sinus into the right atrium.
- The coronary sinus is a continuation of the great cardiac vein and the change is denoted by the valve of Vieussens and entry of the oblique vein of the left atrium (the vein of Marshall).
- Several Thebesian veins and larger anterior veins drain directly into the right atrium, thereby bypassing the coronary sinus.

8   **What are the anatomical locations of the main coronary veins and with which coronary arteries does each vein run (Figure 7; Table 1)?**

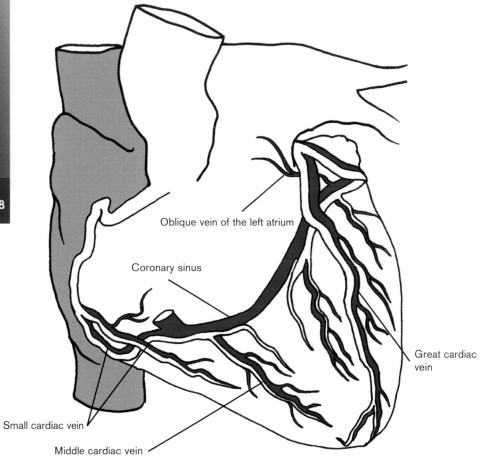

Oblique vein of the left atrium

Coronary sinus

Great cardiac vein

Small cardiac vein

Middle cardiac vein

Figure 7. Coronary venous system.

Coronary vein	Anatomical location	Coronary artery
Table 1. Anatomical location of coronary arteries and veins.		
Coronary vein	**Anatomical location**	**Coronary artery**
Coronary sinus	Left atrioventricular groove	Circumflex artery
Great cardiac vein	Anterior interventricular groove into the left atrioventricular groove	Left anterior descending artery Circumflex artery
Middle cardiac vein	Posterior interventricular groove	Posterior descending artery
Small cardiac vein	Right atrioventricular groove	Right coronary artery Acute marginal artery

9 Describe the conduction system of the heart (Figure 8)

The cardiac conduction system consists of:

a) sino-atrial (SA) node (see below);

b) anterior, middle and posterior internodal tracts in the right atrium as well as Bachmann's bundle in the left atrium;

c) atrioventricular node (see below);

d) bundle of His, which penetrates the central fibrous body to reach the membranous septum to lie on the crest of the muscular ventricular septum just beneath the commissure between the right and non-coronary cusps of the aortic valve;

e) bundle branches:

   i) left bundle branch, which divides into anterior and posterior fascicles that run sub-endocardially down the septal surface of the left ventricle to the apex;

   ii) right bundle branch, which runs on the right side of the ventricular septum towards the base of the medial papillary muscle of the tricuspid valve into the body of the septomarginal trabeculation and traversing the right ventricular cavity through the moderator band;

f) Purkinje fibres.

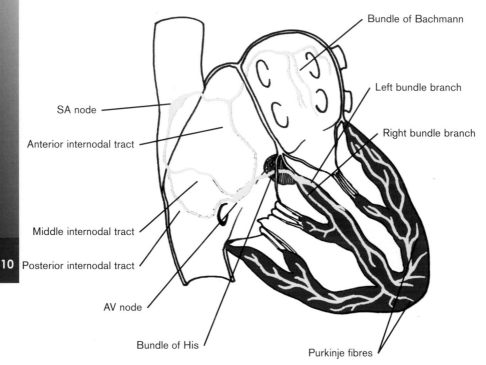

Bundle of Bachmann

Left bundle branch

Right bundle branch

SA node

Anterior internodal tract

Middle internodal tract

10 | Posterior internodal tract

AV node

Bundle of His

Purkinje fibres

Figure 8. Conduction system of the heart. While the conduction fibres originating from the AV node are recognisable anatomic structures surrounded by a capsule of fibrous tissue, the connections between the SA node and the AV node are less defined, therefore they are named tracts rather than bundles. The so-called Bundle of Bachmann propagates the electric impulse to the left atrium through the interatrial septum. SA = sino-atrial; AV = atrioventricular.

10 Describe the location of the sino-atrial node (Figure 9)

- The sino-atrial node is an elliptical or horse-shoe-shaped sub-epicardial structure that lies just lateral to the junction of the superior vena cava and the roof of the right atrium at the superior end of the terminal groove (sulcus terminalis).

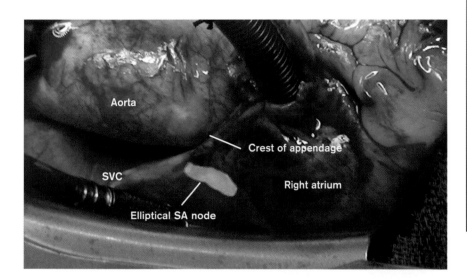

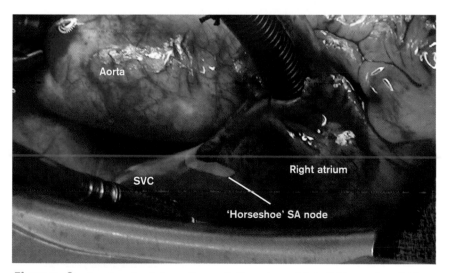

Figure 9. Anatomical location of the sino-atrial (SA) node. SVC = superior vena cava.

11 **What is the blood supply of the sino-atrial node?**

● The sino-atrial nodal artery originates from the RCA in 55% of patients and the circumflex coronary artery in 45% of patients.

● The sino-atrial nodal artery passes in front of the junction between the superior vena cava and right atrial roof in 60% of patients, behind the junction in 33% and around the junction in 7%.

12 **Describe the location of the atrioventricular node (Figures 10 and 11)**

● The atrioventricular node lies within the triangle of Koch.

● The boundaries of the triangle of Koch include:

a)   the tendon of Todaro;

b)   the hinge of the septal leaflet of the tricuspid valve;

c)   the superior margin of the coronary sinus.

● The membranous septum lies just superior to the triangle of Koch and is where the bundle of His penetrates to enter the muscular septum.

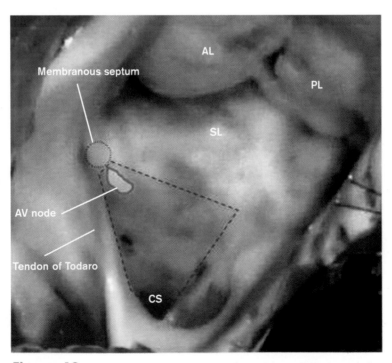

Figure 10. Anatomical location of the atrioventricular node. AL = anterior leaflet of the tricuspid valve; PL = posterior leaflet of the tricuspid valve; SL = septal leaflet of the tricuspid valve; AV = atrioventricular; CS = coronary sinus.

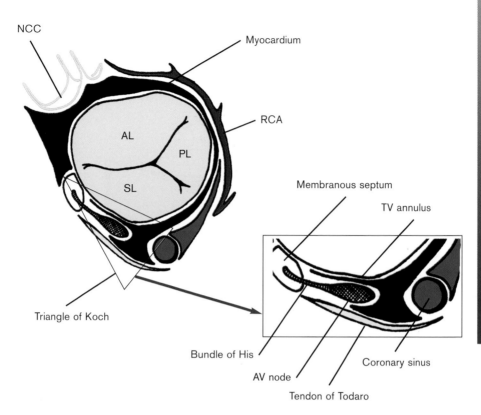

Figure 11. Anatomical location of the atrioventricular node. NCC = non-coronary cusp of the aortic valve; AL = anterior leaflet of the tricuspid valve; RCA = right coronary artery; AV = atrioventricular; PL = posterior leaflet of the tricuspid valve; SL = septal leaflet of the tricuspid valve; TV = tricuspid valve.

13 **What is the blood supply of the atrioventricular node?**

- The atrioventricular nodal artery supplies the node and originates from the RCA in approximately 85-90% of patients with the remaining 10-15% originating from the circumflex coronary artery.

14 Describe the anatomy of the aortic valve (Figures 12 and 13)

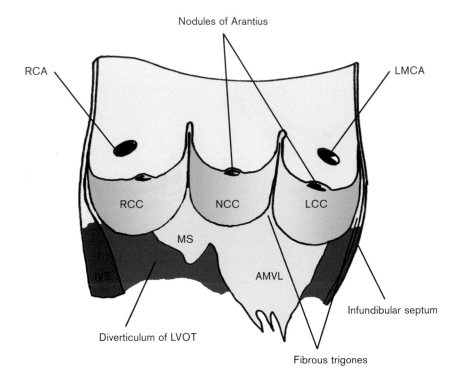

Figure 12. Anatomical relations of the aortic valve. The fibrous trigones provide continuity between the anterior leaflet of the mitral valve and the left coronary and non-coronary cusps of the aortic valve. RCA = right coronary artery; LMCA = left main coronary artery; RCC = right coronary cusp; NCC = non-coronary cusp; LCC = left coronary cusp; AMVL = anterior mitral valve leaflet; MS = membranous septum; IVS = interventricular septum; LVOT = left ventricular outflow tract.

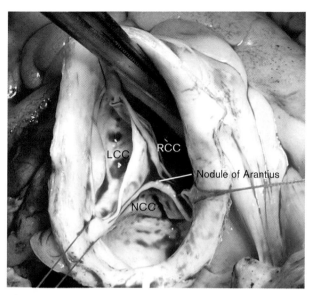

Figure 13. Operative view of the aortic valve. NCC = non-coronary cusp; LCC = left coronary cusp; RCC = right coronary cusp.

- The aortic valve consists of three semilunar leaflets:

  a) right coronary cusp;
  h) left coronary cusp;
  c) non-coronary (posterior) cusp.

- The leaflets are formed by a fibrous core and an endothelial lining.
- The fibrous core is thickened at the free edge of the leaflet, especially centrally, which is known as the nodule of Arantius.
- The leaflets coapt at the free edge of their ventricular surface with three zones of apposition.
- The commissures are the points of contact between the leaflets on the aortic wall.

15 Describe the anatomy of the aortic root (Figure 14)

- Competency of the aortic valve is maintained by several different components of the aortic root working in harmony:

  a) aortic valve leaflets (see above);

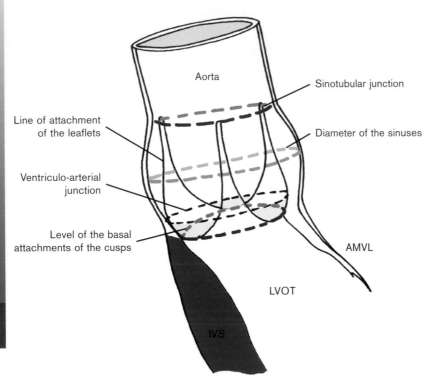

Aorta

Sinotubular junction

Line of attachment of the leaflets

Diameter of the sinuses

Ventriculo-arterial junction

Level of the basal attachments of the cusps

AMVL

LVOT

IVS

Figure 14. Structure of the aortic root. The valve leaflets have been removed. Note how the level of the basal attachment of the cusps is lower than the anatomical ventriculo-arterial junction. LVOT = left ventricular outflow tract; IVS = interventricular septum; AMVL = anterior mitral valve leaflet.

b) sinuses of Valsalva, which allow the aortic valve leaflets to fall back during systole thereby enabling a column of blood to pass unobstructed from the left ventricle into the aorta:
   i)   right coronary sinus;
   ii) left coronary sinus;
   iii) non-coronary sinus;

c) junctions (anatomical and physiological):
   i)   sinotubular junction between the distal part of the sinuses and the proximal part of the ascending aorta;
   ii) anatomical ventriculo-arterial junction between the ventricular myocardium and aortic sinuses;
   iii) basal ring that joins the inferior aspect of the valve leaflets.

● The haemodynamic border between the ventricle and aorta, however, is demarcated by the leaflet attachments and not by the junctions described above.

- As the crown-shaped line of leaflet attachment crosses the anatomical ventriculo-arterial junction, it leaves triangles of arterial wall on the ventricular aspects of the leaflet attachment and semicircular areas of ventricular myocardium within the aortic sinuses.

16 Describe the anatomy of the pulmonary valve
- The pulmonary valve consists of three semilunar leaflets:

   a)   right cusp;
   b)   left cusp;
   c)   anterior cusp.

- Competency of the pulmonary valve is maintained by similar structures to the aortic valve.

17 Describe the anatomy of the mitral valve (Figure 15)
- The mitral valve consists of two leaflets:

   a)   anterior (aortic) mitral valve leaflet;
   b)   posterior (mural) mitral valve leaflet.

- The anterior and posterior mitral valve leaflets are further subdivided by clefts into scallops, known as A1, A2, A3, P1, P2 and P3, respectively.

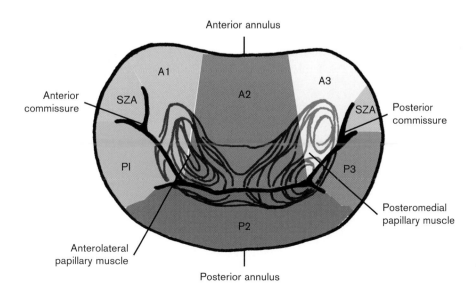

Figure 15. Anatomical view of the mitral valve. SZA = solitary zone of apposition.

- The mitral valve annulus is kidney-shaped with the posterior mitral valve annulus taking up two thirds of the circumference and the anterior mitral valve annulus taking up one third.
- The anterior mitral valve leaflet takes up approximately two thirds of the cross-sectional area of the mitral valve orifice with the posterior mitral valve leaflet taking up one third. Hence, the line of apposition is closer to the posterior mitral valve annulus.

18 Describe the tension apparatus of the mitral valve (Figures 16 and 17)

- Competency of the mitral valve is maintained by several different components of the mitral valve and sub-valvular apparatus acting in harmony:

    a)   leaflets (see above);
    b)   papillary muscles:
        i)   the anterolateral papillary muscle has a single head and takes its blood supply from the circumflex coronary artery;
        ii)   the posteromedial papillary muscle has multiple heads and takes its blood supply from the right coronary artery;

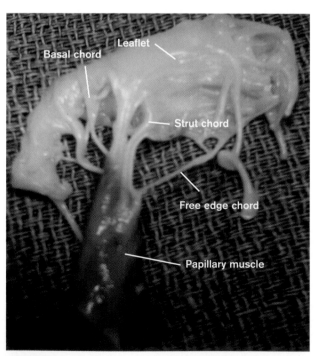

Figure 16. Mitral valve leaflet and sub-valvular apparatus.

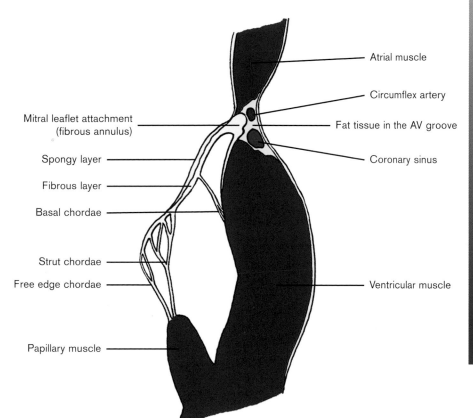

Atrial muscle

Circumflex artery

Mitral leaflet attachment
(fibrous annulus)

Fat tissue in the AV groove

Spongy layer

Coronary sinus

Fibrous layer

Basal chordae

Strut chordae

Free edge chordae

Ventricular muscle

Papillary muscle

19

Figure 17. Structural complex of the mitral valve. The annulus is formed by a ring of fibrous tissue anchoring the leaflets to the interventricular junction. This fibrous body is in direct continuity with the fibrous layer of the leaflet, which is surmounted by the spongy layer. The spongy layer is in continuity with the atrial endocardium. AV = atrioventricular.

- c) chordae tendineae:
  - i) primary (free edge chordae) which run from the papillary muscles to the free edge of the leaflets;
  - ii) secondary (strut chordae) which run from the papillary muscles to the roughened zone on the ventricular surface of each leaflet;
  - iii) tertiary (basal chordae) which run from the papillary muscles or ventricular wall to the base of the leaflets;
- d) mitral valve annulus, which contracts during ventricular systole to reduce the cross-sectional area of the mitral valve orifice by 20-40%;
- e) left ventricle.

19 Describe the anatomy of the tricuspid valve (Figures 18 and 19)

● The tricuspid valve consists of three leaflets:

a) anterior leaflet (largest leaflet);
b) septal leaflet;
c) posterior (mural) leaflet (smallest leaflet).

● Competency of the tricuspid valve is maintained in a similar manner to the mitral valve.

● There are two or three papillary muscles that support the tricuspid valve:

a) anterior papillary muscle (largest) that arises from the moderator band and supports the anterior leaflet of the tricuspid valve and the zone of apposition between the anterior and posterior leaflets;

b) medial papillary muscle (of Lancisi) that supports the septal leaflet of the tricuspid valve and the zone of apposition between the septal and anterior leaflets and through which the right bundle branch passes;

c) posterior papillary muscle (smallest and sometimes indistinct) that supports the posterior leaflet of the tricuspid valve and the zone of apposition between the posterior and septal leaflets.

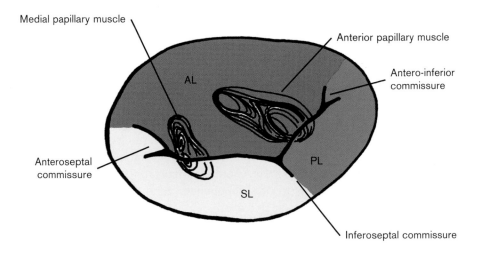

Figure 18. Anatomy of the tricuspid valve. AL = anterior leaflet of the tricuspid valve; PL = posterior leaflet of the tricuspid valve; SL = septal leaflet of the tricuspid valve.

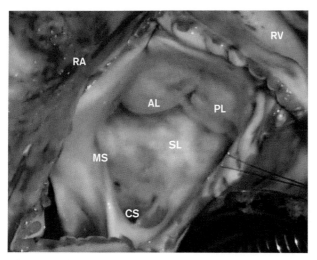

Figure 19. Operative view of the tricuspid valve. AL = anterior leaflet of the tricuspid valve; PL = posterior leaflet of the tricuspid valve; SL = septal leaflet of the tricuspid valve; RA = right atrium; RV = right ventricle; MS = membranous septum; CS = coronary sinus.

20 Describe the structure of the pericardium

- The pericardium consists of two layers:

  a)   fibrous pericardium;
  b)   serous pericardium, which itself has two layers:
      i)   visceral pericardium, which is densely adherent to the epicardium;
      ii)   parietal pericardium, which is densely adherent to the fibrous pericardium.

- The serous pericardial layers are lined by mesothelial cells which secrete and resorb pericardial fluid.
- Approximately 5-10mL of pericardial fluid lies within the pericardial space (between the visceral and parietal pericardium).

21 Describe the location of the oblique and transverse pericardial sinuses (Figure 20)

- The oblique sinus lies posterior to the left atrium, between the four pulmonary veins and medial to the inferior vena cava.
- The transverse sinus lies behind the aorta and pulmonary trunk but in front of the superior vena cava and left atrial appendage.

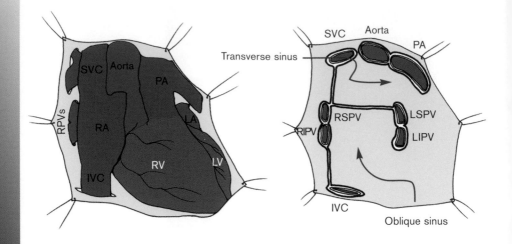

Figure 20. Sinuses of the pericardium. The pericardium has been opened through a longitudinal incision and suspended (left). After complete resection of the heart the posterior pericardium is exposed (right), demonstrating the transverse and oblique pericardial sinuses between the folding of the parietal layer of the pericardium. RPVs = right pulmonary veins; SVC = superior vena cava; IVC = inferior vena cava; RA = right atrium; PA = pulmonary artery; RV = right ventricle; LA = left atrium; LV = left ventricle; RIPV = right inferior pulmonary vein; RSPV = right superior pulmonary vein; LSPV = left superior pulmonary vein; LIPV = left inferior pulmonary vein.

22 Describe the anatomical location of the common femoral artery (Figure 21)

- The common femoral artery is located at the mid-inguinal point, which lies halfway between the anterior superior iliac spine and the symphysis pubis.
- This needs to be distinguished from the deep inguinal ring, which lies at the mid-point of the inguinal ligament, halfway between the anterior superior iliac spine and the pubic tubercle.
- The common femoral artery is a continuation of the external iliac artery and commences just beneath the inguinal ligament.
- The common femoral artery gives off the deep femoral artery (profunda femoris) laterally and then continues as the superficial femoral artery.

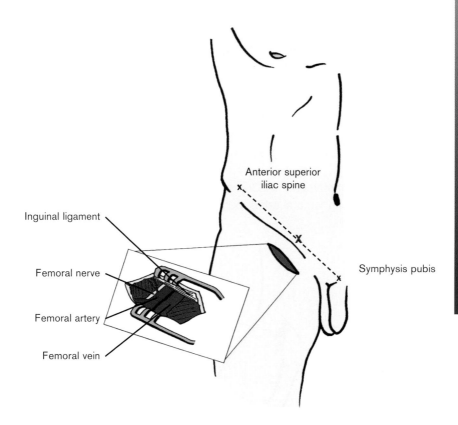

Anterior superior
iliac spine

Inguinal ligament

Femoral nerve

Femoral artery

Femoral vein

Symphysis pubis

Figure 21. Anatomical relations of the common femoral artery.

- The femoral vein lies medial to the femoral artery within the femoral sheath with the femoral nerve lying lateral to the artery but outside the femoral sheath.

23 **Describe the course of the common femoral vein**
- The common femoral vein can be located medial to the femoral artery (see above).
- It is formed from the confluence of the deep and superficial femoral veins just proximal to its junction with the long saphenous vein.
- The common femoral vein continues as the external iliac vein when it passes under the inguinal ligament.

24 Describe the course and landmarks of the long saphenous vein (Figure 22)

- The long saphenous vein commences just anterior and superior to the medial malleolus.
- It continues up the medial aspect of the lower leg (with the saphenous nerve) before turning slightly posteriorly at the superior aspect of gastrocnemius.
- The vein then passes medial to the knee joint (5cm posterior to the medial aspect of the patella).
- From the knee, the vein continues up the medial aspect of the thigh to drain into the common femoral vein at the saphenofemoral junction.
- The saphenofemoral junction can be located 3cm inferior and 3cm medial to the femoral artery pulsation (mid-inguinal point).

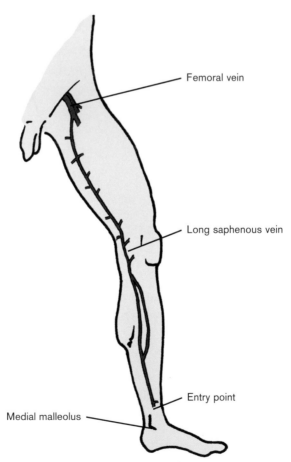

Femoral vein

Long saphenous vein

Entry point

Medial malleolus

Figure 22. Anatomical course of the long saphenous vein.

25 Describe the course and landmarks of the short saphenous vein (Figure 23)

- The short saphenous vein can be located 2cm posterior to the lateral malleolus.
- It courses superiorly superficial to gastrocnemius muscle in the midline of the lower leg and runs in close proximity to the sural nerve.
- It terminates by draining into the popliteal vein just below the knee.

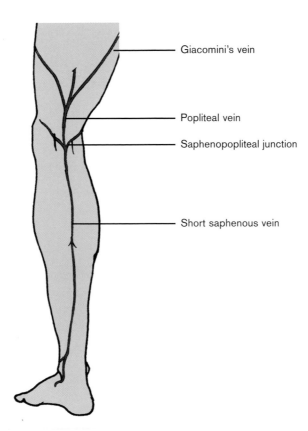

Giacomini's vein

Popliteal vein

Saphenopopliteal junction

Short saphenous vein

Figure 23. Anatomical course of the short saphenous vein.

26 Describe the anatomy of the left internal mammary artery (Figure 24)

- The left internal mammary artery originates from the first part of the subclavian artery medial to scalenus anterior.
- It lies in the neurovascular plane, between the transversus thoracis muscle layer and the internal intercostal muscle layer.

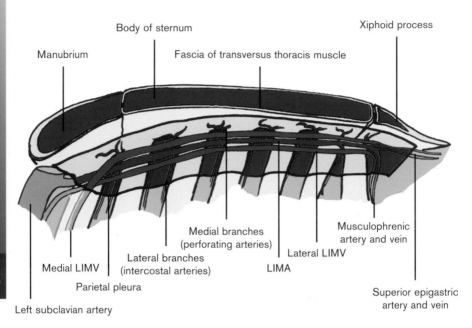

Figure 24. Anatomical course of the left internal mammary artery. LIMA = left internal mammary artery; LIMV = left internal mammary vein.

- The left internal mammary artery courses down the posterior aspect of the chest wall approximately 2cm lateral to the left sternal edge with corresponding left internal mammary veins on either side.
- The branches of the left internal mammary artery include:

  a) intercostal branches, which originate anteriorly into the inter-costal spaces;

  b) perforating branches, which pass anteriorly and supply the overlying muscles including pectoralis major;

  c) sternal branches;

  d) the pericardiophrenic artery, which supplies the phrenic nerve and the lateral aspect of the pericardium.

- The left internal mammary artery terminates around the 6th intercostal space by dividing into:

  a) the superior epigastric artery, which supplies the muscles of the superior aspect of the anterior abdominal wall, including rectus abdominis;

  b) the musculophrenic artery, which supplies branches to the 6th-10th intercostal spaces.

27 Describe the anatomy of the radial artery (Figures 25 and 26)

- The radial artery commences as one of the two terminal branches of the brachial artery, located medial to the biceps tendon.
- It is divided into three parts:

  a) proximal part, which lies between its origin and the distal extent of the antecubital fossa;

  b) middle part, which extends from the antecubital fossa up to the origin of the tendons of brachioradialis, extensor carpi radialis longus and extensor carpi radialis brevis;

  c) distal part, which runs from the origin of these tendons to the wrist crease.

- During its course, the radial artery is situated under the cover of the brachioradialis muscle, with several muscles lying beneath the artery including:

  a) proximal part: brachialis, pronator teres and supinator;

  b) middle part: pronator teres, flexor digitorum superficialis and flexor pollicis longus;

  c) distal part: flexor pollicis longus, flexor digitorum profundus and pronator quadratus.

- Its branches include the recurrent radial artery, superficial palmar artery and muscular branches.
- The radial artery terminates at the level of the radial styloid process and continues as the deep palmar artery.
- The main nerves at risk during harvesting of the radial artery include:

  a) the lateral cutaneous nerve of the forearm (nerve roots C5-6), which carries sensory fibres to the lateral aspect of the forearm;

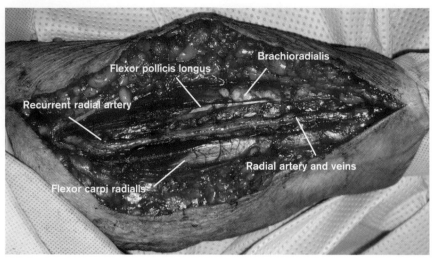

Figure 25. Radial artery.

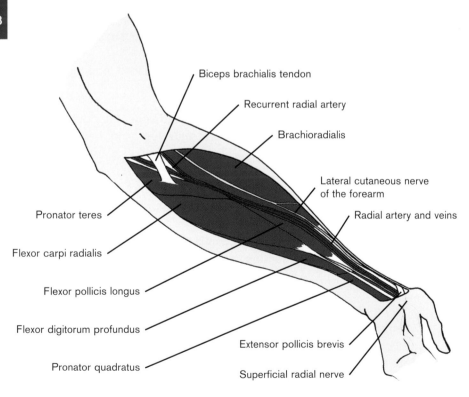

Figure 26. Anatomical course of the radial artery.

b)   the superficial radial nerve (nerve roots C7-8), which crosses the anatomical snuffbox and carries sensory fibres to the thenar eminence.

28 Describe the anatomy of the phrenic nerve (Figure 27)

- The phrenic nerve originates from the C3, C4 and C5 nerve roots.
- It courses down through the neck lying anterior to scalenus anterior.
- It passes posterior to the subclavian artery and medial to the internal mammary artery to lie on the lateral surface of the pericardium.
- The right phrenic nerve passes through the inferior vena caval opening of the diaphragm at the level of T8, whereas the left phrenic nerve pierces the muscular part of the left hemi-diaphragm.

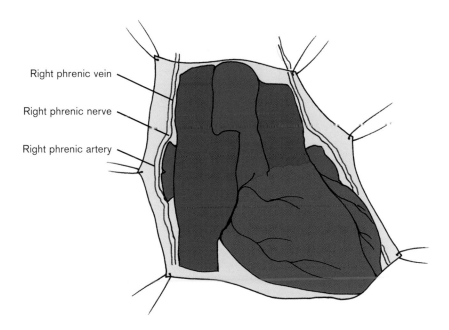

Right phrenic vein

Right phrenic nerve

Right phrenic artery

Figure 27. Intrapericardial course of the phrenic nerve. The pericardium has been opened with a longitudinal incision and suspended. The neurovascular bundle runs along the external surface of the fibrous pericardium.

- The phrenic nerve terminates by branching on the inferior surface of the diaphragm.
- The phrenic nerve supplies:

   a)   motor function to the diaphragm;
   b)   sensory function to the diaphragm and anterior chest and abdominal wall.

29 Describe the anatomy of the descending thoracic aorta (Figure 28)

- The descending thoracic aorta is a direct continuation of the aortic arch and commences just distal to the origin of the left subclavian artery.

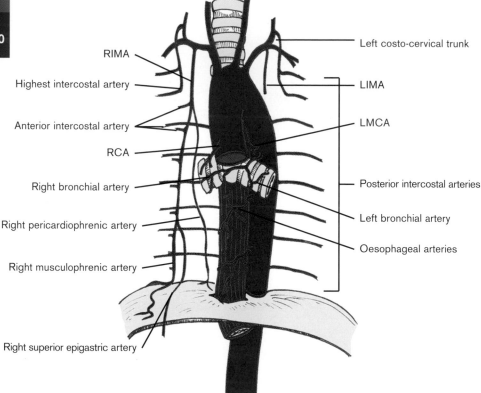

Figure 28. Anatomical course of the descending thoracic aorta. RIMA = right internal mammary artery; LIMA = left internal mammary artery; RCA = right coronary artery; LMCA = left main coronary artery.

- It terminates at the diaphragm where it passes through the aortic hiatus, with the thoracic duct and azygos vein, to continue as the abdominal aorta.
- The descending aorta lies on the posterior thoracic wall, initially to the left of the thoracic vertebrae, gradually moving medially to lie anterior to the vertebral column as it passes through the diaphragm.
- Branches of the descending thoracic aorta include:

  a)   pericardial branches;
  b)   bronchial arteries;
  c)   oesophageal branches;
  d)   mediastinal branches;
  e)   intercostal arteries;
  f)   subcostal arteries;
  g)   superior phrenic arteries.

30 Describe the anatomy of the axillary artery

- The axillary artery is a direct continuation of the subclavian artery and commences at the outer edge of the 1st rib.
- It terminates at the lower border of teres major where it continues as the brachial artery.
- The axillary artery lies within the axillary sheath, with the axillary vein and the brachial plexus, and is divided into three parts by pectoralis major with the 1st part above, 2nd part behind and 3rd part below the muscle.
- Branches of the axillary artery include the:

  a)   highest thoracic artery;
  b)   thoraco-acromial artery;
  c)   subscapular artery;
  d)   lateral thoracic artery;
  e)   anterior humeral circumflex artery;
  f)   posterior humeral circumflex artery.

31 How is the heart formed embryologically?

- The heart tube forms from fusion of the two ventral aortae which originate from the mesodermal layer of the yolk sac.
- Following longitudinal growth and rotation of the heart tube, it divides into three regions: conus truncus, sinus venosus and bulbus cordis.
- Endocardial cushions form the partition between atria and ventricles within the heart tube to create atrioventricular canals and eventually the mitral and tricuspid valves.

- The atrial septum forms from the septum primum and septum secundum, leaving a small opening, the foramen ovale.
- The muscular part of the interventricular septum forms from the ventricular myocardium of both ventricles, whereas the membranous part originates from fusion of the endocardial cushions and the descending truncal cushions.

Recommended reading

1. Muresian H. The clinical anatomy of the mitral valve. *Clin Anat* 2009; 22(1): 85-98.

2. Reyes AT, Frame R, Brodman RF. Technique for harvesting the radial artery as a coronary artery bypass graft. *Ann Thorac Surg* 1995; 59(1): 118-26.

3. Loukas M, Groat C, Khangura R, Owens DG, Anderson RH. The normal and abnormal anatomy of the coronary arteries. *Clin Anat* 2009; 22(1): 114-28.

4. Ho SY. Structure and anatomy of the aortic root. *Eur J Echocardiogr* 2009; 10(1): i3-10.

5. Anderson RH, Yanni J, Boyett MR, Chandler NJ, Dobrzynski H. The anatomy of the cardiac conduction system. *Clin Anat* 2009; 22(1): 99-113.

Chapter 2

Cardiac physiology

1   **Describe the principles of invasive arterial monitoring (Figure 1)**

- The arterial line is usually placed in the non-dominant radial artery but the brachial and femoral arteries can also be cannulated.
- Invasive arterial cannulation allows continuous monitoring of blood pressure and serial arterial blood gas analysis.
- Normal blood gas values include:

   a)   pH - 7.35-7.45;
   b) PaO_2 - 10-13.3kPa; 75-100mmHg;

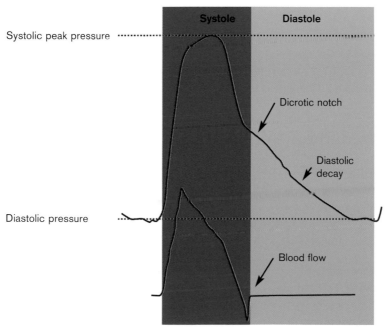

Systole   Diastole

Systolic peak pressure

Dicrotic notch

Diastolic decay

Diastolic pressure

Blood flow

Figure 1. Arterial pressure waveform.

c) $PaCO_2$ - 4.7-6.0kPa; 35-45mmHg;
d) bicarbonate - 22-26mmol/L;
e) base excess - -2 to +2mmol/L;
f) lactate - 0.5-2mmol/L;
g) potassium - 3.5-5mmol/L;
h) ionised calcium - 1.15-1.29mmol/L;
i) glucose - 3.3-5.6mmol/L (fasting).

(For pressures, to convert from kPa to mmHg, multiply by 7.5.)

- The arterial pressure waveform allows determination of:

a) arterial blood pressure;
b) myocardial contractility, which is represented by the slope of the upstroke (dP/dt);
c) systemic vascular resistance, which is represented by the slope of the diastolic decay.

- The dicrotic notch represents closure of the aortic valve and subsequent retrograde flow of blood against the closed valve. It occurs at the end of ventricular systole.
- Complications of arterial line cannulation include bleeding, infection, local ischaemia, thrombosis and damage to nearby nerves.

2 Describe the principles of pulse oximetry

- Pulse oximetry is based on the different absorption characteristics of oxygenated and deoxygenated blood to red and infrared light, thereby allowing continuous non-invasive monitoring of arterial oxygen saturation.
- The pulse oximetry probe is placed on a well perfused digit or ear lobe and has a:

a) source - a pair of light-emitting diodes (LEDs) that produce beams of red (λ660nm) and infrared (λ910nm) light, approximately every 0.03 secs;
b) receiver - a photodetector that measures the intensity of the transmitted light on the opposite side of the probe to the LEDs.

- Oxygenated haemoglobin absorbs more infrared light and transmits more red light than deoxygenated haemoglobin.
- Pulse oximetry is inaccurate in patients with hypothermia, peripheral vasoconstriction, non-pulsatile cardiopulmonary bypass flow, Raynaud's disease, anaemia, hypotension, nail polish, nicotine stains, bright light, electrical interference, high carboxyhaemoglobin levels, jaundice and in the presence of methylene blue.

3 Describe the principles of central venous access (Figure 2)

- Central venous access can be used for:

  a)   monitoring right atrial filling pressures;
  b)   administration of drugs;
  c)   administration of fluids;

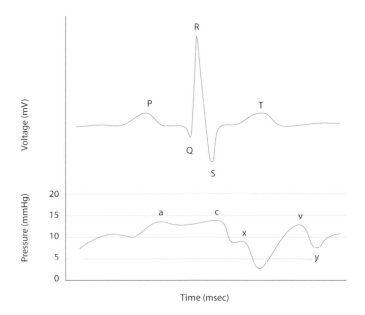

Figure 2. Central venous pressure waveform (below) with corresponding electrocardiogram (above).

Table 1. Central venous pressure waveform.	
a wave	Atrial systole
c wave	Isovolumetric contraction of the right ventricle with bulging of the closed tricuspid valve, resulting in a small rise in right atrial pressure
x descent	Atrial diastole. Relaxation of the atrial muscle results in reduced right atrial pressure
v wave	Venous return against a closed tricuspid valve
y descent	Opening of the tricuspid valve resulting in emptying of the right atrium

d)   parenteral nutrition;
e)   transvenous temporary pacing wires;
f)   pulmonary artery (Swan-Ganz) catheters.

● The tip of the central venous line should sit at the junction of the superior vena cava and right atrium, approximately 15-18cm from the point of entry. Venous catheters can be placed in the:

a)   internal jugular vein, which is located at the:
    i)   midpoint between the mastoid process and suprasternal notch, just lateral to the common carotid artery;
    ii) apex of the triangle of the sternal and clavicular heads of sternocleidomastoid;
b)   subclavian vein, which is located just beneath the junction of the middle and outer third of the clavicle in the deltopectoral groove;
c)   femoral vein, which is located just medial to the femoral artery pulsation at the mid-inguinal point.

● The normal central venous pressure waveform represents the different stages of the cardiac cycle (Table 1).
● Complications of central venous line insertion include bleeding, infection, pneumothorax, damage to adjacent structures (including the common carotid artery and brachial plexus), arrhythmias, haemothorax, chylothorax and air embolism.

4   Describe the principles of a pulmonary artery (Swan-Ganz) catheter (Figure 3)

● Pulmonary artery catheters are usually inserted in patients with low cardiac output to guide inotropic use and optimize left-sided filling pressures. This enables the determination of pulmonary artery pressures, pulmonary artery wedge pressures, systemic vascular resistance, cardiac output and mixed venous saturation.
● The tip of the pulmonary artery catheter is usually 40-45cm from the skin but this can vary considerably.
● Pulmonary artery catheters have four lumens (Figure 4):

a)   proximal lumen, which is located approximately 25-30cm from the tip and lies in the right atrium. It allows for:
    i)   administration of drugs;
    ii)   injection of cold saline for cardiac output measurements;
    iii) central venous pressure measurements;

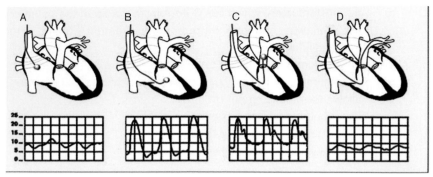

Figure 3. Changing pressure waveforms during flotation of a Swan-Ganz catheter: A) central venous pressure; B) right ventricular pressure, with systolic pressure increasing as the catheter passes across the tricuspid valve; C) pulmonary arterial pressure, with increased diastolic pressure as the catheter passes across the pulmonary valve; and D) pulmonary artery wedge pressure.

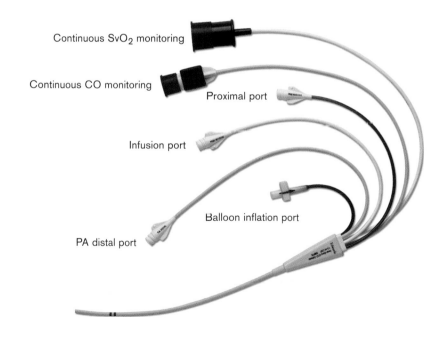

Figure 4. Pulmonary artery (Swan-Ganz) catheter. PA = pulmonary artery; SvO_2 = mixed venous saturations; CO = cardiac output. *Reproduced with permission from Edwards Lifesciences, Irvine, CA, USA.*

b)   thermistor lumen, which lies 3-4cm from the tip of the catheter and allows cardiac output measurement using the thermodilution method;

c)   balloon lumen for inflation and deflation of the flotation balloon;

d)   distal lumen, which is located at the tip of the catheter and allows for measurement of:

  i)   pulmonary artery pressure;
  ii)   mixed venous saturation;
  iii)   pulmonary artery wedge pressure.

- Complications of pulmonary artery catheter insertion include ventricular tachyarrhythmias, knotting of the catheter, pulmonary artery rupture, pulmonary infarction, damage to the tricuspid or pulmonary valves, as well as those attributable to central venous line insertion.

5   Describe the principles of mixed venous oxygen saturation measurement

- Mixed venous saturations represent the difference between oxygen delivered and oxygen consumed by the tissues and hence can be used as an indirect measure of cardiac output.
- Mixed venous saturations should be assessed from blood obtained from the pulmonary artery to ensure adequate mixing of blood from the coronary sinus (maximal oxygen extraction) and the superior and inferior venae cavae.
- Mixed venous saturations can be measured continuously using reflection spectrophotometry or intermittently in a blood gas analyser.
- Normal mixed venous saturations are 60-80%.
- Low mixed venous saturations represent:

a)   decreased oxygen delivery, secondary to:
  i)   low cardiac output;
  ii)   anaemia;
  iii)   reduced arterial oxygen saturation;
b)   increased oxygen consumption, secondary to hyperthermia, pain and shivering.

- High mixed venous saturations may be caused by:

a)   decreased oxygen consumption or extraction, secondary to hypothermia, sepsis or shunting;
b)   increased oxygen delivery (raised inspired oxygen concentration, FiO_2);
c)   a wedged pulmonary artery catheter.

6   **Describe the normal cardiac physiological values measured or calculated in the intensive care unit (Table 2)**

Table 2. Normal cardiac physiological values.

	Abbreviation	Formula	Normal range
Systolic blood pressure	SBP		90-140mmHg
Diastolic blood pressure	DBP		60-90mmHg
Mean arterial blood pressure	MAP	[(SBP - DBP)/3] + DBP	70-105mmHg
Left atrial pressure	LAP		6-12mmHg
Central venous (right atrial) pressure	CVP		2-6mmHg
Arterial oxygen saturation	SaO_2		95-100%
Mixed venous saturation	SvO_2		60-80%
Pulmonary artery systolic pressure	PASP		15-30mmHg
Pulmonary artery diastolic pressure	PADP		5-15mmHg
Mean pulmonary artery pressure	MPAP	[(PASP - PADP)/3] + PADP	10-20mmHg
Pulmonary artery wedge pressure	PAWP		6-12mmHg
Systemic vascular resistance	SVR	80 x (MAP - CVP) / CO	000-1600 dyne/sec/cm^5
Systemic vascular resistance index	SVRI	SVR / BSA	1970-2390 dyne/sec/cm^5/m^2
Pulmonary vascular resistance	PVR	80 x (MPAP - PAWP) / CO	155-255 dyne/sec/cm^5
Pulmonary vascular resistance index	PVRI	PVR / BSA	255-285 dyne/sec/cm^5/m^2
Heart rate	HR		60-100 bpm
Stroke volume	SV		70-90mL (1mL/kg)
Cardiac output	CO	SV X HR	4-8L/min
Cardiac index	CI	CO / BSA	2.5-4L/min/m^2

for resistances, to convert into Wood units, divide dyne/sec/cm^5 by 80

39

7 **What are the normal pressures and oxygen saturations within the cardiac chambers and great vessels (Figure 5)?**

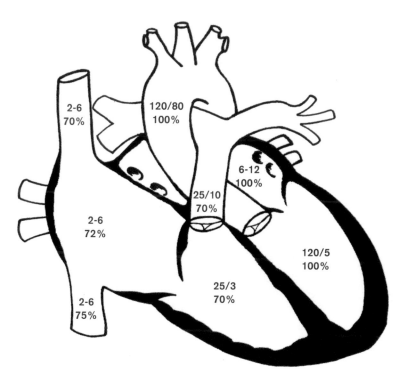

Figure 5. Systemic and pulmonary pressures and oxygen saturations.

8 **Describe the cardiac cycle (Figure 6)**

- The cardiac cycle is divided into systole (ventricular contraction) and diastole (ventricular relaxation).
- Left ventricular systole occurs in four stages:

  a) isovolumetric contraction (0.05s), which occurs when the left ventricle contracts against a closed aortic valve (as the aortic pressures are higher than the ventricular pressures) and the mitral valve is forced closed. During this phase, the ventricular pressure increases, whilst the ventricular volumes remain constant;

  b) rapid ejection phase (0.15s), which occurs once the left ventricular pressure exceeds the aortic pressure, causing the aortic valve to open, ejecting 70% of the stroke volume;

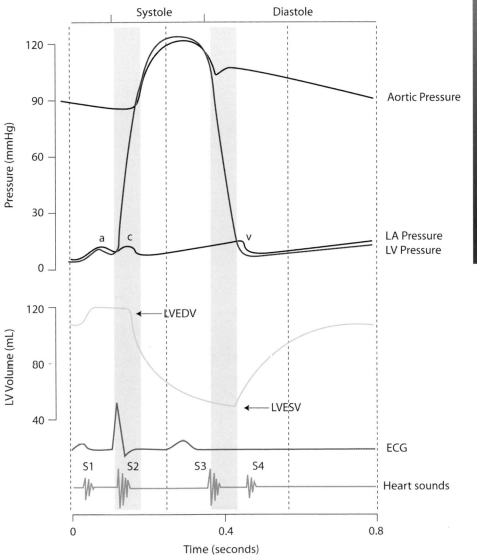

41

Figure 6. Cardiac cycle. LV = left ventricle; LA = left atrium; ECG = electrocardiogram; LVEDV = left ventricular end-diastolic volume; LVESV = left ventricular end-systolic volume.

c)   slow ejection (isotonic contraction phase, 0.10s), during which the remaining 30% of the stroke volume leaves the ventricle, as the force of contraction is reduced at this stage and the aortic and left ventricular pressures begin to fall;

d)   protodiastole (0.05s), which occurs in the transition from the end of systole to the point when the aortic valve closes.

● Left ventricular diastole occurs in four stages:

a)   isovolumetric relaxation (0.05s), which occurs when the ventricular pressure falls rapidly whilst the ventricular volume remains constant, as the aortic and mitral valves are closed;

b)   rapid early ventricular filling (0.10s), which occurs following opening of the mitral valve, causing rapid emptying of the left atrium, thereby increasing the left ventricular pressure and volume;

c)   diastasis (0.20s), during which slow late ventricular filling occurs due to the reduced pressure gradient between the left atrium and left ventricle following early diastolic filling;

d)   atrial systole (0.10s), which occurs with contraction of the left atrium and accounts for up to 30% of ventricular filling. Ejection of blood from the atria causes a small rise in left ventricular pressures.

● The duration of the cardiac cycle depends on the heart rate but in normal healthy individuals lasts approximately 0.8 seconds (with a heart rate of 75 bpm).

● Normal left ventricular end-diastolic volume is 120mL, left ventricular end-systolic volume, 50mL and stroke volume, 70mL (approximately 1mL/kg of body weight).

9 What is left ventricular pre-load (Figure 7)?

● Preload corresponds to the stretching of myocytes within the left ventricle just before initiation of contraction and is represented by the left ventricular end-diastolic volume.

● Preload represents left ventricular filling and is influenced by:

a)   compliance of the left ventricle;
b)   circulating blood volume;
c)   presence of atrial systole;
d)   length of diastole.

10 What is contractility (Figure 8)?

● Myocardial contractility represents the ability of the cardiac muscle to contract at a given preload and afterload.

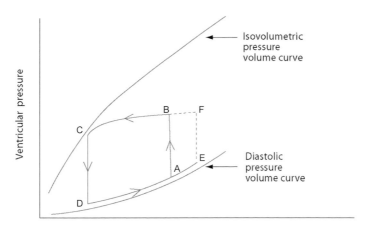

Figure 7. Left ventricular pressure volume loops with changing preload. A = end-diastolic volume. C = end-systolic volume. A to B = isovolumetric contraction, B to C = ventricular ejection, C to D = isovolumetric relaxation, D to A = ventricular filling. If the preload increases with end-diastolic volume at E, the left ventricular ejection (F to C) increases (Frank-Starling law) to restore the end-systolic volume (C) back to baseline.

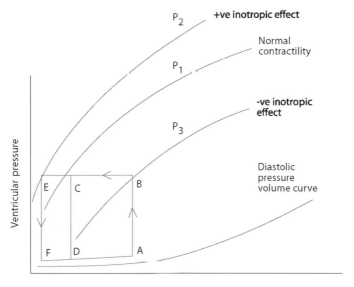

Figure 8. Left ventricular pressure volume loops with changing myocardial contractility. A = end-diastolic volume. C = end-systolic volume. A to B = isovolumetric contraction, B to C = ventricular ejection, C to D = isovolumetric relaxation, D to A = ventricular filling. If the myocardial contractility increases, the left ventricular ejection (B to E) increases, producing an increased stroke volume.

- It is affected by:

  a) the autonomic nervous system, with contractility increased by sympathetic stimulation and decreased by parasympathetic stimulation;

  b) drugs, with contractility increased by inotropes and decreased by β-blockers;

  c) local metabolites, with contractility decreased by hydrogen ions, carbon dioxide and hypoxia;

  d) the Bowditch effect, where an increased heart rate results in increased contractility (force-frequency effect).

11 What is left ventricular afterload (Figure 9)?

- Afterload is the tension generated by the left ventricle during contraction and is represented by the left ventricular end-systolic pressure.

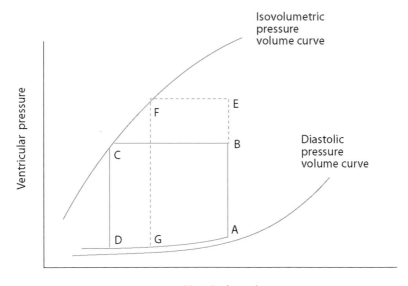

Figure 9. Left ventricular pressure volume loops with changing afterload. A = end-diastolic volume. C = end-systolic volume. A to B = isovolumetric contraction, B to C = ventricular ejection, C to D = isovolumetric relaxation, D to A = ventricular filling. If the afterload increases, the isovolumetric contraction phase (A to E) increases to overcome the increased resistance to ejection, resulting in a reduced ventricular ejection phase (E to F).

- Afterload represents the resistance to left ventricular contraction and is influenced by:

  a) systemic vascular resistance;
  b) area of the aortic valve and left ventricular outflow tract;
  c) left ventricular wall stress (Laplace's law).

12 What is cardiac work?

- Cardiac work of the left ventricle represents the work done by the left ventricle to eject a volume of blood into the aorta.
- It can be calculated by the area within the left ventricular pressure volume loop (Figure 10).

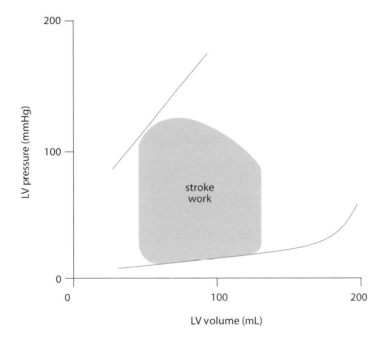

Figure 10. Left ventricular work.

13 What is compliance?

- Compliance is a measure of the change in volume per unit change in pressure.
- Compliance is inversely proportional to the slope of the diastolic component of the left ventricular pressure volume loop (Figure 11).

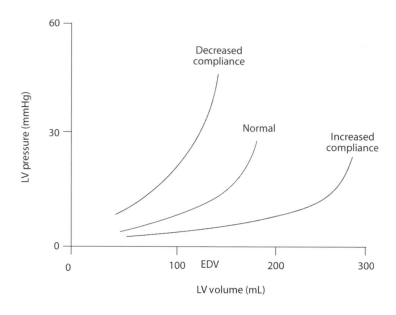

Figure 11. Compliance of the left ventricle (LV).

14 Describe the actions of the adrenergic and dopaminergic receptors (Table 3)

Receptor	Action
Table 3. Actions of the adrenergic and dopaminergic receptors.	
α	Vasoconstriction
β₁	Increased contractility (inotropy)
	Increased heart rate (chronotropy)
	Increased conduction (dromotropy)
β₂	Vasodilation
	Bronchodilation
DA₁	Coronary, renal and splanchnic vasodilation
α = α-adrenergic receptor	
β = β-adrenergic receptor	
DA = dopaminergic receptor	

15 Describe which inotropes act on which receptors (Table 4)

Inotrope	Receptor
Adrenaline	α, β_1, β_2 (depending on dose, see Chapter 3)
Dopamine	α, β_1, β_2, DA_1 (depending on dose, see Chapter 3)
Dopexamine	β_2, DA_1
Dobutamine	β_1, β_2
Isoprenaline	β_1, β_2
Noradrenaline	α, β_1
Metaraminol	α, β_1
Phenylephrine	α

Table 4. Actions of inotropes on adrenergic and dopaminergic receptors.

DA = dopaminergic receptor
α = α-adrenergic receptor
β = β-adrenergic receptor

16 Describe how inotropes increase cardiac contractility

- Most inotropes work by increasing the intracellular cyclic adenosine monophosphate (cAMP) levels, which occurs by:

  a) stimulation of adenylate cyclase, which catalyses the conversion of ATP to cAMP (dopamine, adrenaline, noradrenaline);

  b) inhibition of phosphodiesterase enzyme, which normally converts cAMP to inactive 5' AMP (milrinone, enoximone).

- cAMP augments calcium influx into myocardial cells thereby increasing contractility.

17 Describe how to convert an infusion rate into a dose of intravenous medication

- Dose (μg/kg/min) = $\dfrac{\text{infusion rate (mL/hr) x drug in pump (mg)}}{[\text{Volume in pump(mL)}/1000] \times 60 \times \text{weight (kg)}}$

- Hence, if dopamine is made up with 200mg in 50mL of 5% dextrose:

  dopamine dose (μg/kg/min) = [200/ (50/1000 x 60] x infusion rate / weight
  = 66.67 x infusion rate / weight

- Similarly, if noradrenaline is made up with 4mg in 50mL of 5% dextrose, hence:

  noradrenaline dose (μg/kg/min) = [4/ (50/1000 x 60] x infusion rate / weight
  = 1.33 x rate / weight

- If adrenaline is made up with 2mg in 50mL of 5% dextrose, hence:

  adrenaline dose (μg/kg/min) = [2/ (50/1000 x 60] x infusion rate / weight
  = 0.667 x rate / weight

18 How is stroke volume controlled?

- Stroke volume is determined by preload, contractility and afterload, and is governed by the:

  a) Frank-Starling law, where the force of myocardial contraction is proportional to the initial myocardial fibre length (and therefore to left ventricular end-diastolic volume);
  b) Anrep effect, where the heart autoregulates according to changing afterload. For example, if the afterload increases at a given contractility, the left ventricular end-systolic volume increases, thereby increasing the stroke volume on the next cardiac cycle.

19 How is the heart rate controlled?

- Although the intrinsic heart rate is governed by the automaticity of the sino-atrial node, there are several factors that can influence the cardiac rate, including the:

  a) autonomic nervous system with sympathetic β1 adrenergic stimulation causing an increased heart rate and parasympathetic cholinergic stimulation causing a reduced heart rate;
  b) Bainbridge reflex, where the heart rate increases in response to a sudden increase in venous return.

20 Describe the principles of blood pressure control

- Maintenance of blood pressure is controlled by several different mechanisms:

  a) neural regulation, with afferent inputs from baroreceptors in the aorta and carotid sinus, conveyed by the vagus and glossopharyngeal nerves to the depressor zone of the vasomotor centre in the brainstem. Efferent signals are transmitted to the heart and blood vessels via sympathetic and parasympathetic nerves, which can produce changes in myocardial contraction, heart rate and vasomotor tone;

  b) hormonal regulation, such as with adrenaline and noradrenaline, to control the heart rate, myocardial contraction and vasomotor tone; and renin-angiotensin, which helps to control fluid balance and arteriolar vasomotor tone;

  c) local responses, including intrinsic cardiac responses, such as the Frank-Starling mechanism, Anrep effect, Bainbridge reflex, as well as local vascular autoregulation (see below).

21 Describe the renin-angiotensin system

- The renal juxtaglomerular apparatus releases renin in response to an acute reduction in plasma volume or mean arterial pressure.
- Renin converts circulating angiotensinogen, which is produced in the liver, into inactive angiotensin I.
- Angiotensin I is cleaved into active angiotensin II by a converting enzyme, which is produced by pulmonary and renal endothelium.
- Angiotensin II results in restoration of plasma volume and blood pressure by stimulating:

  a) arteriolar vasoconstriction;

  b) aldosterone release from the adrenal cortex, resulting in sodium and water reabsorption and potassium excretion at the renal distal convoluted tubule;

  c) anti-diuretic hormone (ADH) release from the posterior lobe of the pituitary gland, resulting in water reabsorption at the renal collecting ducts;

  d) thirst via hypothalamic receptors.

- Both angiotensin II and aldosterone negatively feedback on the juxtaglomerular apparatus and renin release.

22 Describe the factors that control local tissue blood flow

- Arteriolar diameter is the principal determinant of local blood flow and is determined by a number of factors:

    a) neural control of vasomotor tone by sympathetic α1-adrenergic receptors causing vasoconstriction and sympathetic β2-adrenergic receptors producing vasodilation;

    b) locally produced vasodilating (nitric oxide, bradykinin, histamine) and vasoconstricting (prostaglandins, angiotensin II, endothelins) agents;

    c) accumulation of metabolites (hydrogen ions, carbon dioxide, potassium ions) locally produces vasodilation;

    d) autoregulation, which is an adaptive mechanism of certain organs (brain, kidney and heart) to maintain constant local blood flow, independently of any changes in the global perfusion pressure.

23 Describe the factors that control coronary blood flow (CBF)

- CBF = coronary perfusion pressure / coronary vascular resistance.
- Coronary perfusion pressure is the difference between diastolic blood pressure and left ventricular end-diastolic pressure.
- Coronary perfusion pressure is reduced when left ventricular end-diastolic pressure increases or systemic blood pressure decreases, especially diastolic blood pressure, as the majority of coronary blood flow to the left ventricle occurs during diastole.
- Similarly, an increase in heart rate shortens the diastolic time period and therefore reduces coronary perfusion.
- Coronary autoregulation attempts to maintain the coronary perfusion pressure within a consistent range during changing systemic blood pressures and is governed by the coronary vascular resistance.
- Coronary vascular resistance is controlled by the pre-capillary resistance vessels which are modified by:

    a) autonomic regulation, with sympathetic stimulation causing vasoconstriction and parasympathetic stimulation causing vasodilation;

    b) endothelial factors, with nitric oxide causing vasodilation and endothelin causing vasoconstriction;

    c) metabolic factors, with adenosine and prostacyclin causing vasodilation.

24 Describe the factors that control myocardial oxygen supply

- Myocardial oxygen supply (MO_2) is determined by arterial oxygen (O_2) content and coronary blood flow (CBF):

MO_2 delivery (mL/min) = CBF (dL/100g/min) x arterial O_2 content (mL/dL).

- Arterial O_2 content =

  (1.34 x Hb [g/dL] x O_2 sats) + dissolved O_2 (0.0031 x PaO_2)

  Each gram of haemoglobin combines with 1.34mL O_2 and only a small amount of oxygen dissolves in blood.

- Hence, the factors that control myocardial oxygen supply include coronary blood flow (left ventricular end-diastolic pressure, diastolic blood pressure, diastolic filling time, coronary vascular resistance), haemoglobin and arterial oxygen saturations.

25 What is Poiseuille's law?

- Poiseuille's law describes the properties that govern flow of a viscous liquid through a vessel with:

$$Flow = \frac{\Delta P \times \pi \times r^4}{8 \times \eta \times L}$$

where ΔP is the change in pressure across the vessel; r is the radius of the vessel; η is the viscosity of the fluid flowing through the vessel; L is the length of the vessel.

- The resistance to flow through the vessel can be calculated by:

$$\frac{8 \times \eta \times L}{\pi \times r^4}$$

- Hence, if the radius of the vessel halves, the resistance increases by a factor of 16 and the flow decreases by a factor of 16.

26 Describe the factors that maintain the resting potential within the cardiomyocyte

- Cardiomyocytes contain voltage-gated ion channels that allow certain charged particles to cross the cell membrane.
- These ion channels maintain a voltage gradient across the cell membrane with sodium and calcium concentrations higher outside the cell and potassium concentration higher inside.

- This concentration gradient is maintained by the Na/K ATP-dependent pump, which pumps potassium ions in and sodium ions out of the cell.
- At rest, cardiomyocytes have potassium channels open whilst sodium and calcium channels are closed, hence potassium ions move out of the cells, leaving negatively charged ions behind and a resting potential of approximately -90mV in ventricular muscle cells.

27 Describe the phases of the cardiomyocyte action potential (Figure 12)

- Depolarisation of a neighbouring cell causes opening of the cardiomyocyte sodium channels. This triggers a series of changes associated with propagation of the cardiac action potential:

   a)   phase 0: influx of sodium ions causes the membrane potential to become transiently positive;

   b)   phase 1: opening of the potassium channels allows potassium to leave the cell, restoring the membrane potential to approximately zero;

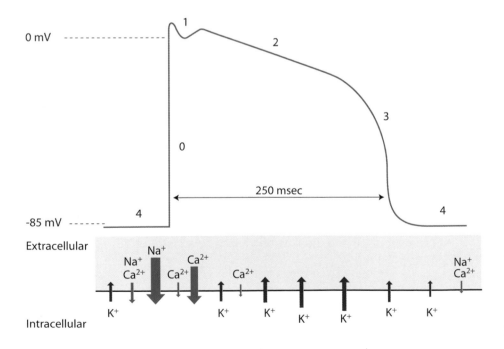

Figure 12. Cardiomyocyte action potential. K+ = potassium ions; Ca2+ = calcium ions; Na+ = sodium ions.

c) phase 2: opening of the calcium channels allows calcium to enter the cell, which balances with the exit of potassium during this plateau phase. The calcium entering during this phase initiates the excitation-contraction coupling process;

d) phase 3: closure of the calcium channels, associated with the exit of potassium, allows repolarisation and restoration of the membrane potential to -90mV;

e) phase 4: resting period which prepares the cell for the next depolarization.

28 How does the cardiac action potential differ in the Purkinje cells and pacemaker cells (Figure 13)?

- Purkinje cells have a more negative resting potential and the upstroke of phase 0 is more rapid.
- The action potential of the pacemaker cells of the sino-atrial node and atrioventricular node differ from normal cardiomyocytes as follows:

a) automaticity, as they are able to depolarize spontaneously in a rhythmic manner without requiring initiation of the action potential by an adjacent cell;

b) phase 0 is less rapid than normal cardiomyocytes;

c) phase 4 progressively increases due to gradual spontaneous depolarization rather than being almost flat with normal cardiomyocytes.

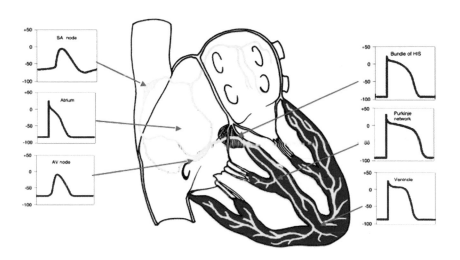

Figure 13. Cardiomyocyte action potential throughout the conduction pathway.

29 What is the refractory period?

- The refractory period refers to the phase of the action potential where the cell cannot be restimulated and acts as a protective mechanism, thereby allowing atrial and ventricular filling and emptying.
- Phase 0-3 of the cardiac action potential represents the absolute refractory period, where the cardiomyocyte is completely unexcitable.
- Ventricular cardiomyocytes have longer refractory periods than atrial cells.

30 Describe the structure of a myofibril (Figure 14)

- Each myofibril contains a series of repeated subunits (sarcomeres) that consist of:

    a)   myosin molecules, which are arranged in thick filaments with thin tails and globular heads (with myosin ATPase);

    b)   actin molecules, which are arranged in thin helical filaments that interdigitate with the thick myosin filaments via cross-bridges.

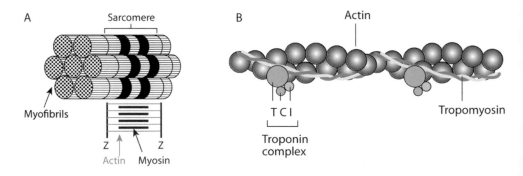

Figure 14. Structure of a myofibril.

- These molecules are responsible for myocardial contraction (with calcium ions acting as the messengers) under the regulatory control of:

  a) tropomyosin (TM), which lies in the grooves between the actin filaments in the relaxed state, thereby blocking the attachment of the myosin cross-bridges and preventing contraction;
  b) troponin (Tp), which is a complex of three subunits:
     i) TpT, which binds to tropomyosin, thereby forming the Tp-TM complex;
     ii) TpI, which binds to actin to keep the Tp-TM complex in place;
     iii) TpC, which binds to the calcium ions to produce the conformational change.

31 Describe the process of cardiac excitation contraction coupling (Figure 15)

- Excitation contraction coupling describes the process where triggering of the cardiac action potential in a cardiomyocyte initiates a series of changes that result in mechanical muscular contraction. These include the following:

  a) calcium ions enter the cells during phase 2 of the cardiac action potential;
  b) an influx of these calcium ions cause a conformational change in the troponin-tropomyosin complex;
  c) this conformational change allows the myosin globular head to form cross-bridges with the actin filaments, interdigitating the thick and thin filaments, to produce mechanical contraction.

- Inotropes increase the concentration of cytosolic calcium ions, resulting in increased ATP being hydrolysed, thereby producing an increased force of myocardial contraction.

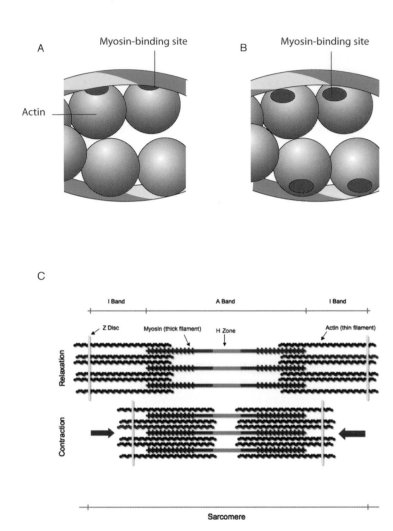

Figure 15. Excitation-contraction coupling. A) Myosin binding sites on the actin molecules are blocked in the relaxed state. B) Conformational change of the troponin-tropomyosin complex (induced by calcium influx) reveals the myosin-binding site allowing cross-bridge formation. C) This induces interdigitation of the myosin and actin molecules and muscular contraction.

32 Draw the oxygen dissociation curve (Figure 16)

- The relationship between arterial oxygen saturation (SaO$_2$) and arterial oxygen partial pressure (PaO$_2$) is non-linear.
- Above a PaO$_2$ of 8kPa (60mmHg), rises and falls in the PaO$_2$ make very little difference to the SaO$_2$.
- Below a PaO$_2$ of 8kPa (60mmHg), however, a small drop in the PaO$_2$ produces a large fall in the SaO$_2$.
- In view of these changes, it is important to keep the PaO$_2$ >10kPa (75mmHg) to leave a margin of safety.

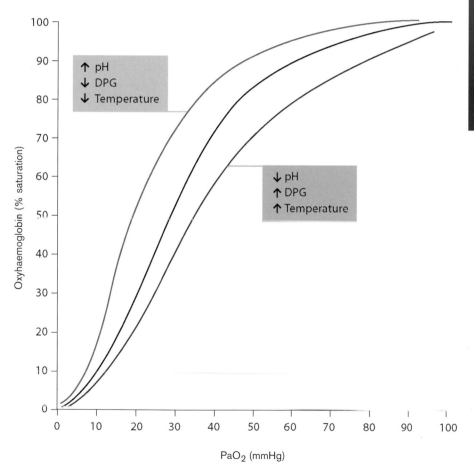

Figure 16. Oxygen dissociation curve. DPG = 2,3-diphosphoglycerate.

33 Describe the Bohr effect

- Factors such as acidosis, hypercapnia and increasing temperature cause a right shift of the oxygen dissociation curve, thereby encouraging oxygen release to the tissues.

34 Describe the principles of Starling's forces (Figure 17)

- Starling's forces govern the movement of water and solutes across a capillary membrane and are principally controlled by:

  a)   capillary hydrostatic pressure;
  b)   plasma colloid oncotic pressure (negatively charged proteins);
  c)   interstitial fluid hydrostatic pressure;
  d)   interstitial fluid colloid oncotic pressure (negatively charged proteins).

- In combination with these forces, fluid movement is also dependent on capillary permeability, the surface area of the capillaries and lymph flow.

58

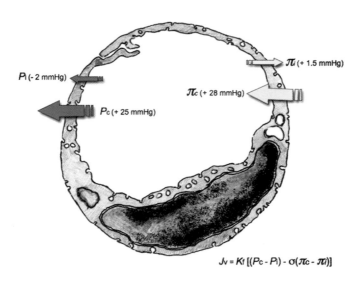

P_i (- 2 mmHg)

π_i (+ 1.5 mmHg)

π_c (+ 28 mmHg)

P_c (+ 25 mmHg)

$$Jv = Kf\,[(Pc - Pi) - \sigma(\pi c - \pi i)]$$

Figure 17. Starling's forces. Pc = capillary hydrostatic pressure; Pi = interstitial fluid hydrostatic pressure; πc = plasma colloid oncotic pressure; πi = interstitial fluid colloid oncotic pressure; Jv = fluid flux; Kf = filtration constant; σ = reflection coefficient.

35 What are the principles of an intra-aortic balloon pump (IABP)(Figures 18 and 19)?

- An IABP acts as a counter-pulsation device that is timed to inflate during diastole thereby augmenting organ perfusion and deflate just prior to systole, thereby reducing left ventricular afterload.
- It is usually placed via the femoral artery and lies in the descending thoracic aorta, with the tip of the balloon position just distal to the origin of the left subclavian artery.
- Malposition of the IABP can result in:

  a) mesenteric or renal ischaemia, if the balloon is too low;
  b) cerebral or left upper limb ischaemia, if the balloon is too high.

- Other complications of IABP insertion include bleeding, infection, thrombo-embolism, leg ischaemia, thrombocytopaenia, balloon rupture and haemolysis.

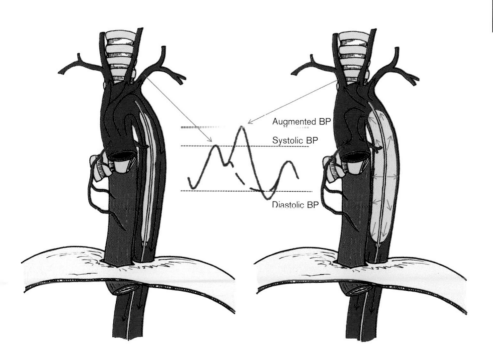

Figure 18. Intra-aortic balloon pump. BP = blood pressure.

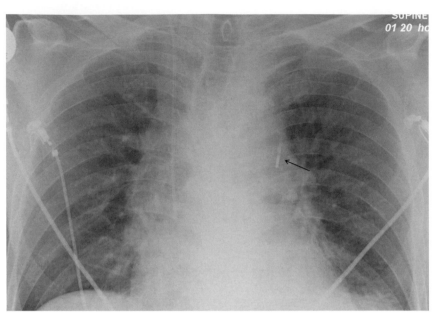

Figure 19. Intra-aortic balloon pump tip (arrow) located on a chest X-ray. Ideally, the IABP tip is placed in the descending aorta, 1-2cm distal to the origin of the left subclavian artery. Radiologically, this can be identified either 2cm below the top of the aortic knuckle or in the 2rd-3rd intercostal space anteriorly.

- An IABP improves the myocardial oxygen supply to demand ratio by:

  a) reducing the tension-time index (systolic wall tension) by reducing the impedance to left ventricular ejection;

  b) increasing the diastolic pressure-time index by increasing coronary flow during diastole.

- IABPs are usually inserted in patients with:

  a) myocardial ischaemia;

  b) low cardiac output syndrome;

  c) volume overload of the left ventricle, such as following acute mitral regurgitation or post-infarct ventricular septal rupture;

  d) acute myocardial deterioration as a bridge to transplantation or left ventricular assist device implantation.

- IABPs are, however, contra-indicated in patients with severe aortic regurgitation, aortic dissection, abdominal aortic aneurysms and severe peripheral atherosclerosis.

36 Describe the stages of haemostasis (Figure 20)

● Haemostasis involves the interaction of several different systems to form a stable clot:

a) vascular phase, which occurs as an immediate response when damage to a vessel wall induces neural reflexes and local myogenic spasm to reduce local blood flow;

b) platelet phase, which occurs when platelets come into contact with endothelial collagen fibres of the damaged vessel. This in turn activates platelet aggregation, mediated by ADP, thromboxane A2, von Willebrand factor, membrane glycoprotein IIb/IIIa receptors, fibrinogen, serotonin (5HT) and platelet activating factor to form a loose platelet plug;

c) clotting phase, which occurs when the intrinsic and extrinsic pathways are activated to convert the loose platelet plug into a stable fibrin clot (see below).

61

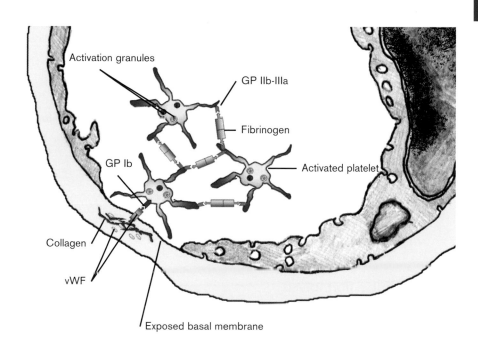

Figure 20. Haemostasis, triggered by endothelial damage inducing activation of platelets followed by fibrinogen cross-bridge formation. vWF = von Willebrand Factor.

37 Describe the clotting cascade (Figure 21)

- The clotting cascade involves activation of a number of coagulation factors (serine proteases) resulting in fibrin (clot) formation. It is controlled by the:

  a)   intrinsic pathway (contact activation pathway);
  b)   extrinsic pathway (tissue factor pathway), which is activated by tissue factor released by the endothelium following vessel damage;
  c)   final common pathway, which is activated by either the intrinsic or extrinsic pathways and results in fibrin formation.

- There are a number of co-factors that play an important role in the coagulation cascade:

  a)   calcium, which is required by tenase and prothrombinase to convert prothrombin into thrombin;
  b)   vitamin K, which is required by the liver for the production of Factors II, VII, IX and X (as well as protein C and protein S).

- There are a number of inherent regulators circulating that control the coagulation cascade:

  a)   protein C, which inactivates Factors Va and VIIIa in the presence of protein S;
  b)   anti-thrombin III, which is a serine protease inhibitor secreted by the endothelium and inhibits thrombin and Factors IXa, Xa and XIa;
  c)   prostacyclin, which inhibits platelet aggregation and causes vasodilation;
  d)   tissue factor pathway inhibitor which is produced by platelets and inhibits Factors Xa and VIIa;
  e)   plasmin (see below).

38 Describe fibrinolysis

- Fibrinolysis is the process of clot breakdown and is primarily controlled by plasmin.
- Plasmin is a serine protease that is synthesised in the liver as inactive plasminogen.
- Its main function is to break down the unstable bonds between fibrin molecules to generate fibrin degradation products.

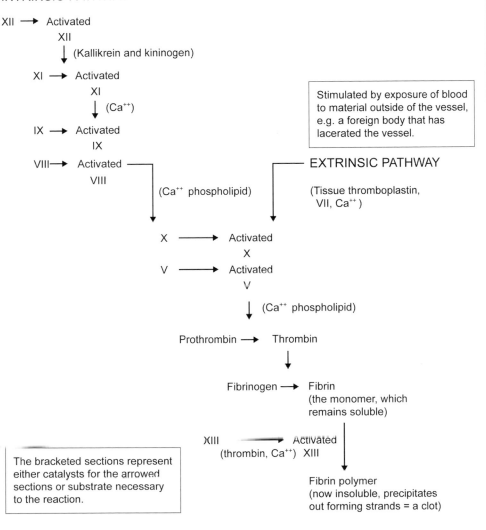

Stimulated by exposure of blood to a negatively charged surface, e.g. in the vessel wall if endothelial lining becomes damaged.

INTRINSIC PATHWAY

XII → Activated XII

(Kallikrein and kininogen)

XI → Activated XI

(Ca^{++})

IX → Activated IX

VIII → Activated VIII

(Ca^{++} phospholipid)

Stimulated by exposure of blood to material outside of the vessel, e.g. a foreign body that has lacerated the vessel.

EXTRINSIC PATHWAY

(Tissue thromboplastin, VII, Ca^{++})

X → Activated X

V → Activated V

(Ca^{++} phospholipid)

Prothrombin → Thrombin

Fibrinogen → Fibrin (the monomer, which remains soluble)

XIII → Activated XIII
(thrombin, Ca^{++})

The bracketed sections represent either catalysts for the arrowed sections or substrate necessary to the reaction.

Fibrin polymer (now insoluble, precipitates out forming strands = a clot)

Figure 21. Coagulation cascade.

- It is activated by tissue plasminogen activator (tPA), urokinase, thrombin, fibrin and Factor XII, and is inactivated by α2-antiplasmin and serpin (serine protease inhibitor).
- It occurs at the same time as fibrin formation to limit thrombus production locally.

39 What is a thrombo-elastogram (TEG)(Figure 22)?

- A thrombo-elastogram allows the measurement of the kinetics and tensile strength (visco-elastic properties) of clot formation and fibrinolysis.
- It assesses several different variables in the coagulation process:

a) R time (normal range 4-8 min), that measures the time to initial fibrin formation;

b) K time (normal range 1-4 min) and alpha angle (normal range 54-67°), which measure fibrinogen-platelet interaction;

c) maximal amplitude (MA) (normal range 59-68mm), that measures platelet aggregation;

d) amplitude 60 minutes after the maximum, which represents the degree of fibrinolysis.

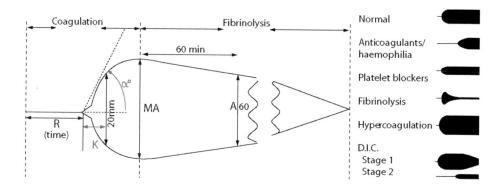

Figure 22. Thrombo-elastogram. MA = maximal amplitude; A_{60} = amplitude at 60 minutes; R = R time; K = K time; α = α angle.

Recommended reading

1.   Bers DM. Cardiac excitation-contraction coupling. *Nature* 2002; 415(6868): 198-205.

2.   Overgaard CB, Dzavík V. Inotropes and vasopressors: review of physiology and clinical use in cardiovascular disease. *Circulation* 2008; 118(10): 1047-56.

Chapter 3

Cardiac pharmacology

1   **What are the pharmacological properties of aspirin?**
- Class of drug: cyclo-oxygenase inhibitor.
- Mechanism of action: aspirin inhibits platelet cyclo-oxygenase thereby reducing the production of thromboxane A2 and platelet adhesiveness.
- Indications: primary and secondary prevention of cardiovascular and cerebrovascular disease.
- Cautions: asthma, peptic ulcer disease and renal impairment.
- Side effects: bronchospasm and gastrointestinal haemorrhage.
- Dose: 75-150mg as prophylaxis and up to 300mg for therapeutic effect in myocardial infarction.

2   **What are the pharmacological properties of clopidogrel?**
- Class of drug: platelet ADP (adenosine diphosphate) receptor antagonist.
- Mechanism of action: clopidogrel irreversibly modifies the platelet ADP receptor thereby directly inhibiting the binding of ADP and subsequent ADP-mediated activation of the glycoprotein IIb/IIIa complex. Platelets exposed to clopidogrel are ineffective for the remainder of their lifetime (5-7 days).
- Indications: primary and secondary prevention of cardiovascular and cerebrovascular disease (CAPRIE trial). It is also used as dual therapy in combination with aspirin for acute coronary syndrome (CURE trial) and long-term anti-thrombotic prophylaxis for drug-eluting stents.
- Cautions: active bleeding.
- Side effects: haemorrhage and neutropaenia.
- Dose: loading dose 300mg followed by 75mg daily maintenance.

3   What are the pharmacological properties of heparin?

- Mechanism of action: heparin is a mucopolysaccharide that:

  a)   inactivates activated Factor X;
  b)   inhibits conversion of prothrombin to thrombin;
  c)   prevents fibrin formation from fibrinogen.

- Indications: treatment and prophylaxis of deep venous thrombosis and pulmonary embolism; unstable angina; anticoagulation during cardiopulmonary bypass; temporary anticoagulation for prosthetic valve patients.
- Cautions: active bleeding.
- Side effects: haemorrhage, hyperkalaemia, osteoporosis, thrombocytopaenia and hypersensitivity.
- Dose:

  a)   prophylactic - 5000U b.d. subcutaneously;
  b)   therapeutic - 5000U (or 75U/kg) IV loading dose followed by an infusion of 18U/kg/hr;
  c)   full cardiopulmonary bypass - 300U/kg bolus; minimal extracorporeal circulation (MECC) - 200U/kg; off-pump CABG - 100U/kg.

- Heparin can be reversed with protamine sulphate.

4   What are the pharmacological properties of low-molecular-weight heparin (LMWH)?

- Mechanism of action: LMWH has similar actions to heparin except:

  a)   LMWH has a longer half-life than heparin;
  b)   LMWH does not require monitoring (APTTR is unaffected);
  c)   LMWH has a greater anti-factor Xa activity;
  d)   LMWH has a lower incidence of thrombocytopaenia and osteoporosis.

- Indications: acute coronary syndrome (FRISC trial, TIMI IIB trial) and prophylaxis for deep vein thrombosis.
- Cautions: active bleeding.
- Side effects: haemorrhage, hyperkalaemia, osteoporosis, thrombocytopaenia and hypersensitivity.
- Dose:

  a)   dalteparin (Fragmin®) -   therapeutic 120U/kg b.d. SC;
                                      -   prophylactic 5000U o.d. SC;

b)   enoxaparin (Clexane®) -   therapeutic 1mg/kg b.d. SC;
                            -   prophylactic 20-40mg o.d. SC.

5   **What are the pharmacological properties of warfarin?**

- Mechanism of action: warfarin is a coumarin derivative that interferes with vitamin K metabolism. Vitamin K is a co-factor in the hepatic production of numerous proteins including coagulation Factors II, VII, IX and X.
- Indications: prophylaxis and treatment for thrombo-embolism with deep vein thrombosis, pulmonary embolism, atrial fibrillation, mechanical prosthetic valves, left ventricular thrombus and transient ischaemic attacks.
- Cautions: hepatic impairment; peptic ulcer disease; warfarin interacts with numerous drugs including amiodarone, antibiotics (such as rifampicin), anticonvulsants, non-steroidal anti-inflammatory drugs and statins.
- Side effects: haemorrhage.
- Dose: dependent on the international normalised ratio (INR) with most indications aiming for an INR of 2.0-3.0, except in patients with mechanical mitral valves (INR 2.5-3.5).
- Warfarin can be reversed with vitamin K, fresh frozen plasma or Beriplex® (human prothrombin complex concentrate).

6   **What are the pharmacological properties of glycoprotein IIb/IIIa blockers?**

- Mechanism of action: glycoprotein IIb/IIIa blockers inhibit platelet aggregation by binding to the glycoprotein IIb/IIIa receptors on platelets thereby preventing these receptors linking to other platelets by fibrinogen cross-bridges.
- Indications: acute coronary syndrome, percutaneous coronary intervention.
- Cautions: active bleeding and hepatic impairment
- Side effects: haemorrhage, thrombocytopaenia and hypersensitivity.
- Dose:

a)   abciximab (ReoPro®) 250μg/kg IV bolus then 125ng/kg/min IV infusion;
b)   tirofibran 400ng/kg/min for 30 minutes then 100ng/kg/min IV infusion.

7   **What are the pharmacological properties of fibrinolytics?**
● Mechanism of action: fibrinolytics convert plasminogen to plasmin, which in turn degrades fibrin-containing thrombi. These drugs are sub-divided into:

a)   non-specific thrombolytic agents (such as streptokinase);
b)   fibrin-specific agents (such as recombinant tissue plasminogen activator and tenecteplase).

● Indications: acute myocardial infarction (MI), acute pulmonary embolism and a thrombosed cardiac valve.
● Cautions: recent stroke, recent gastro-intestinal bleed, recent major surgery, pregnancy, trauma, aortic dissection and if the patient is already on warfarin or has a major bleeding disorder.
● Side effects: haemorrhage, including cerebral haemorrhage, hypersensitivity and systemic emboli (which occurs following clot lysis).
● Dose: streptokinase (for MI) 1.5 million U.

8   **What are the pharmacological properties of aprotinin?**
● Class of drug: anti-fibrinolytic agent.
● Mechanism of action: aprotinin inhibits serine proteases including:

a)   plasmin, thereby inhibiting fibrinolysis;
b)   kallikrein, thereby inhibiting the formation of Factor XIIa in the intrinsic coagulation pathway.

● Indications: prophylaxis to reduce bleeding and the use of blood products following cardiac surgery.
● Cautions: renal impairment and previous aprotinin use (within 6 months).
● Side effects: renal failure, graft patency (in patients with poor distal coronary artery run-off, IMAGE trial) and anaphylaxis.
● Dose: standard Hammersmith regime:

a)   loading dose 2 million KIU (280mg) intravenously;
b)   2 million KIU (280mg) added to the prime volume of the cardiopulmonary bypass circuit;
c)   0.5 million KIU (70mg) per hour infusion.

● Currently, aprotinin has been withdrawn from use, due to results from the BART trial, which has shown an increased risk of death, stroke, renal impairment and heart failure with aprotinin.

9   **What are the pharmacological properties of tranexamic acid?**
- Class of drug: lysine analogue anti-fibrinolytic agent.
- Mechanism of action: tranexamic acid binds to plasminogen, thereby inhibiting fibrinolysis.
- Indications: prophylaxis to reduce bleeding and the use of blood products following cardiac surgery. Tranexamic acid is also used following massive haemoptysis and in haemophiliacs.
- Cautions: renal impairment, disseminated intravascular coagulation and thrombo-embolic disease.
- Side effects: renal function and graft patency.
- Dose: 2g given intravenously at induction of general anaesthesia, followed by 2g added to the prime volume of the cardiopulmonary bypass circuit and 1g at termination of cardiopulmonary bypass.

10   **What are the pharmacological properties of statins?**
- Class of drug: 3-hydroxy-3-methylglutaryl (HMG) CoA reductase inhibitors.
- Mechanism of action: statins competitively inhibit hepatic HMG-CoA reductase, which is involved in cholesterol synthesis.
- Indications: prophylaxis and therapeutic lowering of serum cholesterol; primary and secondary prevention of cardiovascular events.
- Cautions: hepatic impairment and pregnancy.
- Side effects: myalgia, rhabdomyolysis, hepatic dysfunction, nausea, vomiting and abdominal pain.
- Dose: simvastatin, pravastatin, fluvastatin or atorvastatin 10-80mg o.d.

11   **What are the pharmacological properties of beta-blockers?**
- Mechanism of action: β-blockers bind to β-adrenoreceptors to produce negative inotropic and chronotropic effects, thereby reducing myocardial oxygen demand. β-blockers also have a cardiomyocyte membrane stabilizing effect, thereby acting as an anti-arrhythmic agent.
- Indications: angina, hypertension, myocardial infarction, supraventricular tachycardia, primary and secondary prevention of cardiovascular events and heart failure.
- Cautions: asthma, peripheral vascular disease, diabetes mellitus, poor left ventricular function and heart block.

- Side effects: postural hypotension, bradycardia, heart block, peripheral vasoconstriction and bronchospasm.
- Dose:

  a) bisoprolol 1.25-10mg o.d.;
  b) atenolol 25-100mg o.d.;
  c) metoprolol 25-100mg b.d. or t.d.s.;
  d) carvedilol 3.125-50mg o.d. or b.d.

- Cardioselective β-blockers (such as bisoprolol) can be trialled in patients with mild asthma, peripheral vascular disease or diabetes mellitus.
- Certain β-blockers have also been shown to be effective in heart failure, such as carvedilol, bisoprolol and metoprolol.

12 What are the pharmacological properties of labetalol?

- Mechanism of action: labetalol selectively antagonizes α1, β1 and β2-adrenergic receptors, thereby reducing the absolute blood pressure and shear stress forces within the aorta.
- Indications: blood pressure control in patients with acute aortic dissection.
- Cautions: heart block.
- Side effects: hypotension and bradycardia.
- Dose: 15mg/hr increased to 120mg/hr depending on the blood pressure.

13 What are the pharmacological properties of calcium channel blockers?

- Mechanism of action: calcium channel blockers inhibit calcium influx during phase 2 of the cardiac action potential (plateau phase), thereby reducing cardiac contractility and the propagation of cardiac electrical impulses. Calcium channel blockers also relax vascular smooth muscle, thereby dilating coronary and peripheral arteries.
- Indications: angina, hypertension, supraventricular tachycardia, pulmonary hypertension.
- Cautions: poor left ventricular function, heart block and severe aortic stenosis.
- Side effects: flushing, headaches, peripheral oedema, heart block and bradycardia.
- Dose:

  a) amlodipine 5-10mg o.d.;
  b) diltiazem 60-120mg t.d.s. or slow-release preparations 120-360mg o.d.;

c)   nifedipine 5-20mg t.d.s. or slow-release preparations 20-60mg o.d.;
d)   verapamil 40-120mg t.d.s. or slow-release preparations 240-480mg o.d.

14 What are the pharmacological properties of angiotensin-converting enzyme inhibitors (ACEIs)?

● Mechanism of action: angiotensin-converting enzyme inhibitors inhibit the conversion of inactive angiotensin I to active angiotensin II, thereby reducing the vasoconstrictive effects of angiotensin II and reducing the release of aldosterone by the adrenal cortex.
● Indications: hypertension, left ventricular systolic dysfunction, secondary prevention of cardiovascular events.
● Cautions: renal impairment, renal artery stenosis and severe aortic stenosis.
● Side effects: hypersensitivity, hypotension, chronic cough and hyperkalaemia.
● Dose:

a)   ramipril 1.25-10mg o.d.;
b)   perindopril 2-8mg o.d.;
c)   lisinopril 2.5-40mg o.d.;
d)   enalapril 5-20mg o.d. or b.d.;
e)   captopril 6.25-50mg b.d.

15 What are the pharmacological properties of angiotensin II receptor blockers (ARBs)?

● Mechanism of action: angiotensin receptor blockers have similar properties to ACEIs but unlike ACEIs, ARBs do not break down bradykinin, which is thought to be responsible for the persistent cough associated with ACEIs.
● Indications: hypertension and left ventricular systolic dysfunction when ACEIs are not tolerated by the patient (such as chronic cough) or when the patient is on a maximum dose of ACEIs, ARBs can be used synergistically.
● Cautions: renal artery stenosis, renal impairment, aortic stenosis and hypertrophic cardiomyopathy.
● Side effects: hyperkalaemia and hypotension.
● Dose:

a)   candesartan 4-32mg o.d.;
b)   losartan 25-100mg o.d.

16 **What are the pharmacological properties of nitrates?**
- Mechanism of action: nitrates are smooth muscle relaxants that result in:

   a)   coronary vasodilation and reduced coronary spasm;
   b)   reduced preload and afterload, thereby reducing myocardial oxygen demand.

- Indications: angina and left ventricular failure.
- Cautions: hypertrophic cardiomyopathy, aortic stenosis, glaucoma and hypovolaemia.
- Side effects: postural hypotension, tachycardia, headaches, flushing, palpitations and methaemoglobinaemia.
- Dose:

   a)   glyceryl trinitrate infusion 10-200µg/min;
   b)   glyceryl trinitrate sublingual tablet or spray 0.3-0.5mg PRN;
   c)   isosorbide mononitrate 10-60mg b.d. or slow-release 30-120mg o.d.

17 **What are the pharmacological properties of nicorandil?**
- Class of drug: combination of nitrate and potassium channel opener.
- Mechanism of action: nicorandil activates vascular potassium channels, thereby inducing coronary artery and systemic venous dilatation resulting in increased coronary oxygen delivery and reduced preload, respectively.
- Indications: angina.
- Cautions: hypotension and heart failure.
- Side effects: headache, flushing and dizziness.
- Dose: 10-30mg b.d.

18 **What are the pharmacological properties of sodium nitroprusside (SNP)?**
- Mechanism of action: sodium nitroprusside relaxes arterial smooth muscle, thereby reducing systemic and pulmonary afterload.
- Indications: refractory hypertension (following aortic dissection or post-cardiac surgery) and pulmonary hypertension.
- Cautions: hepatic dysfunction; the syringe used to infuse SNP needs to be wrapped in aluminium foil to protect it from the light.
- Side effects: reflex tachycardia, headache, dizziness and cyanide toxicity.
- Dose: 0.5-8µg/kg/min for a maximum of 48 hours.

19 **What are the pharmacological properties of dopamine?**

- Mechanism of action: dopamine is a dopaminergic and adrenergic receptor agonist (see below for effects).
- Indications: low cardiac output state, inotropic support following cardiac surgery or myocardial infarction.
- Cautions: tachyarrhythmias, phaeochromocytoma and patients on mono-amine oxidase inhibitors.
- Side effects: tachycardia, hypertension and peripheral vasoconstriction.
- Dose: dopamine acts on different receptors and has different effects depending on the dose:

  a) between 1-5µg/kg/min, dopaminergic receptors are activated producing vasodilation of coronary, renal, cerebral and splanchnic vasculature;

  b) between 5-10µg/kg/min, dopamine activates β_1 receptors, producing increased myocardial contractility and increased heart rate. At this dose, dopamine also has some β_2 receptor agonist activity producing peripheral vasodilation;

  c) above >10µg/kg/min, dopamine mainly stimulates α-adrenergic receptors, producing systemic vasoconstriction. Although this rise in systemic vascular resistance produces an increase in blood pressure, it may be at the cost of increased myocardial oxygen demand as the heart has to work in the face of increased resistance.

- Dopamine along with all other inotropes (except dobutamine) must be delivered intravenously through a central vein to reduce the risk of peripheral vasoconstriction and subsequent skin necrosis.

20 **What are the pharmacological properties of dobutamine?**

- Mechanism of action: dobutamine is a synthetic inodilator that activates β_1-adrenergic receptors (positive inotropic effects) and also has moderate β_2-adrenergic actions (vasodilation).
- Indications: inotropic support following cardiac surgery, myocardial infarction and cardiogenic shock. Dobutamine is also used for stress echocardiography and magnetic resonance imaging.
- Cautions: tachyarrhythmias, phaeochromocytoma and patients on mono-amine oxidase inhibitors.
- Side effects: tachycardia and hypertension.
- Dose: 2.5-10µg/kg/min IV infusion. It can be given via a peripheral line.

21 What are the pharmacological properties of dopexamine?

- Mechanism of action: dopexamine is a synthetic catecholamine that produces systemic, mesenteric and renal vasodilation by stimulating β_2-adrenergic and DA_1 receptors. It also has mild positive inotropic effects.
- Indications: inotropic support following cardiac surgery or heart failure.
- Cautions: hypertrophic cardiomyopathy, aortic stenosis, thrombocytopaenia and phaeochromocytoma.
- Side effects: tachycardia, nausea, vomiting, headache and thrombocytopaenia.
- Dose: 0.5-6µg/kg/min IV infusion.

22 What are the pharmacological properties of adrenaline?

- Mechanism of action: adrenaline is a potent β_1-adrenergic agonist, producing increased myocardial contractility and increased heart rate. At low doses, adrenaline has β_2 effects of systemic vasodilation and bronchodilation but at higher doses its α-adrenergic vasoconstriction effects predominate.
- Indications: bronchospasm, inotropic support, cardiac arrest.
- Cautions: hypertension, phaeochromocytoma, glaucoma and diabetes mellitus.
- Side effects: tachycardia, arrhythmia, hypertension and metabolic acidosis.
- Dose:

  a)   cardiac arrest: 10mL of 1:10,000 adrenaline (which equates to 1mg);

  b)   inotropic support: 0.01-1.0µg/kg/min IV infusion.

23 What are the pharmacological properties of noradrenaline?

- Mechanism of action: noradrenaline is a potent α_1-adrenergic agonist, producing systemic vasoconstriction, and β_1-adrenergic agonist, producing increased myocardial contractility and increased heart rate.
- Indications: low cardiac output following cardiac surgery or myocardial infarction. Noradrenaline is particularly useful in conditions with low systemic vascular resistance (such as sepsis or anaphylaxis).

- Cautions: hypertension and high systemic vascular resistance.
- Side effects: hypertension, tachyarrhythmias and peripheral ischaemia (e.g. gastro-intestinal tract or renal).
- Dose: 0.01-1.0µg/kg/min intravenous infusion.

24 What are the pharmacological properties of milrinone?

- Class of drug: phosphodiesterase inhibitor.
- Mechanism of action: milrinone acts as an inodilator by reducing systemic and pulmonary vascular resistance as well as having moderate positive inotropic effects.
- Indications: low cardiac output state following cardiac surgery, especially in the presence of pulmonary hypertension or right ventricular failure.
- Cautions: hypertrophic cardiomyopathy and aortic stenosis.
- Side effects: tachyarrhythmias, hypotension and thrombocytopaenia.
- Dose: 0.125-0.75µg/kg/min IV infusion.
- The addition of an α-adrenergic agonist (such as noradrenaline) synergistically is often required to counteract the systemic vascular resistance lowering properties of milrinone.

25 What are the pharmacological properties of phenylephrine?

- Mechanism of action: phenylephrine is a selective α1-adrenergic receptor agonist, which produces systemic vasoconstriction.
- Indications: acute hypotension; to maintain systemic blood pressure whilst on cardiopulmonary bypass.
- Cautions: severe hyperthyroidism.
- Side-effects: hypertension, peripheral ischaemia and headache.
- Dose: 0.5-3.0µg/kg/min IV infusion, 0.5-1mg IV boluses whilst on cardiopulmonary bypass.

26 What are the pharmacological properties of isoprenaline?

- Mechanism of action: isoprenaline is a selective β_1- and β_2-adrenergic agonist, which produces positive inotropic, chronotropic and bronchodilatory effects.
- Indications: bradycardia, unresponsive to atropine.
- Cautions: tachycardia.
- Side effects: cardiac dysrhythmias.
- Dose: 0.02-0.2µg/kg/min IV infusion.

27 What are the pharmacological properties of thiazide diuretics?

- Mechanism of action: thiazide diuretics inhibit sodium reabsorption at the distal convoluted tubule.
- Indications: hypertension, peripheral oedema.
- Cautions: nephrotic syndrome and hyperaldosteronism.
- Side effects: postural hypotension, hypokalaemia, hyponatraemia and gout.
- Dose:

  a)   bendroflumethiazide 2.5mg o.d. to 10mg t.d.s.;
  b)   metolazone 5-80mg o.d.

28 What are the pharmacological properties of loop diuretics?

- Mechanism of action: loop diuretics inhibit water and electrolyte reabsorption from the ascending limb of the loop of Henle.
- Indications: pulmonary oedema, heart failure, hyperkalaemia, peripheral oedema and oliguria associated with renal impairment.
- Cautions: hypovolaemia and renal failure.
- Side effects: hypokalaemia, gout, hyponatraemia and deafness.
- Dose:

  a)   furosemide 10-80mg o.d. or b.d., oral or IV infusion at a rate of 2-10mg/hr;
  b)   bumetanide 1-5mg o.d. or b.d., oral or IV.

29 What are the pharmacological properties of mannitol?

- Mechanism of action: mannitol is a potent osmotic diuretic and a weak renal vasodilator.
- Indications: cerebral oedema, fluid overload associated with cardiopulmonary bypass.
- Cautions: congestive cardiac failure.
- Side effects: fever.
- Dose: 0.5g/kg given as a bolus with the cardiopulmonary bypass circuit prime volume.

30 What are the pharmacological properties of amiloride?

- Class of drug: potassium-sparing diuretic.
- Mechanism of action: amiloride blocks sodium reabsorption at the distal convoluted tubules and collecting ducts, thereby promoting the loss of sodium and water, whilst preserving potassium.

- Indications: diuresis with potassium conservation.
- Cautions: potassium supplementation and concurrent ACEI administration.
- Side effects: hyperkalaemia, hyponatraemia and postural hypotension.
- Dose: 5-10mg o.d.

31 What are the pharmacological properties of spironolactone?

- Class of drug: aldosterone antagonist.
- Mechanism of action: spironolactone inhibits the action of aldosterone at the distal convoluted tubule, thereby promoting the loss of sodium and water, whilst preserving potassium.
- Indications: oedema and ascites caused by cardiac failure, hepatic cirrhosis or nephrotic syndrome, Conn's syndrome.
- Cautions: potassium supplementation, concurrent ACEI administration and Addison's disease.
- Side effects: hyperkalaemia, hyponatraemia, postural hypotension and gynaecomastia.
- Dose: 25-400mg o.d.

32 What are the pharmacological properties of digoxin?

- Mechanism of action: digoxin inhibits the action of the sarcolemmal membrane Na-K-ATPase, thereby inhibiting the sodium pump. This results in a greater influx of sodium and displacement of bound intracellular calcium producing a weak inotropic effect. Digoxin also prolongs the atrioventricular node refractory period and conduction, as well as stimulating vagal function, thereby slowing down the ventricular rate.
- Indications: atrial fibrillation, heart failure.
- Cautions: heart block, Wolff-Parkinson-White syndrome and ventricular tachyarrhythmias.
- Side effects: nausea, vomiting, gynaecomastia, paraesthesia, convulsions and confusion.
- Dose:

    a) loading dose 1000-1500µg over 24 hours IV or oral;
    b) maintenance 62.5-250µg o.d. depending on heart rate and renal function;
    c) therapeutic plasma levels are 0.8-2ng/mL (1-2.5nmol/L) from blood taken 6-8 hours after the last dose.

- Digibind® is used to reverse the effects of digoxin in cases of toxicity.

33 What are the pharmacological properties of lidocaine?

- Class of drug: class Ib anti-arrhythmic medication.
- Mechanism of action: lidocaine shortens the duration of the cardiac action potential.
- Indications: ventricular arrhythmias, local anaesthesia.
- Cautions: hepatic dysfunction and heart block.
- Side effects: dizziness, paraesthesia, confusion, convulsions, hypotension and bradycardia.
- Dose:

    a)   anti-arrhythmic dose (intra-venous):
        i)   100mg over 5 minutes followed by;
        ii)   4mg per minute over 30 minutes followed by;
        iii)   2mg per minute for 2 hours followed by;
        iv)   1mg per minute;
    b)   local anaesthetic maximum dose:
        i)   plain lidocaine 5mg/kg;
        ii)   lidocaine with adrenaline 7mg/kg.

For a 70kg patient, the maximum dose of plain lidocaine is 350mg. Using 1% lidocaine, which represents 1g of lidocaine per 100mL, a maximum volume of 35mL can be used.

34 What are the pharmacological properties of amiodarone?

- Mechanism of action: amiodarone increases the action potential duration throughout the cardiac conduction system, thereby reducing the excitability of both atrial and ventricular myocytes.
- Indications: atrial and ventricular arrhythmias.
- Cautions: hepatic impairment, thyroid dysfunction, hypokalaemia, bradycardia and drug interactions with warfarin and digoxin.
- Side effects: hypotension (when given intravenously), photosensitivity, slate-grey skin, peripheral neuropathy, nausea, vomiting, pulmonary fibrosis, hypothyroidism and hepatic dysfunction.
- Dose:

    a)   loading dose 1.2g over 24 hours:
        i)   300mg IV over 1 hour followed by 900mg over 23 hours;
            or
        ii)   400mg PO t.d.s.;
    b)   maintenance regime: 200mg t.d.s. for 1 week, then 200mg b.d. for 1 week, then 200mg o.d.

35 **What are the pharmacological properties of magnesium?**

- Mechanism of action: magnesium prolongs atrial and atrioventricular nodal refractory periods.
- Indications: atrial and ventricular tachyarrhythmias.
- Cautions: myasthenia gravis.
- Side effects: hypotension and flushing.
- Dose: 5g magnesium sulphate IV over 10-15 minutes.

Recommended reading

1. Alderman EL, Levy JH, Rich JB, Nili M, Vidne B, Schaff H, Uretzky G, Pettersson G, Thiis JJ, Hantler CB, Chaitman B, Nadel A. Analyses of coronary graft patency after aprotinin use: results from the International Multicenter Aprotinin Graft Patency Experience (IMAGE) trial. *J Thorac Cardiovasc Surg* 1998; 116(5): 716-30.

2. Fergusson DA, Hébert PC, Mazer CD, Fremes S, MacAdams C, Murkin JM, Teoh K, Duke PC, Arellano R, Blajchman MA, Bussières JS, Côté D, Karski J, Martineau R, Robblee JA, Rodger M, Wells G, Clinch J, Pretorius R; BART Investigators. A comparison of aprotinin and lysine analogues in high-risk cardiac surgery. *N Engl J Med* 2008; 358(22): 2319-31.

3. The CAPRIE Steering Committee. A randomised, blinded trial of clopidogrel versus aspirin in patients at risk of ischemic events (CAPRIE). *Lancet* 1996; 348: 1329-39.

4. The Clopidogrel in Unstable angina to prevent Recurrent Events trial Investigators. Effects of clopidogrel in addition to aspirin in patients with acute coronary syndromes without ST-segment elevation. *N Engl J Med* 2001; 345: 494-502.

5. Klein W, Buchwald A, Hillis SE, Monrad S, Sanz G, Turpie AG, van der Meer I, Olaisson E, Undeland S, Ludwig K. Comparison of low-molecular-weight heparin with unfractionated heparin acutely and with placebo for 6 weeks in the management of unstable coronary artery disease. Fragmin in unstable coronary artery disease study (FRISC). *Circulation* 1997; 96: 61-8.

6. Antman EM, McCabe CH, Gurfinkel EP, Turpie AG, Bernink PJ, Salein D, Bayes De Luna A, Fox K, Lablanche JM, Radley D, Premmereur J, Braunwald E. Enoxaparin prevents death and cardiac ischemic events in unstable angina/non-Q-wave myocardial infarction: results of the thrombolysis in myocardial infarction (TIMI) 11B trial. *Circulation* 1999; 100: 1593-601.

7. Randomised trial of cholesterol lowering in 4444 patients with coronary heart disease: the Scandinavian Simvastatin Survival Study (4S). *Lancet* 1994; 344(8934): 1383-9.

8. Yusuf S, Sleight P, Pogue J, Bosch J, Davies R, Dagenais G. The Heart Outcomes Prevention Evaluation Study Investigators. Effects of an angiotensin-converting-enzyme inhibitor, ramipril, on cardiovascular events in high-risk patients. *N Engl J Med* 2000; 342: 145-53.

Chapter 4

Electrocardiography

1 What is an electrocardiogram (ECG)(Figure 1)?

- An electrocardiogram is a graphical representation of the heart's electrical activity measuring the electrical potential between different

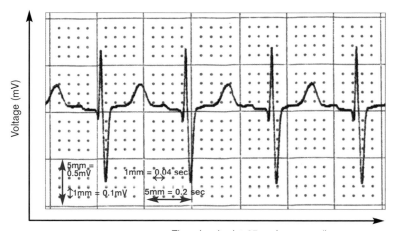

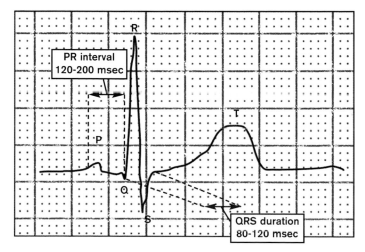

Figure 1. Electrocardiogram.

parts of the body with a positive deflection representing the electrical vector moving towards the positive electrode.

- The typical ECG paper speed is 25mm/sec but can be increased to 50mm/sec in order to assess the morphology of the complexes more clearly.
- The width of the small squares represents 0.04 sec and large squares 0.2 sec (at 25mm/sec).
- The height of the small squares represents 0.1mV and large squares 0.5mV.

2 Where are the ECG electrodes placed (Figure 2)?

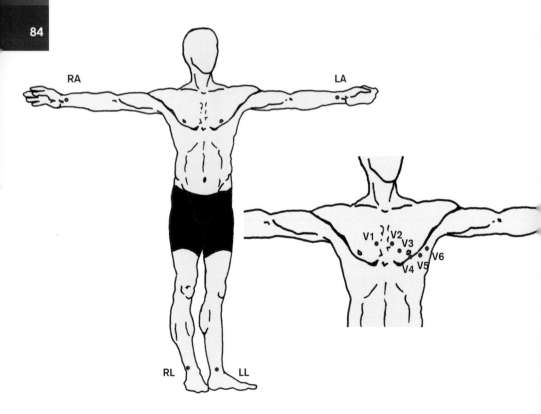

Figure 2. Positioning of the ECG electrodes.

- RA (right arm), LA (left arm), RL (right leg), and LL (left leg) electrodes are placed on the appropriate limb.
- V1 is placed in the 4th intercostal space at the right sternal edge.
- V2 is placed in the 4th intercostal space at the left sternal edge.
- V3 is placed between V2 and V4.
- V4 is placed in the 5th intercostal space in the midclavicular line.
- V5 is placed between V4 and V6.
- V6 is placed in the 5th intercostal space in the midaxillary line.

3 What are the limb leads and augmented limb leads (Figure 3)?

- Limb leads:

  a) I: negative electrode on the right arm and positive electrode on the left arm;
  b) II: negative electrode on the right arm and positive electrode on the left leg;
  c) III: negative electrode on the left arm and positive electrode on the left leg.

- Augmented limb leads:

  a) aVR (augmented vector right): positive electrode on the right arm with a negative electrode combination of the left arm and left leg;
  b) aVL (augmented vector left): positive electrode on the left arm with a negative electrode combination of the right arm and left leg;
  c) aVF (augmented vector foot): positive electrode on the left leg with a negative electrode combination of the right arm and left arm.

- The augmented limb leads are unipolar whereas the limb leads are bipolar.
- The RL acts as the ground lead.

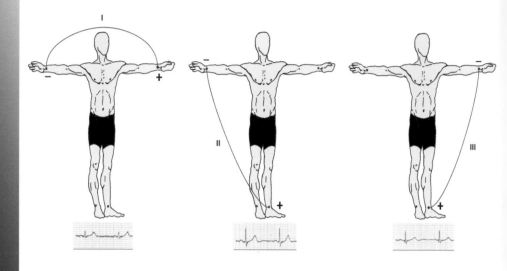

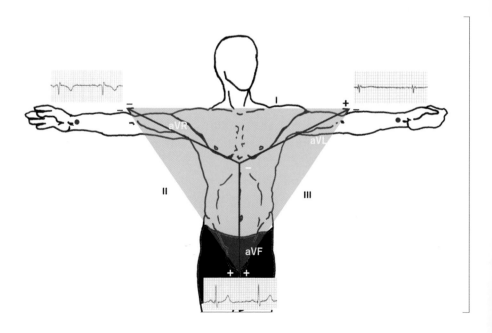

Figure 3. Limb leads and augmented limb leads demonstrating Einthoven's triangle.

4 **What are the important components when assessing an ECG?**

- Rate:

    a) normal heart rate is 60-100 beats per minute (bpm) with <10% variation (Figure 4);
    b) sinus bradycardia is a heart rate of <60 bpm (Figure 5);
    c) sinus tachycardia is a heart rate of >100 bpm (Figure 6);
    d) sinus arrhythmia is a heart rate variation of >10% (Figure 7).

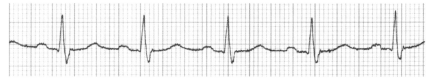

Figure 4. Normal sinus rhythm.

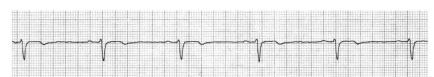

Figure 5. Sinus bradycardia.

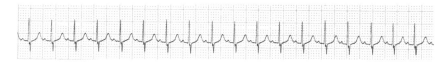

Figure 6. Sinus tachycardia.

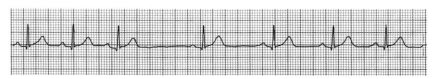

Figure 7. Sinus arrhythmia.

- Rhythm:

    a) normal sinus rhythm - the P wave precedes each QRS complex;
    b) supraventricular ectopics;
    c) supraventricular tachycardia:
        i)   I: atrial fibrillation - absence of P waves, replaced by irregular, chaotic fibrillatory (F) waves with an irregular ventricular response (often >100 bpm) (Figure 8);

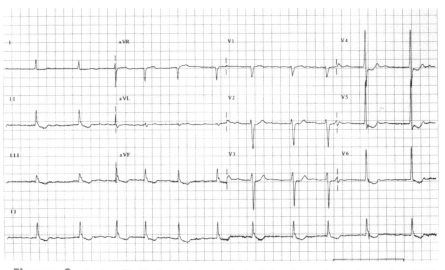

Figure 8. Atrial fibrillation demonstrated by irregularly irregular QRS complexes and the absence of P waves.

        ii) II: atrial flutter - flutter waves (most prominent in V1) with an atrial rate typically 300 bpm and a ventricular response of 150 bpm (2:1 block), although the block may be variable (Figure 9);
        iii) III: atrioventricular nodal (junctional) tachycardia (Figure 10);
    d) ventricular ectopics, including bigeminy and trigeminy (Figure 11);
    e) ventricular tachycardia - broad QRS complexes (>0.12 sec), a ventricular rate of >100 bpm and atrioventricular discordance (Figure 12);
    f) ventricular fibrillation - coarse or fine fibrillatory waves (Figure 13).

- Axis:

    a) normal QRS axis -30° to +90°;
    b) left axis deviation -30° to -90°;

4:1 block

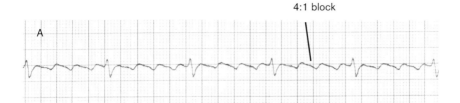

Variable block

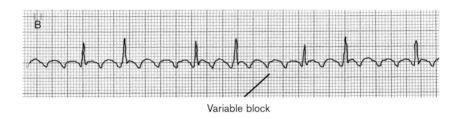

Figure 9. Atrial flutter with: A) 4:1 block; and B) variable block.

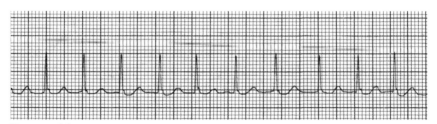

Figure 10. Junctional tachycardia.

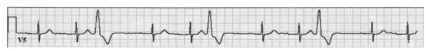

Figure 11. Ventricular ectopics every third beat (trigeminy).

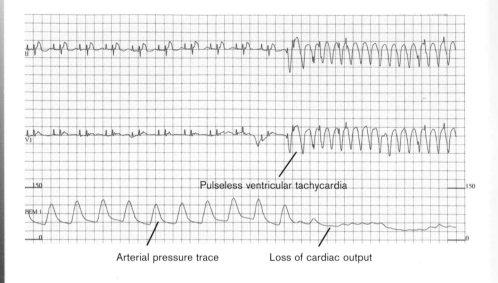

Figure 12. Ventricular tachycardia demonstrated by a broad complex tachycardia associated with loss of cardiac output on the arterial pressure trace.

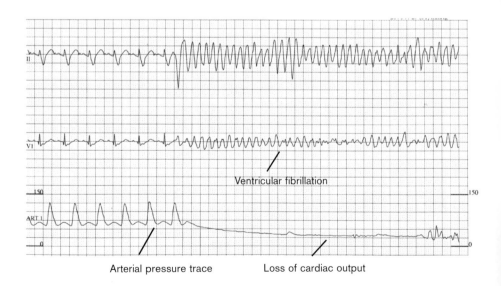

Figure 13. Ventricular fibrillation demonstrated by coarse fibrillatory waves associated with loss of cardiac output on the arterial pressure trace.

c)   right axis deviation +90° to +180°;
d)   extreme axis deviation ('No man's land') -90° to -180°.

● P-wave morphology:

a)   normal P wave height <2.5mm and width <0.11 sec in lead II;
b)   tall P wave (P pulmonale) - right atrial hypertrophy;
c)   wide P wave (P mitrale) - left atrial hypertrophy.

● PR interval:

a)   normal duration 0.12-0.2 sec (3-5 small squares);
b)   short PR interval - Wolff-Parkinson-White syndrome, Lown-Ganong-Levine syndrome;
c)   prolonged PR interval - heart block.

● QRS duration and morphology:

a)   normal QRS duration 0.08-0.12 sec with normal Q wave <0.04 sec and <25% of total QRS complex;
b)   wide QRS complexes - right or left bundle branch block;
c)   tall QRS complexes - left or right ventricular hypertrophy;
d)   pathological Q waves - myocardial infarction.

● ST segment morphology:

a)   normally isoelectric ST segment;
b)   ST elevation - myocardial infarction, pericarditis, left bundle branch block;
c)   ST depression - myocardial ischaemia, digoxin toxicity, left ventricular hypertrophy.

● T-wave morphology:

a)   normal T wave;
b)   tall T wave - hyperkalaemia, hyperacute myocardial infarction, left bundle branch block;
c)   small T wave - hypokalaemia;
d)   flattened or inverted T wave - myocardial ischaemia, digoxin toxicity, left ventricular hypertrophy.

● U wave:

a)   normally absent;
b)   U wave present - hypokalaemia.

- QT interval:

  a) corrected QT interval (QTc) = QT interval /(√RR interval);
  b) normal QTc ≤0.42 sec;
  c) long QTc - myocardial infarction, hypocalcaemia, sotalol, amiodarone, Romano-Ward syndrome.

5 How is the heart rate assessed on an ECG?

- With each small square representing 0.04 sec, the RR interval can be measured to obtain the time interval between each cardiac cycle. The heart rate can be calculated using the formula (Figure 14):

Heart rate (bpm) = 60 / RR interval

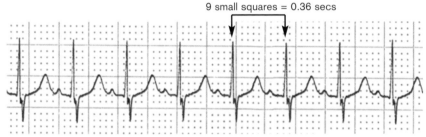

9 small squares = 0.36 secs

RR interval = 0.36 secs
HR = 60 / RR interval
HR = 60 / 0.36 = 167 bpm

Figure 14. Calculating the heart rate using the RR interval.

- An alternative is to count the number of large squares between each R wave and then use the formula (Figure 15):

Heart rate (bpm) = 300 / number of large squares

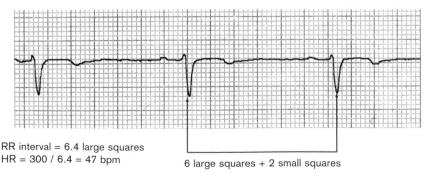

RR interval = 6.4 large squares
HR = 300 / 6.4 = 47 bpm

6 large squares + 2 small squares

Figure 15. Calculating the heart rate using the number of large squares method.

6 How is the cardiac axis assessed on an ECG?

• The degree of net amplitude displacement is determined in leads I and aVF on a cardiac axis plot (Figure 16).

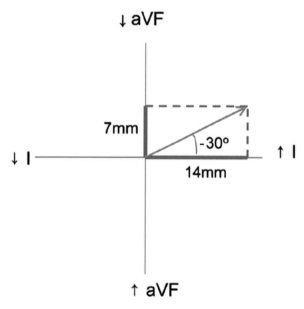

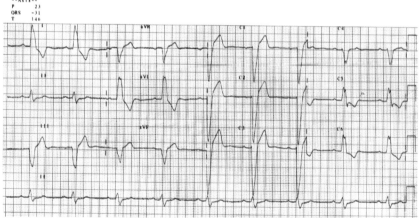

Figure 16. Electrical axis calculated by plotting the net amplitude in leads I and aVF.

• Other simple methods include:

  a) finding the isoelectric lead and the QRS axis is at 90° to it (Figure 17);

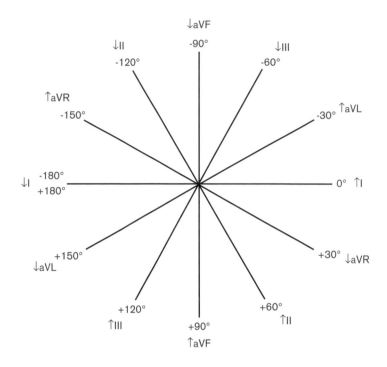

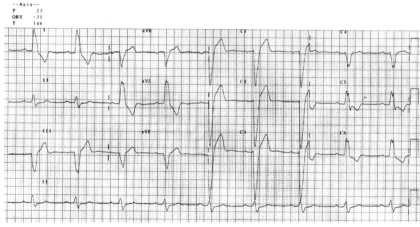

Figure 17. Electrical axis calculated using the isoelectric lead method. In the above ECG, the most isolelectric lead is II. The lead perpendicular to II is aVL. As the predominant deflection in aVL is positive, the QRS axis is approximately -30°.

b) checking the deflection of the QRS complexes in leads I and aVF (Table 1 and Figure 18).

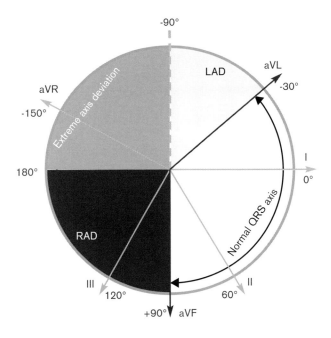

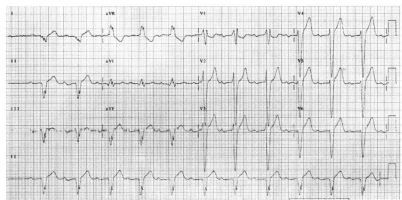

Figure 18. Electrical axis calculated by assessing the predominant vectors in leads I and aVF, demonstrating extreme axis deviation with downward deflection in both leads I and aVF. RAD = right axis deviation; LAD = left axis deviation.

Table 1. Deflection of the QRS complexes to assess cardiac axis.			
	Lead I	Lead aVF	Lead II
Normal axis	↑	↑	
Normal axis	↑	↓	↓
Left axis deviation	↑	↓	↑
Right axis deviation	↓	↑	
Extreme axis deviation	↓	↓	

7 What are the causes of left axis deviation?

- Left bundle branch block.
- Left anterior hemiblock.
- Left atrial hypertrophy.
- Inferior myocardial infarction.
- Hyperkalaemia.
- Wolff-Parkinson-White syndrome.
- Ostium primum atrial septal defect.
- Emphysema / chronic obstructive pulmonary disease.
- Left ventricular hypertrophy.

8 What are the causes of right axis deviation?

- Normal variant in children and tall thin adults.
- Right bundle branch block.
- Left posterior hemiblock.
- Right atrial hypertrophy.
- Right ventricular hypertrophy.
- Anterolateral myocardial infarction.
- Wolff-Parkinson-White syndrome.
- Ostium secundum atrial septal defect.
- Pulmonary embolus.
- Emphysema / chronic obstructive pulmonary disease.

9 What are the causes of extreme axis deviation?

- Emphysema.
- Hyperkalaemia.
- Ventricular tachycardia.
- Pacemaker.
- Lead malposition.

10 What are the ECG findings of left ventricular hypertrophy (LVH)(Figure 19)?

- Sokolow criteria - S in V1 + R in V5 or V6 (whichever is taller) >35mm.
- Other criteria used to diagnose left ventricular hypertrophy include:

  a) S in V1 or R in V5 or R in V6 >25mm;
  b) R in I + S in III >25mm;
  c) R in I or R in aVL >14mm.

- Lateral (I, aVL, V5 and V6) T-wave inversion may also be present as part of a left ventricular 'strain' pattern.
- It is important to appreciate the different factors that affect electrocardiographic voltage: left ventricular cavity size and muscle mass, the presence of pericardial fluid, lung volume in front of the heart and chest wall thickness.

V1 S wave + V6 R wave = 55mm

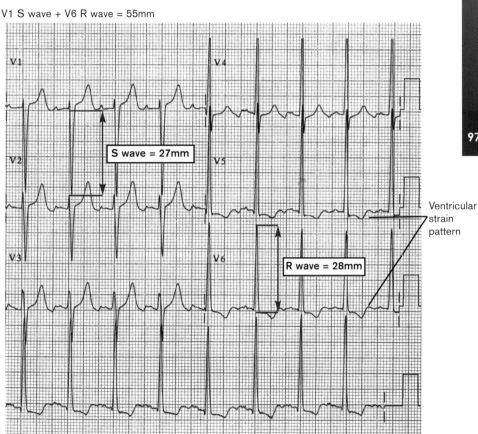

Figure 19. Left ventricular hypertrophy demonstrated by large S waves in V1, large R waves in V6 and a strain pattern in V5-6.

11 What are the ECG findings of right ventricular hypertrophy (RVH)(Figure 20)?

R in C1 (V1) + S in C6 (V6) >11mm
R in C1 (V1) >7mm

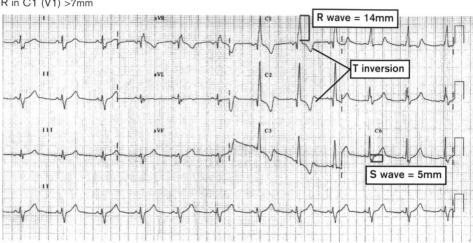

R wave = 14mm

T inversion

S wave = 5mm

Figure 20. Right ventricular hypertrophy demonstrated by a large R wave in V1 and large S wave in V6.

- The different criteria used to diagnose right ventricular hypertrophy include:

  a)   R in V1 + S in V6 >11mm;
  b)   R in V1 or S in V6 >7mm;
  c)   R/S ratio in V1 >1 or R/S ratio in V6 <1.

- Anterior T-wave inversion may also be present as part of RVH.
- As neonates have RV predominance, their ECG shows a dominant R in V1 and S in V6.
- The axis moves towards the left with an adult configuration by the age of 15 with S in V1 and R in V6.

12 What are the ECG findings of left atrial enlargement (Figure 21)?

- Left atrial dilation or hypertrophy is signified by P mitrale (>0.11 sec):

  a)   m-shaped P wave in lead II; or
  b)   biphasic P wave in lead V1.

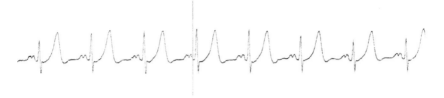

Figure 21. Left atrial enlargement demonstrated by P mitrale in lead II.

13 What are the ECG findings of right atrial enlargement (Figure 22)?

- Right atrial dilation or hypertrophy is signified by P pulmonale in leads II and V1 with a pointed P wave >2.5mm tall.

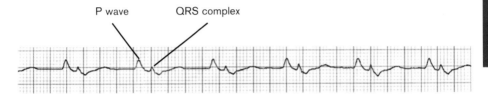

Figure 22. Right atrial enlargement demonstrated by P pulmonale in lead II.

14 What are the ECG findings of myocardial ischaemia and infarction?

- Myocardial ischaemia - ST depression with T-wave flattening or inversion (Figure 23).
- Myocardial infarction:

    a) ST elevation and peaked T wave;
    b) Q waves >0.04 sec or >25% of total QRS complex;
    c) Inverted T waves.

- Changes occur in respective leads:

    a) inferior (right coronary artery) - II, III and aVF (Figure 24);
    b) anterior (left anterior descending artery) - V2-4 (Figure 25);
    c) lateral (circumflex and left anterior descending artery) - I, aVL, V5, V6 (Figure 26);

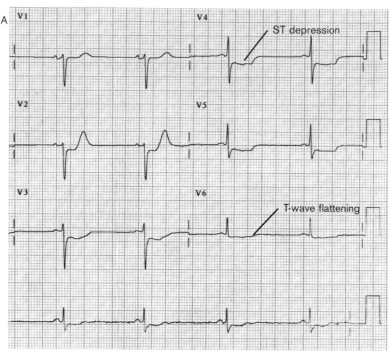

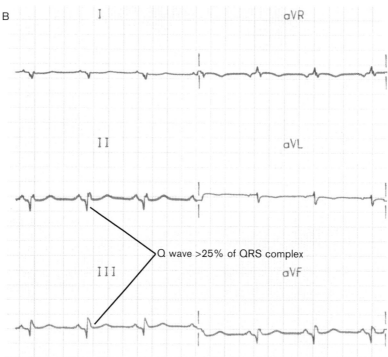

Figure 23. A) Myocardial ischaemia demonstrated by ST depression and T-wave flattening. B) Old myocardial infarction demonstrated by Q waves.

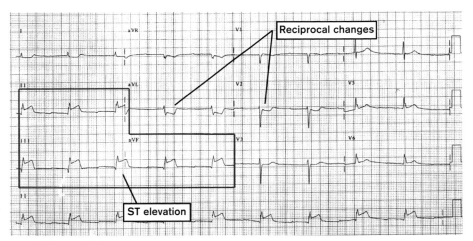

Figure 24. Inferior myocardial infarction demonstrated by ST elevation in leads II, III and aVF.

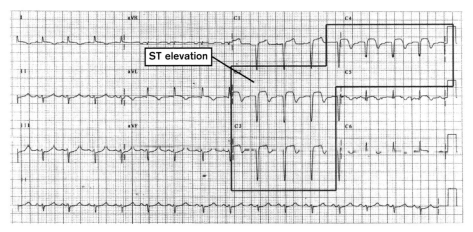

Figure 25. Anterior myocardial infarction demonstrated by ST elevation in leads V2-4.

  d) posterior (circumflex artery) - mirror image in leads V1-3 (Figure 27).

• In acute myocardial infarction, reciprocal changes may be seen in the opposite territories.

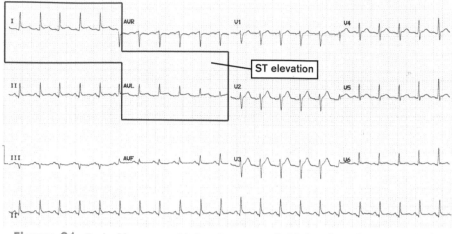

Figure 26. Early changes of lateral myocardial infarction demonstrated by mild ST elevation in leads I and aVL.

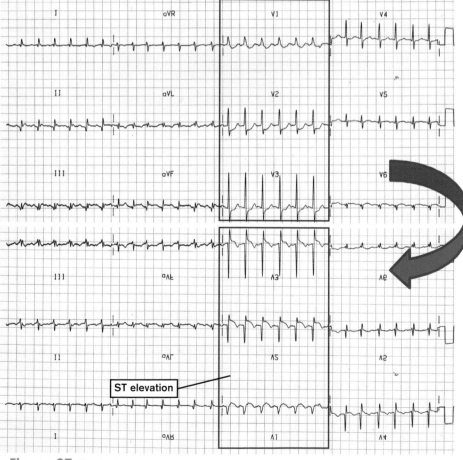

Figure 27. Posterior myocardial infarction demonstrated by ST elevation on leads V1-3 when the ECG is turned over to produce a mirror image.

15 What are the ECG findings of pericarditis (Figure 28)?

- Stage I: global concave upwards ST elevation.
- Stage II: pseudonormalisation of the ST segment with T-wave flattening.
- Stage III: inverted T waves.
- Stage IV: normal ECG.

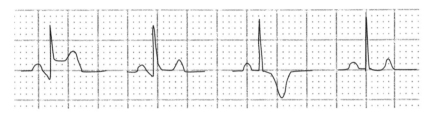

Figure 28. Pericarditis (stages I-IV).

16 How is broad complex supraventricular tachycardia differentiated from ventricular tachycardia on the ECG?

- The arrhythmia is more likely to be ventricular in origin if there is:

    a) a QRS complex duration >0.14s;
    b) concordance throughout the chest leads;
    c) QRS morphology changing with time;
    d) left or right axis deviation;
    e) atrioventricular dissociation;
    f) a presence of fusion or capture beats;
    g) a regular ventricular rhythm (as opposed to atrial fibrillation with aberrant conduction).

17 What is torsade de pointes (Figure 29)?

- Torsade de pointes is a form of ventricular tachycardia characterised by broad QRS complexes with multiple morphologies (changing QRS axis) and varying RR intervals.
- Common causes include heart block, hypokalaemia, hypomagnesaemia, drugs (e.g. sotalol, amiodarone, erythromycin), and long QT syndrome.

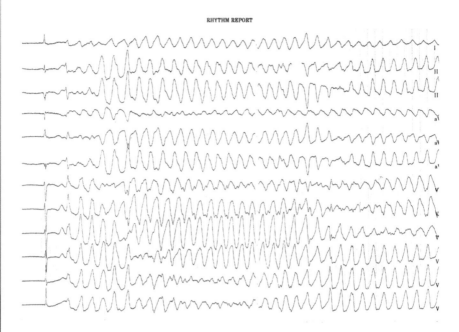

RHYTHM REPORT

Figure 29. Torsade de pointes demonstrated by ventricular tachycardia with changing QRS axes on all the leads.

18 What are the ECG findings of hyperkalaemia (Figure 30)?

- Small or absent P waves.
- Widening of the QRS complex, which may lead to ventricular fibrillation.
- Shortened or absent ST segment.
- Wide, tall, peaked T waves.

19 What are the ECG findings of hypokalaemia (Figure 31)?

- Atrial fibrillation.
- First or second degree heart block.
- Small or absent T waves.
- Prominent U waves.

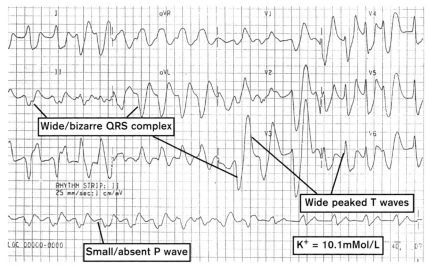

Figure 30. Hyperkalaemia demonstrated by the absent P waves, wide QRS complexes and peaked T waves.

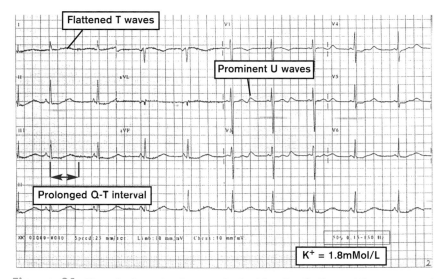

Figure 31. Hypokalaemia demonstrated by the flattened T waves and prominent U waves.

20 What are the ECG findings of hypercalcaemia?

- Prolonged PR interval.
- Short QTc interval.

21 What are the ECG findings of hypocalcaemia?

- Long QTc interval.
- Small T wave.
- Cardiac dysrhythmias.

22 What are the ECG findings of acute pulmonary embolism (Figure 32)?

- Sinus tachycardia.

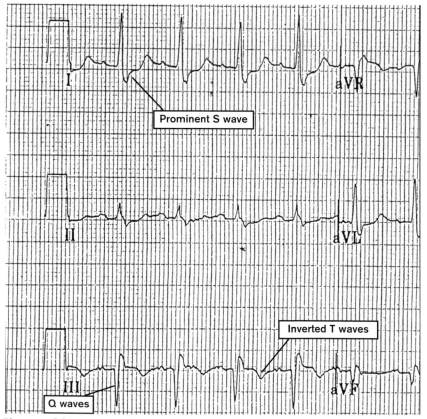

Figure 32. Pulmonary embolism demonstrated by an S wave in lead I, Q wave in lead III and T-wave inversion in lead III (S1, Q3, T3).

- Classic S1Q3T3 pattern (not always present):

  a)   prominent S wave in lead I;
  b)   Q wave in lead III;
  c)   inverted T wave in lead III.

- Right heart strain:

  a)   right axis deviation;
  b)   right bundle branch block;
  c)   T-wave inversion in leads V1-V3;
  d)   P pulmonale (peaked P waves in V1).

23 What are the ECG features of heart (atrioventricular) block?

- First degree heart block - PR interval >0.2 sec (Figure 33).

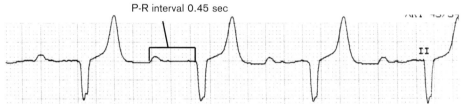

P-R interval 0.45 sec

II

Figure 33. 1° heart block demonstrated by a prolonged PR interval.

- Second degree heart block:

  a)   Mobitz Type I (Wenckebach phenomenon): progressive lengthening of the PR interval until a P wave is not conducted, followed by a QRS complex with a shortened PR interval (Figure 34);

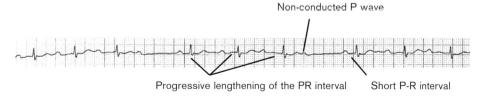

Non-conducted P wave

Progressive lengthening of the PR interval   Short P-R interval

Figure 34. 2° heart block - Mobitz Type I demonstrated by progressive lengthening of the PR interval followed by a non-conducted P wave.

b) Mobitz Type II: fixed PR interval with failure of conduction of the atrial impulse, e.g. 2:1 block, 3:1 block, etc (Figure 35).

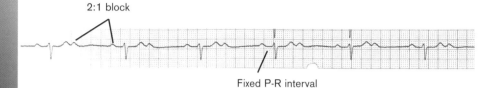

2:1 block

Fixed P-R interval

Figure 35. 2° heart block - Mobitz Type II demonstrated by a 2:1 block.

- Third degree (complete) heart block - P waves are not conducted through the AV node resulting in complete dissociation with QRS complexes. The ventricles are depolarised by a ventricular escape rhythm (Figure 36).

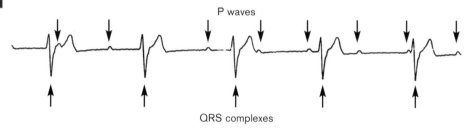

P waves

QRS complexes

Figure 36. 3° heart block demonstrated by complete atrio-ventricular dissociation.

- Pacemakers should be considered for Mobitz Type II secondary heart block and third degree complete heart block.

24 What are the ECG features of right bundle branch block (RBBB)(Figure 37)?

- Wide QRS >120ms.
- rSR' or rR' pattern in V1 and S waves in V6.
- T-wave discordance (T-wave inversion in V1-3).
- Right axis deviation (not always present).

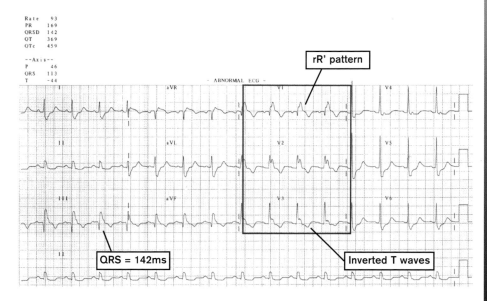

Figure 37. Right bundle branch block demonstrated by a prolonged QRS duration (>120ms) and a predominant R wave in lead V1.

25 What are the ECG features of left bundle branch block (LBBB)(Figure 38)?

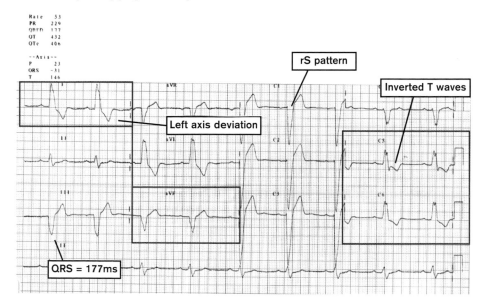

Figure 38. Left bundle branch block demonstrated by a prolonged QRS duration (>120ms), a predominant S wave in lead V1, left axis deviation and inverted T waves in leads V5-6.

- Wide QRS >120ms.
- QS or rS complex in V1 and R waves in V6.
- T-wave discordance (T-wave inversion in V5-6).
- Left axis deviation.

26 What are the ECG features of left anterior hemiblock (LAHB)(Figure 39)?

- Left axis deviation (in the absence of other causes).
- QRS <120ms (incomplete bundle branch block).
- qR complex in the lateral limb leads (I and aVL).
- rS pattern in the inferior leads (II, III, and aVF).

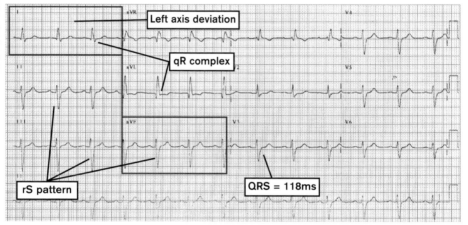

Figure 39. Left anterior hemiblock demonstrated by qR complexes in leads I and aVL; rS pattern in leads II, III and avF; left axis deviation and incomplete bundle branch block (QRS 100-120ms).

27 What are the ECG features of left posterior hemiblock (LPHB)?

- Right axis deviation (in the absence of other causes).
- QRS <120ms (incomplete bundle branch block).
- S in lead I and Q in lead III.

28 What is bifascicular block (Figure 40)?

- When two of the main three fascicles are blocked:

    a)   RBBB and LAHB;
    b)   RBBB and LPHB;
    c)   LAHB and LPHB (i.e. LBBB).

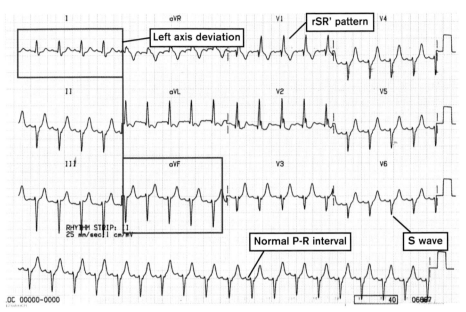

Figure 40. Bifascicular block demonstrated by left anterior hemiblock (left axis deviation), right bundle branch block (QRS duration >120ms and predominant R wave in V1) and a normal PR interval.

29 What is trifascicular block (Figure 41)?

- Traditionally, trifascicular block includes:

    a)   RBBB;
    b)   LAHB or LPHB;
    c)   First degree heart block.

- Technically however, the three fascicles are the right bundle branch, the left anterior branch and the left posterior branch. Hence, trifascicular block by definition actually represents right bundle branch block, left anterior hemiblock and left posterior hemiblock, i.e. complete AV block.

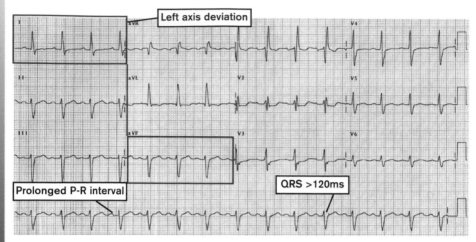

Figure 41. Trifascicular block demonstrated by left anterior hemiblock (left axis deviation), right bundle branch block (QRS duration >120ms and predominant R wave in V1) and 1° heart block (PR interval >200ms).

30 What is Wolff-Parkinson-White (WPW) syndrome (Figure 42)?

- WPW syndrome causes ventricular pre-excitation due to an accessory atrioventricular pathway (bundle of Kent).
- The ECG findings of WPW syndrome include:

  a) short PR interval <120ms;
  b) delta wave - slurred upstroke from the P wave to the QRS complex (delta wave in V1 is positive in Type A WPW syndrome and negative in Type B WPW syndrome);
  c) widened QRS complex (pre-excitation via the bundle of Kent followed by normal excitation via the AV node, thus resulting in a broad QRS complex);
  d) ST and T-wave changes.

31 What is Lown-Ganong-Levine (LGL) syndrome?

- Ventricular pre-excitation caused by an accessory atrioventricular pathway (James fibres).
- The ECG findings of LGL syndrome include:

  a) a short PR interval <120ms;
  b) the absence of delta waves;
  c) a normal QRS complex width;
  d) ST and T-wave changes.

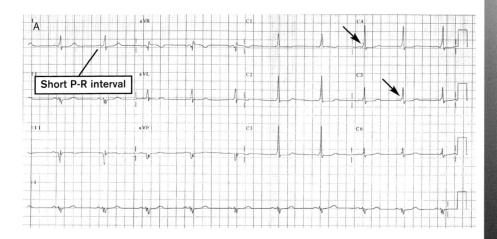

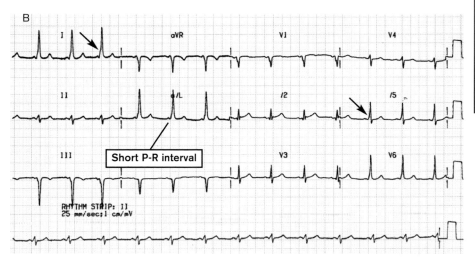

113

Figure 42. Wolff-Parkinson-White (WPW) syndrome demonstrated by delta waves (arrows) and a short PR interval. A) Type A WPW with a predominant R wave in V1 and B) Type B WPW with a predominant S wave in V1.

32 What is long QT syndrome (Figure 43)?

- Long QT syndrome is defined as a corrected QT interval (QTc) >0.46 sec (normal ~0.42 sec).
- It represents prolongation of ventricular repolarisation and is associated with syncope, ventricular arrhythmias (including torsades de pointes) and death.
- Primary causes include genetic mutations of myocyte ion channels (e.g. Romano-Ward syndrome - autosomal dominant inherited form).
- Secondary causes include myocardial infarction, electrolyte disturbances (hypocalcaemia), drugs (sotalol, amiodarone), and hypothyroidism.

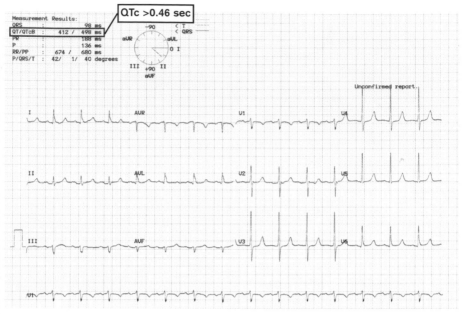

Figure 43. Long QT syndrome demonstrated by a prolonged QTc (>0.46 sec).

33 What is electric alternans?

● Electric alternans is a QRS axis or amplitude that alternates between beats.

● It may be caused by a pericardial effusion or tamponade where the heart is moving within fluid.

34 What are the indications for an exercise ECG?

● Patients with an atypical chest pain history to determine the aetiology.

● Evaluation of cardiac function and exercise capacity.

● Prognosis following myocardial infarction.

● Detection of exercise-induced arrhythmias.

● Detection of symptoms in equivocal patients with aortic stenosis.

● Exercise ECG testing has a sensitivity of 80%, specificity of 75% and an associated mortality of 0.01%.

35 What are the contra-indications for an exercise ECG?

● Severe aortic stenosis.

● Acute myocarditis or pericarditis.

● Unstable angina.

- Uncontrolled hypertension.
- Severe left main stem stenosis or left main equivalent.
- Heart failure.
- Certain arrhythmias - fast atrial fibrillation, heart block, ventricular arrhythmias.
- Orthopaedic or neurological impairment.
- Acute myocardial infarction - but it is possible to perform an exercise ECG prior to discharge.

36 What is the Bruce protocol?

- The Bruce protocol is a diagnostic exercise ECG test with seven stages on the treadmill (each lasting 3 minutes) with the speed and incline progressively increased (Table 2).

Table 2. The Bruce protocol.

Stage	1	2	3	4	5	6	7
Speed (mph)	1.7	2.5	3.4	4.2	5.0	5.5	6.0
Incline (%)	10	12	14	16	18	20	22

- The modified Bruce protocol starts with a 0% incline at 1.7 mph for stage I, 5% incline at 1.7 mph for stage 2, then as per the Bruce protocol.

37 What are the endpoints for an exercise ECG?

- Attainment of the target heart rate - commonly this is 85% of the predicted maximum for the patient's age:

    a) males predicted maximum = 220 - age;
    b) females predicted maximum = 210 - age.

- Symptoms - angina pectoris, undue dyspnoea, faintness, fatigue.
- Cardiac arrhythmias - heart block, atrial fibrillation, supraventricular tachycardia.
- Severe hypertension.
- Positive test (see below).

38 What is a positive exercise ECG test (Figure 44)?

- ST depression >2mm in several leads (down-sloping and persisting >5 minutes into the recovery period).
- ST elevation.
- Chest pain (in association with ST changes predicts an 85% sensitivity of coronary artery disease).
- Increased R-wave voltage (normally R-wave voltage decreases during exercise).
- Inverted U waves.
- Failure of systolic blood pressure to rise with exercise.
- Ventricular arrhythmias (including >10 ventricular ectopics per minute).
- New mitral regurgitation auscultated immediately after completion of the exercise test.

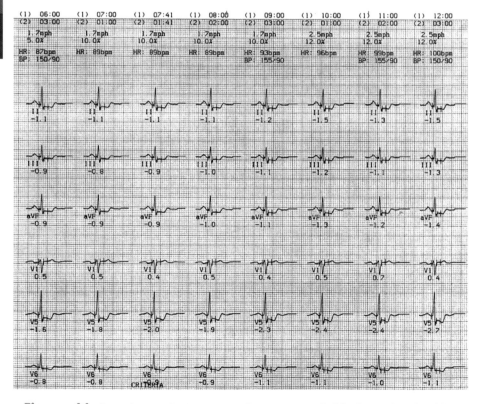

Figure 44. Exercise ECG demonstrating myocardial ischaemia with ST depression in leads II, III and aVF (inferior) and leads V5-6.

Recommended reading

1. Meek S, Morris F. ABC of clinical electrocardiography. Introduction. I - leads, rate, rhythm, and cardiac axis. *BMJ* 2002; 324(7334): 415-8.

2. Channer K, Morris F. ABC of clinical electrocardiography: myocardial ischaemia. *BMJ* 2002; 324(7344): 1023-6.

3. Morris F, Brady WJ. ABC of clinical electrocardiography: acute myocardial infarction - Part I. *BMJ* 2002; 324(7341): 831-4.

4. Edhouse J, Brady WJ, Morris F. ABC of clinical electrocardiography: acute myocardial infarction - Part II. *BMJ* 2002; 324(7343): 963-6.

5. Edhouse J, Morris F. ABC of clinical electrocardiography: broad complex tachycardia - Part II. *BMJ* 2002; 324(7340): 776-9.

6. Esberger D, Jones S, Morris F. ABC of clinical electrocardiography: junctional tachycardias. *BMJ* 2002; 324(7338): 662-5.

7. Goodacre S, Irons R. ABC of clinical electrocardiography: atrial arrhythmias. *BMJ* 2002; 324(7337): 594-7.

Chapter 5

Echocardiography

1 What is echocardiography?

- Echocardiography is a non-invasive cardiac imaging modality, which uses piezo-electric crystals that emit and receive ultrasound waves at a rate of 1000 per second.
- These crystals convert electrical oscillations into mechanical oscillations (sound).
- When the ultrasound waves reach an interface between two different mediums, part of the ultrasound wave is reflected back towards the probe. The echocardiogram can measure two entities:

  a) the distance from the probe, which is calculated by the time delay between the transmission and reception of the reflected sound wave;

  b) the density of the tissue, which is calculated by the intensity of the reflected signal.

- Echocardiography is usually carried out with the patient in the left lateral decubitus position, using a 2.25MHz probe in adults and a 5MHz probe in children.
- The quality of the echocardiography images is affected by the structures between the heart and the probe. Hence, poor images are obtained in patients with lung disease, obesity and chest wall deformities.

2 What is Doppler echocardiography?

- Doppler echocardiography uses the principles of the Doppler effect, where the relative velocity and direction of a sound source to the observer determines the received frequency of the sound.
- The Doppler probe acts as the transmitter (usually 2MHz) and receiver of the ultrasound waves.

- If blood moves towards the Doppler probe the received frequency of ultrasound wave increases and if blood moves away from the probe the frequency decreases.

- Doppler echocardiography images plot velocity against time, with flows above the line representing blood moving towards the probe and below the line for blood moving away from the probe (Figure 1).

- There is also a densitometric dimension of the image as turbulent flow has a wide range of velocities, and is represented by the Doppler flow signal 'filled in' compared to normal laminar flow which has all the blood cells travelling at similar velocity, represented as a single line on the Doppler flow signal.

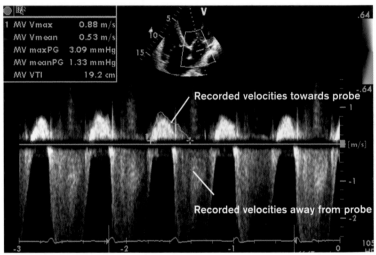

Figure 1. Doppler echocardiography with flow towards the probe (across the mitral valve) above the line and flow away from the probe (across the aortic valve) below the line.

3 What is aliasing?

- Aliasing refers to the phenomenon when the Nyquist limit of maximum velocity is exceeded, resulting in 'wrapping around' of the Doppler signal and an abnormally low velocity (Figure 2).

- Aliasing only occurs with pulsed-wave Doppler. In view of this, high velocity jets need to be assessed using continuous-wave Doppler, where aliasing does not occur.

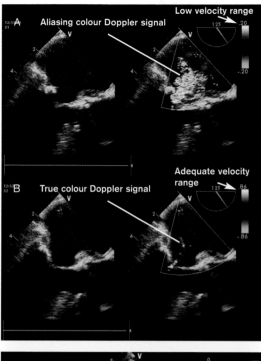

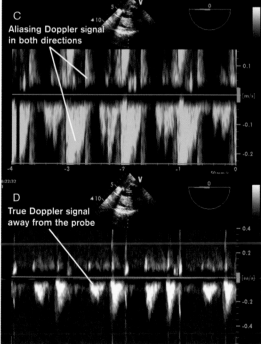

Figure 2. Aliasing.

4   What are the different modes of echocardiography?

- M (motion) mode - uses a single beam of ultrasound and produces a one-dimensional moving image of the heart (Figure 3).
- 2D echocardiography - cross-sectional imaging (see below).
- 3D echocardiography.
- Doppler echocardiography (see below).

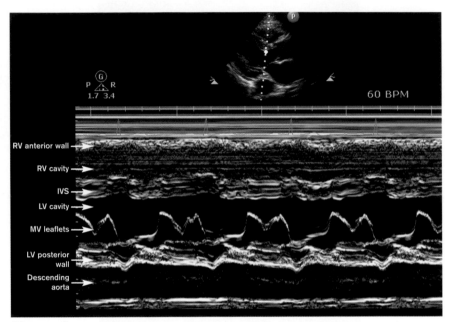

Figure 3. M-mode echocardiography. IVS = interventricular septum; RV = right ventricle; LV = left ventricle; MV = mitral valve.

5   What are the standard 2D echocardiography views?

- Parasternal long axis view, where the probe is placed at the left sternal edge in the second to fourth intercostal space with the probe marker pointing towards the right shoulder (Figure 4).
- Parasternal short axis view, where the probe is placed at the left sternal edge in the second to fourth intercostal space with the probe marker pointing towards the left shoulder. Images are taken at the level of the aortic valve, mitral valve leaflet tips, papillary muscles and apex (Figure 5A-D).

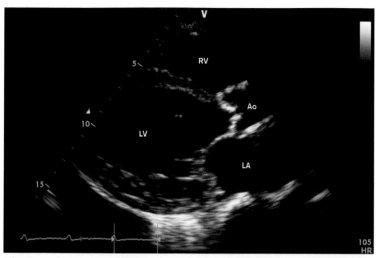

Figure 4. Parasternal long axis view. RV = right ventricle; LV = left ventricle; LA = left atrium; Ao = ascending aorta.

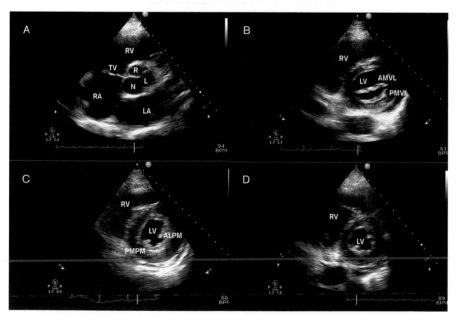

Figure 5. Parasternal short axis views at the level of the: A) aortic valve; B) mitral valve leaflet tips; C) papillary muscles; and D) apex. LV = left ventricle; LA = left atrium; RV = right ventricle; RA = right atrium; TV = tricuspid valve; N, R, L = non, right, left coronary cusps of the aortic valve; PMVL = posterior mitral valve leaflet; AMVL = anterior mitral valve leaflet; PMPM = posteromedial papillary muscle; ALPM = anterolateral papillary muscle.

- Apical four-chamber view, where the probe marker is pointing towards the left shoulder (Figure 6).
- Apical five-chamber view, where the probe is angulated anteriorly from the four-chamber view (Figure 7).

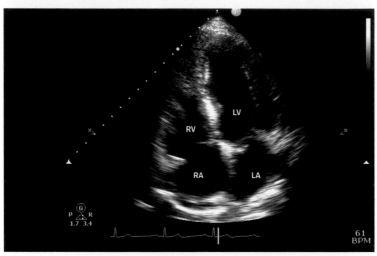

Figure 6. Apical 4-chamber view. RV = right ventricle; RA = right atrium; LV = left ventricle; LA = left atrium.

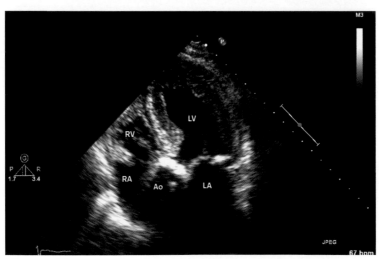

Figure 7. Apical 5-chamber view. RV = right ventricle; RA = right atrium; LV = left ventricle; LA = left atrium; Ao = ascending aorta.

- Apical long axis two-chamber view (Figure 8).
- Subcostal view, where the probe is placed just below the xiphoid process (Figure 9).

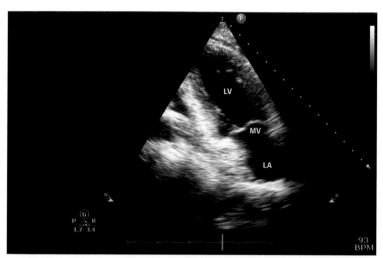

Figure 8. Apical long axis 2-chamber view. LV = left ventricle; LA = left atrium; MV = mitral valve.

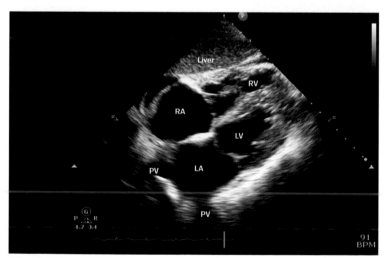

Figure 9. Subcostal view. RV = right ventricle; RA = right atrium; LV = left ventricle; LA = left atrium; PV = pulmonary vein.

- Suprasternal view, where the probe is placed in the suprasternal notch.
- Right parasternal view, where the probe is placed at the right sternal edge in the second to fourth intercostal space.

6 What are the different modes of Doppler echocardiography?

- Continuous-wave Doppler, where the transmitter continuously emits ultrasound waves, thereby allowing the probe to measure high velocities. It is, however, unable to localise the signal, as it can originate from any point along the ultrasound beam (Figure 10).

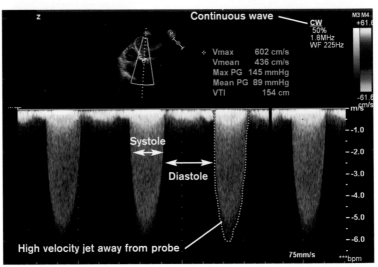

Figure 10. Continuous-wave Doppler.

- Pulsed-wave Doppler, which allows the flow to be localised or sampled from a small region but is only useful for velocities up to 2m/s, otherwise it may result in aliasing (see earlier) (Figure 11).
- Colour-flow mapping Doppler, which uses colour-encoded pulsed-wave Doppler superimposed over the 2D echo image, demonstrating blood velocity and the direction of flow (Figure 12):

  a) blue colour represents flow away from the probe, whilst red colour represents flow towards the probe (BART);

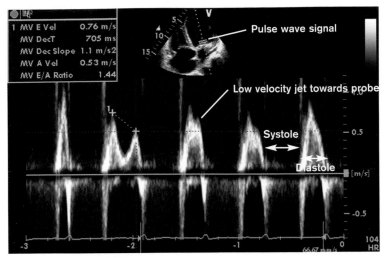

1 MV E Vel	0.76 m/s	
MV DecT	705 ms	
MV Dec Slope	1.1 m/s2	
MV A Vel	0.53 m/s	
MV E/A Ratio	1.44	

Figure 11. Pulsed-wave Doppler.

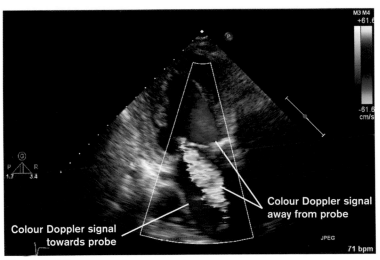

Figure 12. Colour-flow Doppler.

b)   as flow velocities increase, the colour becomes progressively lighter;

c)   as colour-flow mapping uses pulsed-wave Doppler, colour reversal (aliasing) occurs at higher velocities.

7   What are the normal echocardiographic cardiac chamber sizes and function?

- The normal dimensions are influenced by age, sex, height and physical training (athletes)(Table 1).

Table 1. Normal echocardiographic cardiac chamber sizes and function.

	Diastole	Systole
Left ventricular internal diameter (cm)	3.5-5.6	2.0-4.0
Posterior wall thickness (cm)	0.6-1.2	0.9-1.8
Interventricular septum (cm)	0.6-1.2	0.9-1.8
Right ventricle (cm)	1.9-2.6	1.2-1.8
	Normal range	
Left ventricular ejection fraction (%)	50-80	
Fractional shortening (%)	25-45	
Left ventricular mass index (g/m^2)	44-102	
Right ventricular ejection fraction (%)	45-60	
Aortic root (cm)	2.0-4.0	
Left atrium (cm)	2.0-4.0	
Left ventricular end-diastolic volume (mL)	80-140	
Left ventricular end-systolic volume (mL)	25-65	

128

8   What are the normal values for cardiac valve areas and peak velocities (Table 2)?

Table 2. Normal values for cardiac valve areas and peak velocities.

	Valve area (cm^2)	Peak velocity (m/s)
Aortic valve	2.5-3.5	0.9-1.7
Mitral valve	4.0-6.0	0.6-1.3
Tricuspid valve	5.0-8.0	0.3-0.7
Pulmonary valve	2.5-4.0	0.5-1.0

9 **How is left ventricular function assessed echocardiographically?**

● Regional wall motion abnormality:

    a)   normal;
    b)   hypokinetic (decreased motion);
    c)   akinetic (absent movement);
    d)   dyskinetic (paradoxical movement);
    e)   aneurysmal.

● Global left ventricular function is assessed visually as good, moderate or poor.

● Ejection fraction (EF) and fractional shortening (FS) can be calculated using the formulae:

$$EF (\%) = 100 \times (LVIDd^3 - LVIDs^3) / LVIDd^3$$
$$FS (\%) = 100 \times (LVIDd - LVIDs) / LVIDd$$

where LVIDd = left ventricular internal diameter in diastole, LVIDs = left ventricular internal diameter in systole.

● The left ventricular cavity and wall measurements are taken with M-mode echocardiography from the parasternal long axis view with the beam through the tips of the mitral valve leaflets at end-diastole (R wave) and end-systole (T wave) (Figure 13).

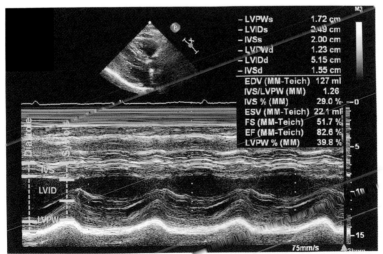

Figure 13. Left ventricular cavity and wall measurements in diastole and systole. IVSd/IVSs = interventricular septal thickness in diastole/systole; LVIDd/LVIDs = left ventricular internal diameter in diastole/systole; LVPWd/LVPWs = left ventricular posterior wall thickness in diastole/systole.

- The ejection fraction can also be calculated by Simpson's method, where the left ventricle is divided into multiple slices of known thickness and diameter along the short axis. The left ventricular volume can then be calculated by the sum total of the volume of each slice (area x thickness = $\pi(D/2)^2$ x T) in systole and diastole. Ejection fraction and cardiac output can then be calculated using the formulae:

Ejection fraction (%) = 100 x (LVEDV - LVESV) / LVEDV
Stroke volume = LVEDV - LVESV
Cardiac output = stroke volume x heart rate

where D = diameter of left ventricle cavity in each slice, T = thickness of each slice, LVEDV = left ventricular end-diastolic volume, LVESV = left ventricular end-systolic volume.

10 How are pressure gradients across a valve calculated (Figure 14)?

- Using the modified Bernoulli equation, two different pressure gradients can be calculated across a cardiac valve:

$$\Delta P = 4v^2$$

where ΔP = change in pressure (mmHg), v = velocity (m/sec).

a) peak gradient, which is calculated from the peak velocity;
b) mean gradient, which is calculated from the mean velocity (i.e. velocity time integral).

- These Doppler-calculated gradients represent actual instantaneous physiological gradients. The peak-to-peak gradient which is calculated at cardiac catheterisation is measured by the withdrawal of the catheter from the left ventricle to the aorta. The peak gradient across the aortic valve, the peak left ventricular pressure and peak aortic pressure, however, do not occur at the same time.
- The main limitations of Doppler-calculated gradients are:

a) using the modified Bernoulli equation to calculate gradients from measured velocities is governed by a number of assumptions including that of linear flow. Valvular stenosis, however, produces turbulent flow;
b) the ultrasound beam must be parallel to the direction of blood flow, otherwise the peak velocity and, hence, peak gradient will

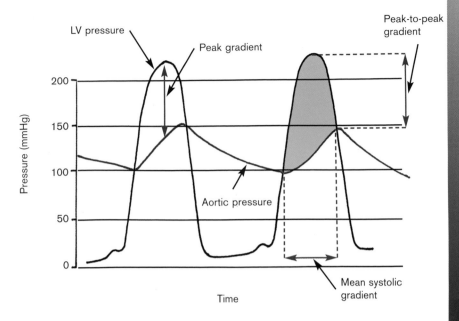

Figure 14. Mean and peak pressure gradient calculated by Doppler in comparison to peak-to-peak gradient calculated by cardiac catheterisation. LV = left ventricle.

be underestimated and this can be a problem with the eccentric flow of aortic stenosis.

11 What is the continuity equation?

- The continuity equation is based on the principle of conservation of mass, hence the flow of blood across the outflow tract of a chamber must be the same as the flow of blood across the valve of that chamber (Figure 15).
- Volume of blood flow = cross-sectional area (A) x velocity of blood (V).
- Hence, as regards the aortic valve:

Blood flow across the aortic valve = Blood flow across the left ventricular outflow tract

$$Area_{AoV} \times VTI_{AoV} = Area_{LVOT} \times VTI_{LVOT}$$
$$Area_{AoV} = \frac{Area_{LVOT} \times VTI_{LVOT}}{VTI_{AoV}}$$

where LVOT = left ventricular outflow tract, VTI = velocity time integral, AoV = aortic valve.

- If the peak velocity across the aortic valve is <2m/s, the continuity equation is not accurate.

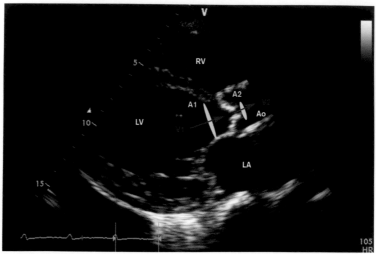

Figure 15. Continuity equation demonstrating that the total flow (area x velocity) of blood that passes through the left ventricular outflow tract (LVOT) is the same as the total flow of blood passing through the aortic valve. A1 = LVOT area; V1 = LVOT flow velocity; A2 = aortic valve area; V2 = intra-aortic flow velocity; RV = right ventricle; LV = left ventricle; LA = left atrium; Ao = ascending aorta.

12 What is the aortic dimensionless index?

- Dimensionless index = $\dfrac{VTI_{LVOT}}{VTI_{AoV}}$
- Normal = 1, severe aortic stenosis <0.25.

13 How is valvular stenosis quantified on echocardiography?

- Valvular stenosis can be quantified using the following:

  a) peak velocity across the valve;
  b) peak gradient across the valve;
  c) mean gradient across the valve;
  d) valve area, which can be calculated by:

    i) planimetry - direct measurement of the valve in the short axis view (Figure 16);

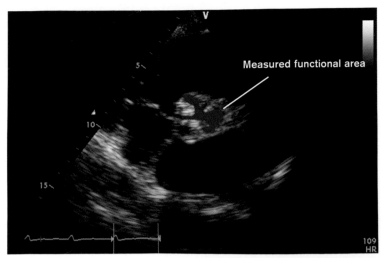

Figure 16. Measurement of aortic valve area by planimetry on the short axis view.

    ii)   continuity equation - applicable to both the aortic and mitral valves.

- Additional techniques used for measuring aortic stenosis include (see Chapter 12):

a)   dimensionless index = $\dfrac{VTI_{LVOT}}{VTI_{AoV}}$ (see above);

b)   maximal aortic cusp separation (MACS), which is measured using M-mode echocardiography with the cursor across the aortic valve leaflet tips. Normal MACS is >2cm and severe aortic stenosis is <0.8cm (Figure 17).

- Additional techniques used to aid quantification of mitral stenosis include (see Chapter 13):

a)   the pressure half-time, where the:

$$\text{mitral valve area (cm}^2) = \frac{220}{\text{pressure half-time (ms)}} \text{ (see below),}$$

b)   pulmonary artery systolic pressure (see below).

- It is also important to assess the aetiology of the valvular stenosis, valve morphology, degree of leaflet movement, changes in left ventricular and left atrial function and size, and the presence of other valvular lesions.

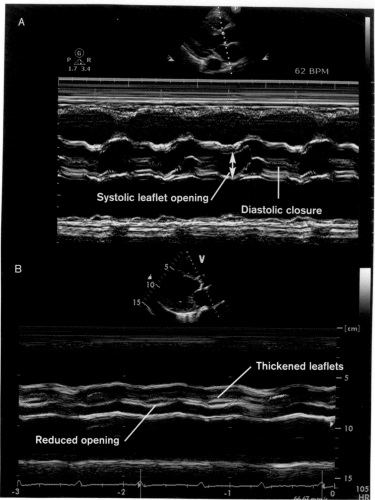

Figure 17. Maximal aortic cusp separation demonstrating: A) normal aortic valve; and B) severe aortic stenosis.

14 How is pulmonary artery systolic pressure measured by echocardiography (Figure 18)?

- Most normal hearts have a small degree of tricuspid regurgitation (TR) present.

- Using the modified Bernoulli equation for the pressure gradient across the tricuspid valve:

RVSP - RAP = 4 v^2

where v = peak velocity across tricuspid valve, RVSP = right ventricular systolic pressure, RAP = right atrial pressure (normally 0-10mmHg) = JVP (jugular venous pressure).

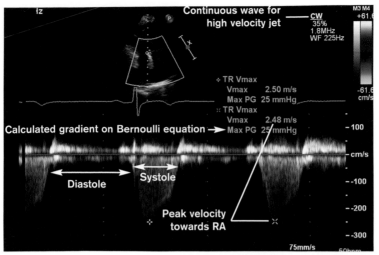

Figure 18. Measurement of pulmonary artery systolic pressure. Using the small degree of tricuspid regurgitation present in most normal hearts, the right ventricular systolic pressure (RVSP) can be calculated. If no pulmonary stenosis is present, the RVSP also represents the pulmonary artery systolic pressure. RA = right atrium.

135

- Hence RVSP = 4 v^2 + JVP.
- Assuming there is no pulmonary stenosis, RVSP also represents the pulmonary artery systolic pressure (normally <25mmHg).
- If no TR is present, the pulmonary artery pressures cannot be calculated using this method.

15 How is valvular regurgitation quantified on echocardiography?

- Jet size - colour-flow mapping (see below).
- Vena contracta width (width of the narrowest part of the regurgitant jet).
- Proximal isovelocity surface area (PISA) or proximal isosurface acceleration to calculate:

  a) regurgitant volume;
  b) regurgitant fraction;
  c) effective regurgitant orifice area.

- Flow reversal:

  a)   systolic flow reversal in the pulmonary veins for mitral regurgitation;
  b)   diastolic flow reversal in the descending aorta for aortic regurgitation.

- Additional techniques used for measuring aortic regurgitation include (Figure 19):

  a)   deceleration rate - with severe aortic regurgitation >3m/s^2;
  b)   pressure half-time - with severe aortic regurgitation <300ms.

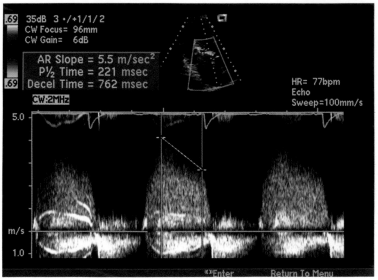

Figure 19. Deceleration rate and pressure half-time measurements to quantify the severity of aortic regurgitation.

- It is also important to assess for the aetiology of the valvular regurgitation, valve morphology, degree of leaflet movement, changes in left ventricular and left atrial function and size, and the presence of other valvular lesions.

16 How is valvular regurgitation quantified on colour-flow Doppler (Figure 20 and Table 3)?

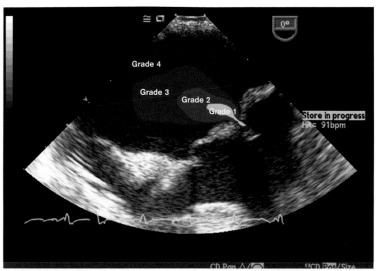

Figure 20. Quantification of valvular regurgitation on colour flow Doppler.

Table 3. Quantification of valvular regurgitation on colour-flow Doppler.		
Grade 0	Nil	No regurgitation
Grade 1	Mild	Regurgitant flow immediately adjacent to the valve (not on every beat)
Grade 2	Mild-moderate	Regurgitant flow filling up to 1/3 of the cross-sectional area of the receiving chamber, on every beat
Grade 3	Moderate-severe	Regurgitant flow filling up to 2/3 of the cross-sectional area of the receiving chamber, on every beat
Grade 4	Severe	Regurgitant flow filling up to almost all of the receiving chamber, on every beat, with distal flow reversal

17 What is the vena contracta (Figure 21)?

● The vena contracta is defined as the narrowest segment of regurgitant flow stream and typically occurs just beyond the regurgitant orifice.

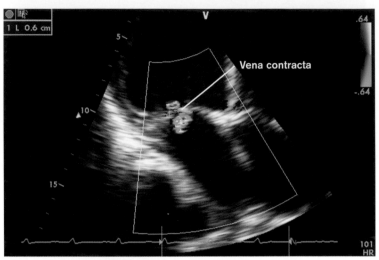

Figure 21. Vena contracta.

18 What is the proximal isovelocity surface area (PISA) (Figure 22)?

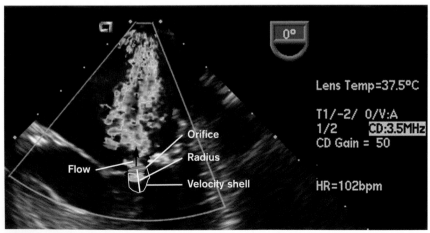

Figure 22. Proximal isovelocity surface area (PISA).

- PISA is based on the haemodynamic principles of flow converging on an orifice in hemispheric layers of equal velocity.
- The effective regurgitant orifice area (EROA) can be calculated by measuring the surface area of the converging hemisphere.
- The regurgitant volume can be calculated by multiplying the EROA by the flow velocity.

19 What are the components of the mitral valve inflow pattern?

- Using pulsed-wave Doppler:

   a)   the E (early) wave represents the rapid early diastolic left ventricular filling phase;

   b)   the A (atrial) wave represents the late diastolic left ventricular filling phase, associated with left atrial contraction and, hence, is lost in patients with atrial fibrillation;

   c)   the acceleration time (AT) occurs from the onset of mitral diastolic flow to the peak of the E wave;

   d)   the deceleration time (DT) occurs from the peak of the E wave to the end of early mitral flow (Figure 23).

- The normal EA ratio is 1-2.
- Abnormal EA ratios occur in patients with diastolic dysfunction (see below), restrictive cardiomyopathy and constrictive pericarditis.

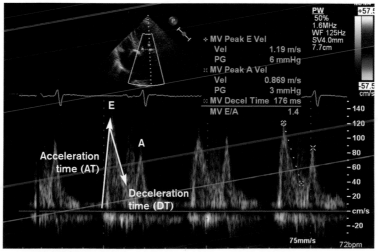

Figure 23. Mitral valve inflow pattern.

20 What are the characteristics of diastolic dysfunction found on echocardiography (Figure 24)?

- Diastolic dysfunction is characterised by increased chamber stiffness and impaired relaxation following ventricular contraction resulting in impaired diastolic flow from the left atrium to ventricle due to increased resistance to flow.
- There are four echocardiographic grades of diastolic dysfunction:

a)   Grade I - abnormal relaxation (E<A);
b)   Grade II - pseudonormal filling (E>A);
c)   Grade III - reversible restrictive filling (E>>A);
d)   Grade IV - fixed restrictive filling (E>>>A).

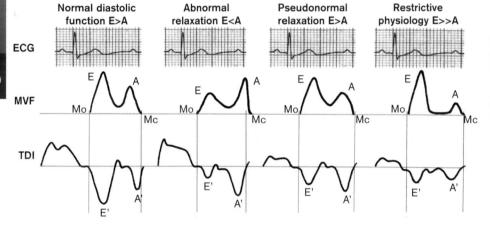

Figure 24. Grades I - III of diastolic dysfunction demonstrated on mitral valve inflow (MVF) patterns and tissue Doppler indices (TDI). ECG = electrocardiogram; E = E wave; A = A wave; Mo = opening of the mitral valve; Mc = closing of the mitral valve.

21 How is the pressure half-time (PHT) determined to calculate the area of the mitral valve (Figure 25)?

- The angle of the slope of the E wave on the mitral valve inflow pattern represents the rate at which the left atrial and left ventricular pressures equalise following opening of the mitral valve.
- In mitral stenosis, the rate of decline of pressure equalisation is slower and this is represented on the E wave slope as a more shallow angle.

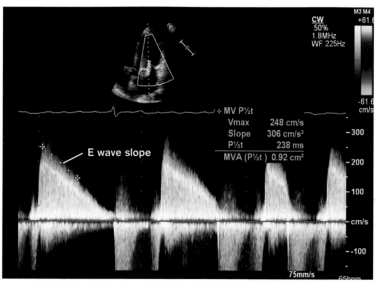

Figure 25. Mitral valve area measurement using pressure half-time. P½t = pressure half-time.

- This phenomenon can be quantified using pressure half-time (PHT) measurements allowing the mitral valve area (MVA) to be calculated indirectly:

$$MVA\ (cm^2) = \frac{220}{PHT\ (msec)}$$

- As the graph actually depicts change in velocity, the PHT is actually when velocity falls to 0.7 of its peak value (calculated by the Bernoulli equation):

velocity is proportional to the square root of pressure (0.7 = √0.5).

22 How is a pericardial effusion differentiated from a pleural effusion on echocardiography (Figure 26)?

- In comparison to pleural effusions, pericardial effusions:

  a) terminate at the atrioventricular groove;

  b) do not extend beyond the level of the descending aorta.

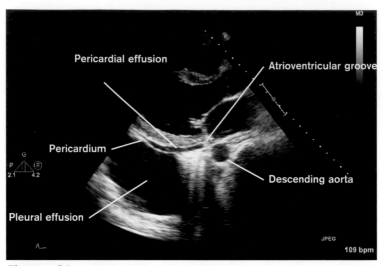

Figure 26. Differentiating a pericardial effusion from a pleural effusion on echocardiography.

23 What are the echocardiographic characteristics of left ventricular hypertrophy (Figure 27)?

- Left ventricular hypertrophy is defined as a left ventricular mass index >136g/m² in men and >112g/m² in women.

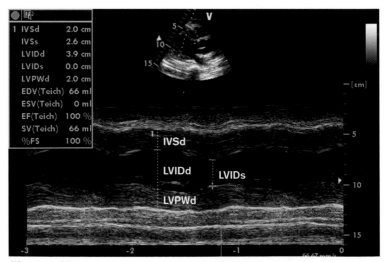

Figure 27. Left ventricular hypertrophy. IVSd = inter-ventricular septal thickness in diastole; LVIDd/LVIDs = left ventricular internal diameter in diastole/systole; LVPWd = left ventricular posterior wall thickness in diastole.

- The left ventricular mass index can be calculated using a series of formulae:

  LVM (g) = 1.04 [(LVIDd + IVSd + LVPWd)^3 - LVIDd^3] - 14
  BSA (m^2) = [height (cm) x weight (kg) / 3600] $^{1/2}$
  LVMI (g/m^2) = LVM / BSA

  where LVM = left ventricular mass, LVIDd = left ventricular internal diameter in diastole, IVSd = interventricular septal thickness in diastole, LVPWd = left ventricular posterior wall thickness in diastole, BSA = body surface area, LVMI = left ventricular mass index.

- Asymmetrical septal hypertrophy is defined as an IVSd: LVPWd ratio >1.5 and occurs more commonly in elderly women and in patients with hypertrophic cardiomyopathy (Figure 28).

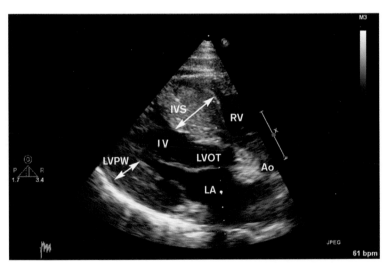

Figure 28. Asymmetrical septal hypertrophy. IVS = interventricular septum; RV = right ventricle; LVPW = left ventricular posterior wall; LV = left ventricle; LVOT = left ventricular outflow tract; LA = left atrium; Ao = ascending aorta.

24 How is the aortic valve assessed on echocardiography?

- 2D echocardiography:

  a)   aortic valve leaflets - motion (normal, excessive, restricted), thickening, calcification, bicuspid aortic valve, planimetry for aortic valve area, vegetation;

b)   aortic root - dilation, dissection, abscess.

● M-mode:

a)   cardiac function and size - left ventricular hypertrophy, left ventricular dilation, left ventricular dysfunction.

● Doppler echocardiography:

a)   colour-flow Doppler - jet width, vena contracta, regurgitant fraction, regurgitant volume, effective regurgitant orifice area;

b)   pulsed-wave Doppler - descending aorta diastolic flow reversal;

c)   continuous-wave Doppler - peak velocity, peak pressure gradient, mean pressure gradient, pressure half-time, continuity equation.

25 How is the mitral valve assessed on echocardiography?

● 2D echocardiography:

a)   mitral valve leaflets and subvalvar apparatus - motion (normal, excessive, restricted), thickening, calcification, planimetry for mitral valve area, vegetations, flail segment, chordal elongation, papillary muscle dysfunction and left atrial thrombus.

● M-mode:

a)   cardiac function and size - left ventricular dilation, left ventricular dysfunction, left atrial dilation.

● Doppler echocardiography:

a)   colour-flow Doppler - jet width, vena contracta, regurgitant fraction, regurgitant volume, effective regurgitant orifice area;

b)   pulsed-wave Doppler - pulmonary vein flow reversal, mean pressure gradient, pressure half-time, pulmonary artery systolic pressure.

26 What are the characteristics of pericardial tamponade on echocardiography (Figure 29)?

- Large-volume pericardial effusion.
- Right atrial and ventricular diastolic collapse.
- Exaggerated respiratory variations in transmitral and transtricuspid flows, normally seen in inspiration and expiration.

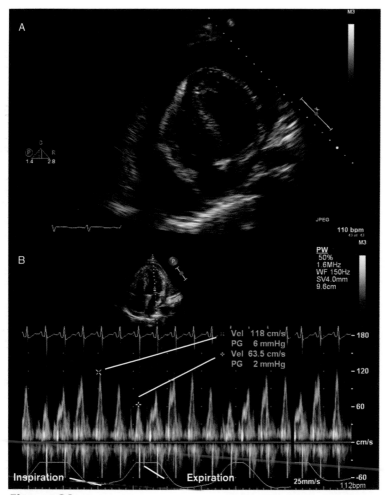

Figure 29. Pericardial tamponade, demonstrated by: A) large pericardial effusion and right ventricular collapse on an apical 4-chamber view; and B) marked respiratory transmitral inflow variation.

27 What are the characteristics of constrictive pericarditis on echocardiography (Figure 30)?

- Thickened and calcified echobright pericardium.
- Abrupt cessation of left ventricular filling in early diastole (due to a non-compliant pericardium) resulting in a septal bounce pattern.
- Posterior left ventricular wall flattening during late diastole (due to a non-compliant pericardium restricting diastolic filling).
- Dilated superior and inferior venae cavae and hepatic veins due to raised systemic venous pressures.
- Abnormal mitral inflow pattern reflecting left ventricular diastolic dysfunction.
- Exaggerated respiratory variation of the mitral and tricuspid valve inflow patterns, with >25% increase in transtricuspid and >25% decrease in transmitral flow during inspiration.

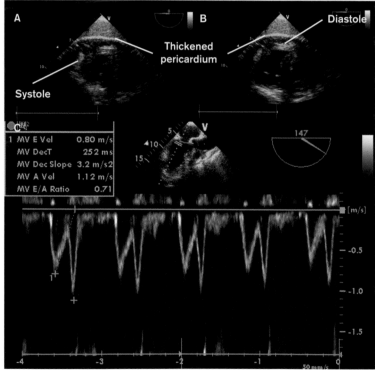

Figure 30. Echocardiographic features of constrictive pericarditis. 2D echocardiography in: A) systole; and B) diastole, demonstrating restricted ventricular filling and thickened echobright pericardium. C) M-mode echocardiography demonstrating grade I diastolic dysfunction with E:A reversal on the mitral valve inflow pattern.

28 What are the characteristics of hypertrophic cardiomyopathy on echocardiography?

- Asymmetrical septal hypertrophy (ASH) with an IVSd: LVPWd ratio >1.5.
- Systolic anterior motion (SAM) of the mitral valve, which may result in mitral regurgitation.
- Left ventricular outflow tract obstruction (LVOTO).
- Mid-systolic fluttering or closure of the aortic valve.
- Diastolic dysfunction.

29 What are the characteristics of restrictive cardiomyopathy on echocardiography?

- Diastolic dysfunction.
- Systolic dysfunction.
- Concentric thickening of the posterior wall and interventricular septum.
- Reduced left and right ventricular cavity dimensions.
- Reduced septal wall motion.
- Endomyocardial fibrosis may also be present resulting in cavity obliteration and an echobright endocardium.

30 What are the important features to assess on echocardiography in patients with coronary artery disease?

- Global left ventricular systolic function.
- Regional wall motion abnormalities (attributable to coronary artery territories).
- Complications of myocardial infarction - ventricular septal rupture, papillary muscle rupture, left ventricular free wall aneurysm or rupture.
- Ischaemic mitral regurgitation.
- Associated valvular disease.
- Pericardial effusion.
- Left ventricular thrombus.

31 What are the characteristics of an atrial myxoma on echocardiography (Figure 31)?

- Atrial myxomas usually present as a heterogenous mass often with cystic areas and areas of calcification.

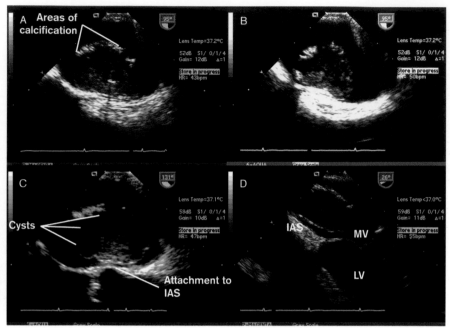

Figure 31. Echocardiographic features of a left atrial myxoma. IAS = inter-atrial septum; MV = mitral valve; LV = left ventricle.

● These tumours are often mobile with a stalk attached to the intra-atrial septum and may be visualised prolapsing into the left ventricle.

32 What are the main indications for stress echocardiography?

● Viability studies in the presence of hibernating myocardium (see Chapter 7).

● Low-flow low-gradient aortic stenosis (see Chapter 12).

● Left ventricular outflow tract obstruction to determine the need for intervention (resting gradient >30mmHg, stress-induced gradient >100mmHg).

● Stress can be induced by:

    a)   exercise;
    b)   pacing;
    c)   pharmacology (dobutamine or adenosine).

33 What are the main indications for transoesophageal echocardiography (TOE)?

- Ascending aortic dissection, with a specificity approaching 100% and a sensitivity of 98%. There is, however, a blind spot at the distal ascending aorta.
- Mitral valve regurgitation, to further delineate the aetiology of the regurgitation.
- Infective endocarditis, especially with prosthetic valves and to identify peri-annular abscesses.
- Intra-operatively to assess:

  a)   the success of aortic or mitral valve repair;
  b)   de-airing following an open heart procedure;
  c)   left ventricular function.

- Intracardiac masses including tumours and thrombus.
- Atrial and ventricular septal defects.

34 What are the contra-indications to TOE?

- Oesophageal disease including neoplasia, varices, webs and fistulae.
- Upper gastrointestinal bleeding.
- Severe cervical arthritis or instability.

35 What are the main views on transoesophageal echocardiography (Figures 32-35)?

See overleaf

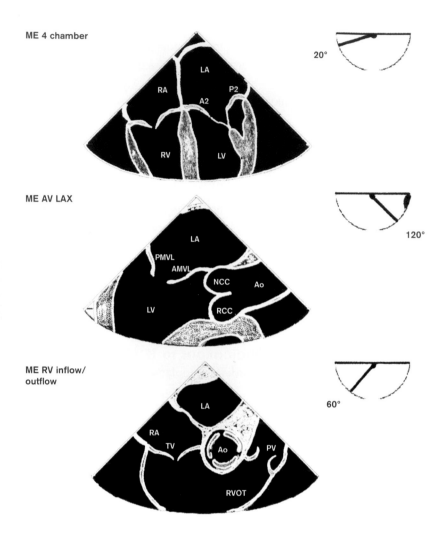

Figure 32. Standard transoesophageal echocardiographic views demonstrating a mid-oesophageal (ME) 4-chamber view (upper image), a mid-oesophageal aortic valve (AV) long axis (LAX) view (middle image) and a mid-oesophageal right ventricular (RV) inflow/outflow view (lower image). RV = right ventricle; RA = right atrium; LV = left ventricle; LA = left atrium; A2, P2 = scallops of the anterior (A) or posterior (P) mitral valve leaflets; AMVL = anterior mitral valve leaflet; PMVL = posterior mitral valve leaflet; Ao = ascending aorta; NCC = non-coronary cusp of the aortic valve; RCC = right coronary cusp of the aortic valve; TV = tricuspid valve; RVOT = right ventricular outflow tract; PV = pulmonary valve.

ME mitral
commissures

ME AV SAX

ME bicaval

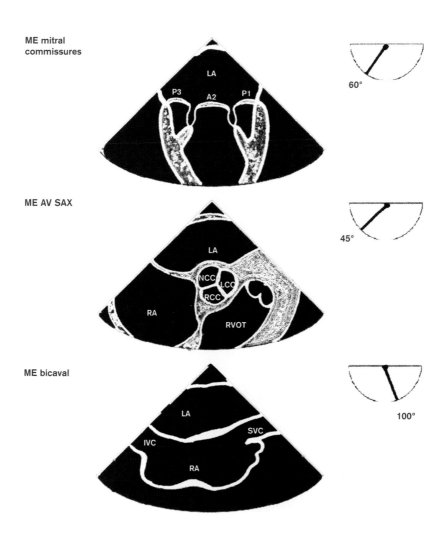

Figure 33. Standard transoesophageal echocardiographic views demonstrating a mid-oesophageal (ME) mitral commissural view (upper image), a mid-oesophageal aortic valve (AV) short axis (SAX) view (middle image) and a mid-oesophageal bicaval view (lower image). LA = left atrium; P1, A2, P3 = scallops of the anterior (A) or posterior (P) mitral valve leaflets; RA = right atrium; RVOT = right ventricular outflow tract; NCC = non-coronary cusp of the aortic valve; RCC = right coronary cusp of the aortic valve; LCC = left coronary cusp of the aortic valve; IVC = inferior vena cava; SVC = superior vena cava.

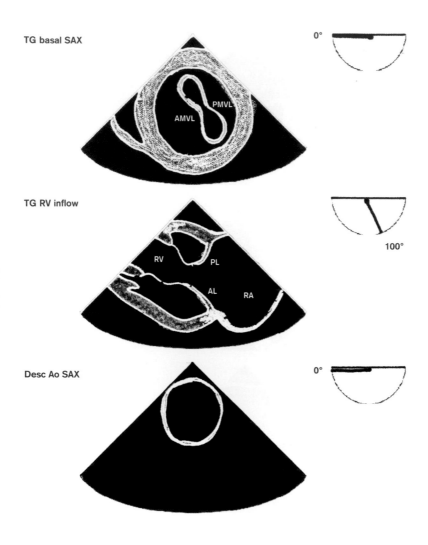

Figure 34. Standard transoesophageal echocardiographic views demonstrating a transgastric (TG) basal short axis (SAX) view (upper image), a transgastric right ventricular (RV) inflow view (middle image) and a descending aortic short axis (SAX) view (lower image). PMVL = posterior mitral valve leaflet; AMVL = anterior mitral valve leaflet; RV = right ventricle; RA = right atrium; PL = posterior tricuspid valve leaflet; AL = anterior tricuspid valve leaflet; Desc Ao = descending aorta.

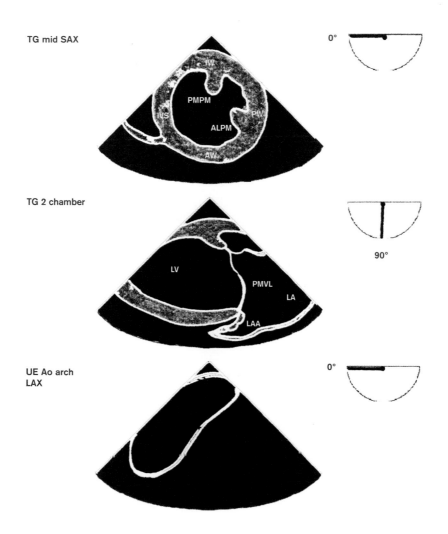

TG mid SAX

0°

TG 2 chamber

90°

UE Ao arch
LAX

0°

153

Figure 35. Standard transoesophageal echocardiographic views demonstrating a transgastric (TG) mid short axis (SAX) view (upper image), a transgastric 2-chamber view (middle image) and an upper oesophageal (UE) aortic arch long axis (LAX) view (lower image). IVS = interventricular septum; AW = anterior wall of left ventricle; PW = posterior wall of left ventricle; IW = inferior wall of left ventricle; PMPM = posteromedial papillary muscle; ALPM = anterolateral papillary muscle; LV = left ventricle; LA = left atrium; LAA = left atrial appendage; PMVL = posterior mitral valve leaflet; Ao = aorta.

Recommended reading

1.   Shanewise JS, Cheung AT, Aronson S, Stewart WJ, Weiss RL, Mark JB, Savage RM, Sears-Rogan P, Mathew JP, Quiñones MA, Cahalan MK, Savino JS. ASE/SCA guidelines for performing a comprehensive intraoperative multiplane transesophageal echocardiography examination. *J Am Soc Echocardiogr* 1999; 12(10): 884-900.

2.   Lang RM, Bierig M, Devereux RB, Flachskampf FA, Foster E, Pellikka PA, Picard MH, Roman MJ, Seward J, Shanewise JS, Solomon SD, Spencer KT, Sutton MS, Stewart WJ; Chamber Quantification Writing Group; American Society of Echocardiography's Guidelines and Standards Committee; European Association of Echocardiography. Recommendations for chamber quantification. *J Am Soc Echocardiogr* 2005; 18(12): 1440-63.

3.   Stout K, Otto CM. Quantification of valvular aortic stenosis. *ACC Current Journal Review* 2003; 12(2): 54-8.

4.   Baumgartner H, Hung J, Bermejo J, Chambers JB, Evangelista A, Griffin BP, Lung B, Otto CM, Pellikka PA, Quiñones M; American Society of Echocardiography; European Association of Echocardiography. Echocardiographic assessment of valve stenosis. *J Am Soc Echocardiogr* 2009; 22(1): 1-23.

5.   Zoghbi WA, Enriquez-Sarano M, Foster E, Grayburn PA, Kraft CD, Levine RA, Nihoyannopoulos P, Otto CM, Quinones MA, Rakowski H, Stewart WJ, Waggoner A, Weissman NJ; American Society of Echocardiography. Recommendations for evaluation of the severity of native valvular regurgitation with two-dimensional and Doppler echocardiography. *J Am Soc Echocardiogr* 2003; 16(7): 777-802.

Chapter 6

Cardiac catheterisation

1 **What is coronary angiography?**
- Coronary angiography is an invasive cardiological investigation where radio-opaque dye is injected through the coronary ostia to delineate coronary artery anatomy using multiple 2D cine images.

2 **How is coronary angiography performed?**
- The patient is kept fasted for 4 hours prior to the procedure and given a premedication, including a benzodiazepine and an opiate.
- The patient is placed supine on a radiolucent mobile screening table.
- Access to the aortic root is gained via the femoral, brachial, radial or ulnar artery by placing an arterial sheath using a percutaneous modified Seldinger technique.
- The coronary ostia are engaged with a variety of pre-formed catheters (such as a Judkins left or Judkins right) and non-ionic radio-opaque dye is injected into the left and right coronary arteries under fluoroscopic guidance.
- As a 6Fr (2mm) catheter is often used, it is possible to judge the size of the vessels relative to the catheter.
- As well as the coronary arteries, the left ventricle, mitral valve, aortic valve and ascending aorta can all be assessed during the same procedure.
- The different views obtained of the coronary arteries are described by the position of the X-ray detector:

  a) right anterior oblique (RAO),
  b) left anterior oblique (LAO);
  c) anteroposterior (AP).

  These views will have different degrees of associated cranial and caudal tilt.
- On completion of the procedure, the arterial sheath is removed and haemostasis can be achieved using a collagen plug (AngioSeal®).

3   **What are the standard views of the left coronary system during coronary angiography (Figures 1-5)?**

- RAO 20° caudal 20°.
- AP 0° caudal 30°.
- AP 0° cranial 40°.
- LAO 50° cranial 30°.
- LAO 50° caudal 30° ('spider' view).
- On the RAO view, the ribs descend down to the right side of the image with the thoracic spine on the left side of the image.
- On the LAO view, the ribs descend down to the left side of the image with the thoracic spine on the right side of the image.
- The left anterior descending artery descends towards the apex. It is usually the longest vessel and has septal arteries branching off at 90°.
- The circumflex artery is the closest artery to the thoracic spine and the descending aorta.
- If the procedure has been performed via the femoral route, the catheter will be visible in the descending aorta, close to the thoracic spine.

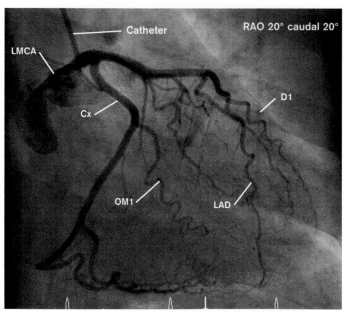

Figure 1. Right anterior oblique (RAO) view of the left coronary system. LMCA = left main coronary artery; Cx = circumflex artery; D1 = 1st diagonal artery; OM1 = 1st obtuse marginal artery; LAD = left anterior descending artery.

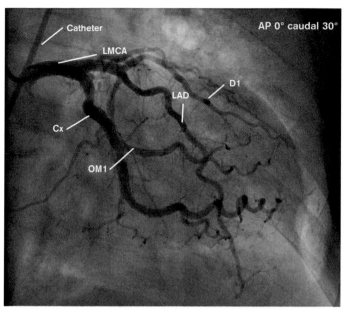

Figure 2. Anteroposterior (AP) caudal view of the left coronary system. LMCA = left main coronary artery; Cx = circumflex artery; D1 = 1st diagonal artery; OM1 = 1st obtuse marginal artery; LAD = left anterior descending artery.

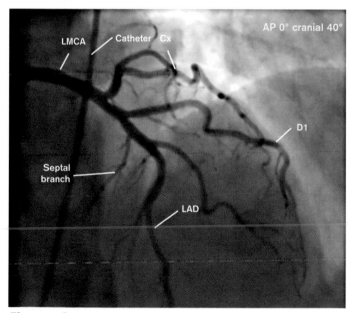

Figure 3. Anteroposterior (AP) cranial view of the left coronary system. LMCA = left main coronary artery; Cx = circumflex artery; D1 = 1st diagonal artery; OM1 = 1st obtuse marginal artery; LAD = left anterior descending artery.

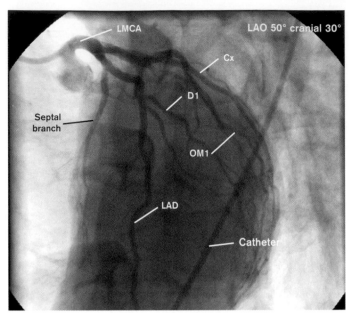

Figure 4. Left anterior oblique (LAO) cranial view of the left coronary system. LMCA = left main coronary artery; Cx = circumflex artery; D1 = 1st diagonal artery; OM1 = 1st obtuse marginal artery; LAD = left anterior descending artery.

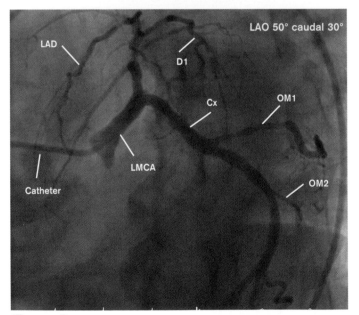

Figure 5. Left anterior oblique (LAO) caudal view ('spider view') of the left coronary system. LMCA = left main coronary artery; Cx = circumflex artery; D1 = 1st diagonal artery; OM1 = 1st obtuse marginal artery; OM2 = 2nd obtuse marginal artery; LAD = left anterior descending artery.

4   **What are the standard views of the right coronary system during coronary angiography (Figures 6 and 7)?**

● LAO 30° cranio-caudal 0°.
● RAO 30° cranio-caudal 0°.

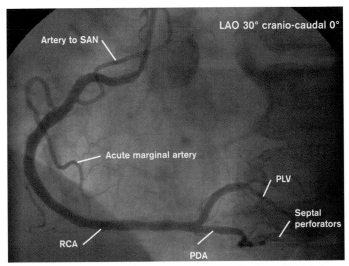

Figure 6. Left anterior oblique (LAO) view of the right coronary system. SAN = sino-atrial node; RCA = right coronary artery; PDA = posterior descending artery; PLV = posterior left ventricular artery.

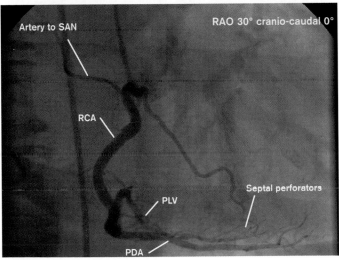

Figure 7. Right anterior oblique (RAO) view of the right coronary system. SAN = sino-atrial node; RCA = right coronary artery; PDA = posterior descending artery; PLV = posterior left ventricular artery.

5   **What are the standard views of the left ventricle during cardiac catheterization (Figures 8 and 9)?**
- RAO view, which demonstrates global and regional left ventricular function (anterobasal, anterior, apical, inferior and inferobasal).
- LAO view, which demonstrates regional left ventricular function (lateral, septal and inferior).

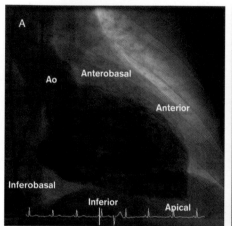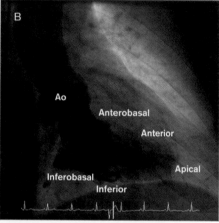

Figure 8. Right anterior oblique (RAO) view of the left ventricle in: A) diastole; and B) systole. Ao = ascending aorta.

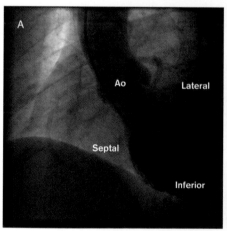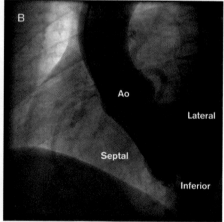

Figure 9. Left anterior oblique (LAO) view of the left ventricle in: A) diastole; and B) systole. Ao = ascending aorta.

6   **What are the indications for coronary angiography?**
- Chronic stable angina.
- Acute coronary syndrome - unstable angina, non-ST elevation myocardial infarction, ST elevation myocardial infarction.

- Positive exercise tolerance test (ETT).
- Ischaemic cardiomyopathy.
- Pre-operative assessment in patients undergoing valve or aortic surgery, if aged >40 years old or with multiple risk factors.
- Survivors of cardiac arrest.
- Patients with multiple risk factors for coronary artery disease where the diagnosis is important for occupation, e.g. airline pilot.

7 What are the relative contra-indications for coronary angiography?

- Acute Type A aortic dissection.
- Aortic valve infective endocarditis with a vegetation present.
- Decompensated heart failure or acute pulmonary oedema.
- Active infection.
- Renal dysfunction, due to the risk of contrast nephropathy.
- Allergy to radio-opaque contrast.

8 What are the complications of coronary angiography?

- Local vascular complication 3%.
- Contrast nephropathy 0.5%.
- Emergency surgery for pericardial tamponade, coronary artery dissection (Figure 10), retained fragment of wire or ongoing coronary ischaemia 0.1%.

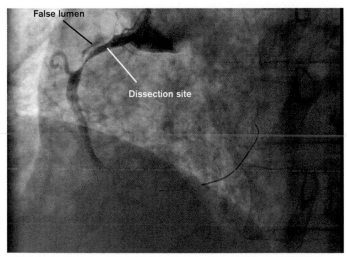

Figure 10. Coronary artery dissection following coronary angiography.

- Cerebrovascular accident 0.05%.
- Myocardial infarction 0.05%.
- Mortality <0.05%.

9 What are the important features that can be assessed during cardiac angiography (Figure 11)?

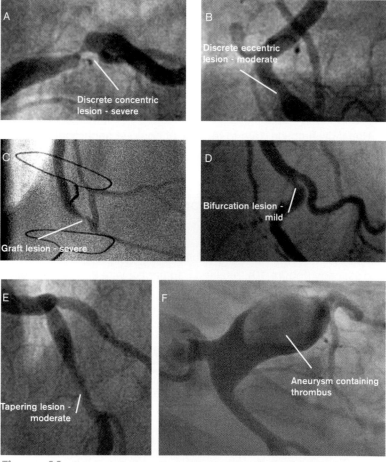

Figure 11. Coronary artery lesions: A) discrete concentric lesion; B) discrete eccentric lesion; C) saphenous vein graft lesion; D) bifurcation lesion; E) tapering lesion; F) aneurysm containing thrombus.

- Left main stem.
- Left anterior descending (LAD) artery system - LAD artery, diagonal arteries, septal arteries.
- Circumflex coronary artery system - atrioventricular circumflex artery, obtuse marginal arteries, intermediate artery.

- Right coronary artery (RCA) system - RCA, posterior descending artery, posterior left ventricular branch.
- Coronary artery dominance.
- Retrograde filling of occluded vessels.
- Global left ventricular function with regional wall motion abnormalities.
- Mitral valve - regurgitation, annular calcification.
- Aortic valve - regurgitation, calcification, dilated aortic root.

10 **How is mitral regurgitation classified by angiography?**
- According to the Sellers' classification (Figure 12):

   a) I: incomplete opacification of the left atrium that clears with each beat;
   b) II: complete opacification of the left atrium that does not clear with each beat;
   c) III: complete opacification of the left atrium with a similar density to the left ventricle;
   d) IV: complete opacification of the left atrium in one beat, that becomes progressively more dense with each beat, with contrast refluxing into the pulmonary veins.

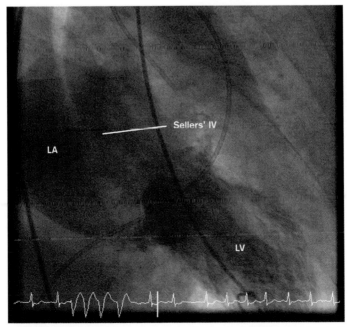

Figure 12. Sellers' grade IV mitral regurgitation. LA = left atrium; LV = left ventricle.

11 **How is aortic regurgitation classified by angiography (Figure 13)?**

● According to the Sellers' classification:

a) 1+: small regurgitant jet across the aortic valve but without opacification of the left ventricle;

b) 2+: regurgitant jet across the aortic valve with faint opacification of the left ventricle;

c) 3+: dense opacification of the left ventricle with no distinct jet across the aortic valve usually visualized;

d) 4+: opacification of the left ventricle greater than the aorta.

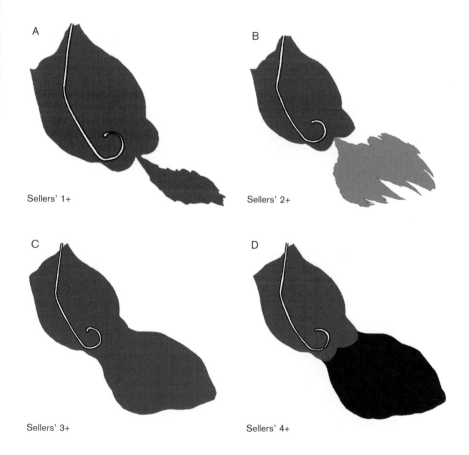

Figure 13. Sellers' angiographic classification of aortic regurgitation.

12 How is left ventricular function classified by ventriculography?

• Global left ventricular function:

  a) good: >50% left ventricular ejection fraction;
  b) moderate: 30-50% left ventricular ejection fraction;
  c) poor: <30% left ventricular ejection fraction.

• Regional wall motion abnormalities based on five areas of the left ventricle on the RAO view (anterobasal, apex, anterior, inferior, inferobasal) and three areas on the LAO view (lateral, septal, inferior):

  a) normal;
  b) hypokinetic;
  c) akinetic;
  d) dyskinetic;
  e) aneurysmal.

13 What is a significant stenosis of a coronary artery (Figure 14)?

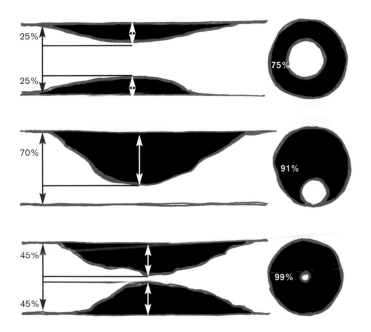

Figure 14. Coronary artery stenosis as classified by luminal diameter and cross-sectional area.

- The correlation between luminal stenosis and cross-sectional area (CSA) stenosis is governed by the formula:

  area = πr^2 (where r = radius of vessel, π = 3.14) hence:

  a)   50% luminal diameter reduction = 75% CSA reduction;
  b)   70% luminal diameter reduction = 91% CSA reduction;
  c)   90% luminal diameter reduction = 99% CSA reduction.

- Significant stenosis is defined as >60% luminal diameter (84% CSA reduction).
- Left main stem significant stenosis is defined as >50% luminal diameter (75% CSA reduction).
- It is important to assess each lesion in several views as the inter-observer error is low for mild (<50%) and severe (>80%) luminal stenoses but the error is significant for stenoses 50-80%.
- More recently, fractional flow reserve (FFR) is being increasingly used to determine the haemodynamic significance of a coronary stenosis. FFR is calculated by the ratio of the coronary pressure distal to the lesion compared to the pressure proximal to the lesion. FFR in a normal coronary artery is 1.0, with an FFR <0.80 indicating an ischaemic coronary lesion (>90% accuracy). Data from the FAME study suggest that FFR-guided revascularisation, in comparison to angiography-guided revascularisation, results in improved freedom from death, myocardial infarction and repeat revascularisation.

14 What is TIMI flow?

- TIMI (thrombolysis in myocardial infarction) derives its name from a trial of similar name and describes the different grades of coronary flow:

  a)   grade 0: no contrast flow;
  b)   grade 1: reduced flow and incomplete opacification of the distal vessel;
  c)   grade 2: slow distal filling but complete opacification of the distal vessel;
  d)   grade 3: prompt antegrade contrast flow with rapid clearing.

15 How are systemic-pulmonary shunt ratios calculated?

- Using the Fick principle:

  $$\text{Flow} = \frac{O_2 \text{ consumption}}{\text{arteriovenous } O_2 \text{ concentration difference}}$$

$$\text{Flow} = \frac{O_2 \text{ consumption}}{\text{arteriovenous } O_2 \text{ sats difference} \times Hb \times 1.34 \times 10}$$

$$\text{Pulmonary flow} = \frac{O_2 \text{ consumption}}{(PV\ O_2 \text{ sats} - PA\ O_2 \text{ sats}) \times Hb \times 1.34 \times 10}$$

$$\text{Systemic flow} = \frac{O_2 \text{ consumption}}{(Ao \text{ sats} - RA \text{ sats}) \times Hb \times 1.34 \times 10}$$

As O_2 consumption and Hb are the same in both equations

Pulmonary flow: systemic flow ratio =
(shunt ratio)
$$\frac{PV\ O_2 \text{ sats} - PA\ O_2 \text{ sats}}{Ao \text{ sats} - RA \text{ sats}}$$

$PV\ O_2$ sats usually assumed to be 100%
$$RA \text{ sats} = \frac{(3 \times SVC \text{ sats}) + (1 \times IVC \text{ sats})}{4}$$

where PV = pulmonary vein, PA = pulmonary artery, Ao = aorta, RA = right atrium, SVC = superior vena cava, IVC = inferior vena cava, Hb = haemoglobin, sats = saturations.

16 How is cardiac output calculated at cardiac catheterisation?

- Using the direct Fick method:

$$\text{Cardiac output} = \frac{O_2 \text{ consumption}}{AV\ O_2 \text{ concentration difference}}$$

O_2 content = (Hb $\times$ 1.34 $\times$ O_2 sats) + plasma O_2 content
1g of Hb when 100% saturated combines with 1.34mL O_2
Plasma O_2 content in 100mL plasma ~0.3mL

$$CO = \frac{O_2 \text{ consumption}}{\{[(Ao \text{ sats} - PA \text{ sats}) \times Hb \times 1.34] + 0.3\} \times 10}$$

where CO = cardiac output, AV = arteriovenous, Hb = haemoglobin, Ao = aorta, PA = pulmonary artery.

- Any systemic artery can be used for systemic saturations but the pulmonary artery must be used for the mixed venous content.
- Oxygen consumption is measured by the respiratory gas monitor on a ventilator.
- Cardiac output can also be measured using the indirect Fick method with dye dilution (similar to the thermodilution method used with pulmonary artery catheters).

17 How is the aortic valve area calculated by cardiac catheterisation (Figure 15)?

- Using the Gorlin equation:

$$AoV\ area = \frac{AoV\ flow}{44.5 \times \sqrt{mean\ aortic\ gradient}}$$

and as $AoV\ flow = \dfrac{cardiac\ output}{systolic\ ejection\ period}$

$$AoV\ area = \frac{CO}{44.5 \times SEP \times \sqrt{mean\ aortic\ gradient}}$$

and as SEP = left ventricular ejection time x heart rate

$$AoV\ area = \frac{CO}{44.5 \times LVET \times HR \times \sqrt{mean\ aortic\ gradient}}$$

where AoV = aortic valve, CO = cardiac output, SEP = systolic ejection period, LVET = left ventricular ejection time, HR = heart rate.

- The same formula and constant can be used for the pulmonary valve.
- Although this formula can be used with prosthetic valves, the calculations are dependent on 'forward flow', which is inaccurate in the presence of regurgitation.

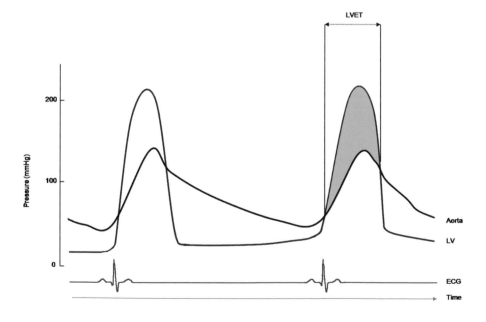

Figure 15. Gorlin method of calculating aortic valve area.

18 How is the mitral valve area calculated by cardiac catheterisation?

- Using the Gorlin equation:

$$\text{MV area} = \frac{\text{MV flow}}{31 \times \sqrt{\text{mean mitral gradient}}}$$

and as $\text{MV flow} = \dfrac{\text{cardiac output}}{\text{diastolic filling period}}$

$$\text{MV area} = \frac{\text{CO}}{31 \times \text{DFP} \times \sqrt{\text{mean mitral gradient}}}$$

where MV = mitral valve, CO = cardiac output, DFP = diastolic filling period.

- The same formula and constant can be used for the tricuspid valve.

19 What is coronary artery intravascular ultrasound (IVUS)(Figure 16)?

- IVUS is a transcatheter ultrasound probe that is introduced into the coronary artery over an angioplasty wire.
- It allows direct imaging of the luminal diameter and vessel wall giving a visual assessment of atheroma and calcification.
- It is useful in patients with equivocal stenosis and vessels with marked endoluminal calcification.

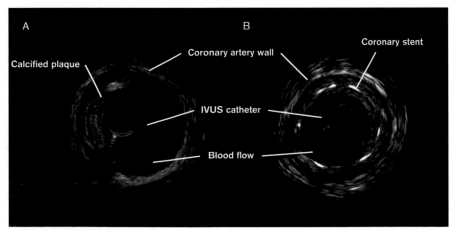

Figure 16. Intravascular ultrasound demonstrating: A) calcification and stenosis of the right coronary artery; B) presence of a coronary stent.

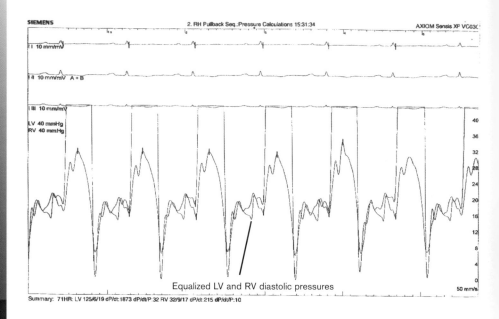

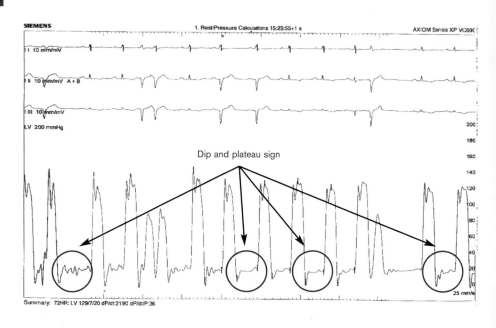

Figure 17. Dip and plateau pressure waveform associated with constrictive pericarditis.

20 What is intracoronary pressure wire monitoring?

- Using a fine wire pressure transducer, the intracoronary pressure can be measured, thereby allowing a comparison of the pressure distal to the lesion with the pressure proximal to the lesion. This allows the fractional flow reserve (FFR) to be calculated to determine the haemodynamic significance of a lesion. The normal FFR should be approximately 1.0, whereas an FFR <0.8 indicates a significant flow limiting lesion.
- Flow limitation can also be assessed by measuring the pressure gradient after administering a vasodilator, e.g. adenosine.

21 What is the square root sign ('dip and plateau' pressure waveform)(Figure 17)?

- The square root sign is defined as an abnormal ventricular diastolic filling pattern caused by rapid early ventricular filling followed by a sudden halt in ventricular filling.
- This occurs at the end of the first third of diastole onwards as the ventricle is unable to distend any further.
- The square root sign is associated with constrictive pericarditis and restrictive cardiomyopathy but not with pericardial tamponade.

171

Recommended reading

1. Scanlon PJ, Faxon DP, Audet AM, Carabello B, Dehmer GJ, Eagle KA, Legako RD, Leon DF, Murray JA, Nissen SE, Pepine CJ, Watson RM, Ritchie JL, Gibbons RJ, Cheitlin MD, Gardner TJ, Garson A Jr, Russell RO Jr, Ryan TJ, Smith SC Jr. ACC/AHA guidelines for coronary angiography. A report of the American College of Cardiology/American Heart Association Task Force on practice guidelines (Committee on Coronary Angiography). Developed in collaboration with the Society for Cardiac Angiography and Interventions. *J Am Coll Cardiol* 1999; 33(6): 1756-824.

2. Tonino PA, De Bruyne B, Pijls NH, Siebert U, Ikeno F, van't Veer M, Klauss V, Manoharan G, Engstrøm T, Oldroyd KG, Ver Lee PN, MacCarthy PA, Fearon WF; FAME Study Investigators. Fractional flow reserve versus angiography for guiding percutaneous coronary intervention. *N Engl J Med* 2009; 360(3): 213-24.

3. Sellers RD, Levy MJ, Amplatz K, Lillehei CW. Left retrograde cardioangiography in acquired cardiac disease: technic, indications and interpretations in 700 cases. *Am J Cardiol* 1964; 14: 437-47.

Chapter 7

Radiological imaging

1 **What are the principles of chest radiography (Figure 1)?**

- A chest radiograph is a non-invasive investigation that demonstrates thoracic anatomy by using small doses (0.1mSv) of ionizing radiation (X-rays).
- Different views, including anteroposterior (AP), postero-anterior (PA) and lateral, can be obtained depending on the projection of the X-ray

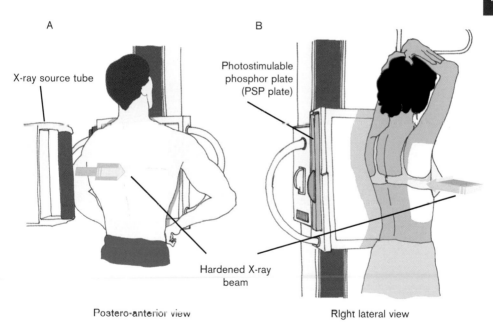

A

B

X-ray source tube

Photostimulable
phosphor plate
(PSP plate)

Hardened X-ray
beam

Postero-anterior view

Right lateral view

Figure 1. A) PA chest radiograph obtained with the X-ray source posteriorly and photostimulable phosphor plate anteriorly. B) Right lateral chest radiograph with the X-ray source on the right side and photostimulable phosphor plate to the left.

beam. For example, a PA chest radiograph is produced when the X-rays are emitted posteriorly and detected anteriorly.

● Other views include inspiration, expiration and decubitus films.

2   What are the important technical features to assess on a chest radiograph (Figure 2)?

● Penetration - the vertebral bodies should only just be visible with optimal penetration.

● Projection - the position of the scapula can be used to distinguish PA from AP. The PA projection gives a more accurate assessment of cardiac size.

● Orientation - the left and right side markings should be checked.

● Rotation - the medial ends of the left and right clavicles should be equidistant from the spinous processes of the thoracic vertebrae.

● Inspiratory effort - the anterior 6th right rib and posterior 10th right rib should be visible above the diaphragm.

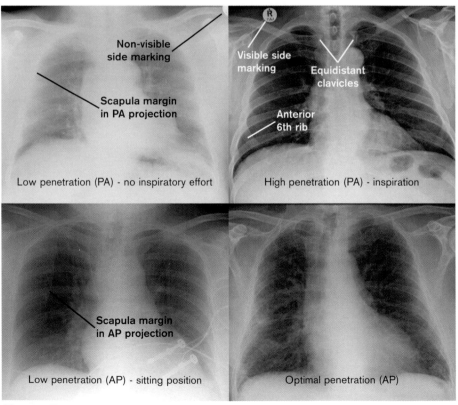

Figure 2. Technical features assessed on a chest radiograph. PA = postero-anterior; AP = anteroposterior.

3   **What are the important anatomical features to assess on a chest radiograph (Figure 3)?**

● Airway:

a)   trachea. Assess the position of the trachea, which should be central or slightly deviated to the right due to the presence of the aortic knuckle.

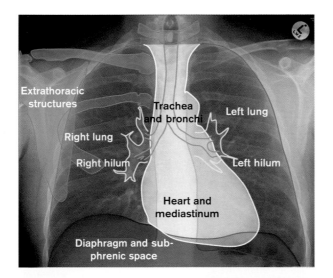

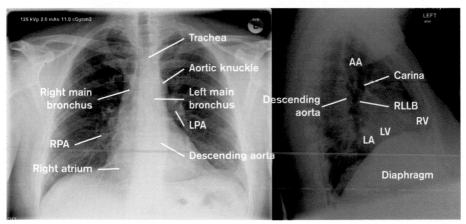

Figure 3. Anatomical features assessed on a PA and lateral chest radiograph. RPA = right pulmonary artery; LPA = left pulmonary artery; AA = aortic arch; RLLB = right lower lobe bronchus; RV = right ventricle; LV = left ventricle; LA = left atrium.

- Breathing:

  a) lungs. Check for the presence of radio-opaque lesions, pneumothorax, haemothorax, volume loss and the position of the horizontal fissure;
  b) hila. The left hilum should be <2.5cm higher than the right with a normal concave shape.

- Circulation:

  a) heart. Assess the cardiac size and shape for the presence of any chamber enlargement or pericardial effusion (globular enlargement of the cardiac silhouette);
  b) mediastinum. Assess the great vessels which lie within the mediastinum.

- Diaphragm:

  a) position of the diaphragm. The right diaphragm is usually <3cm higher than the left;
  b) sub-phrenic space. Check for air under the diaphragm or the presence of a gastric bubble or dilated loops of bowel;
  c) costophrenic angles. Assess for pleural effusions.

- Extrathoracic structures:

  a) sternum, ribs, clavicles, scapulae and vertebrae. Check for any fractures or displacement.
  b) prosthetic materials - valves, sternal wires, stents, catheters.

4   **What are the features of a pleural effusion on a chest radiograph (Figure 4)?**
- Pleural effusions can usually be identified as a concave density in place of the normally convex diaphragm.
- On the lateral decubitus films, layering of the free fluid can be seen.

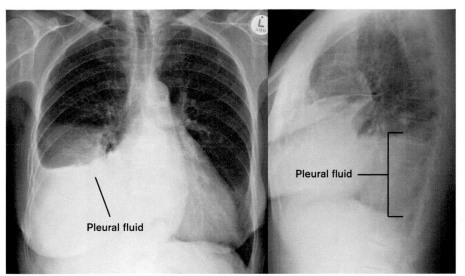

Figure 4. Chest radiographical features of a pleural effusion on PA and lateral films.

5   **What are the features of pulmonary oedema on a chest radiograph (Figure 5)?**
- Marked prominence of the pulmonary vasculature.
- Increased opacification of the peripheral alveolar spaces.
- Small, linear septal densities (Kerley B lines).

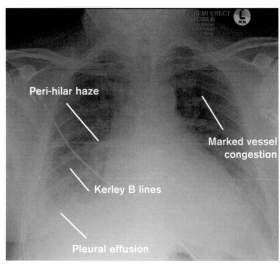

Figure 5. Chest radiographical features of pulmonary oedema.

6   **What are the features of a pericardial effusion on a chest radiograph (Figure 6)?**

●   Globular enlargement of cardiac shape.

●   Since pericardial fluid is roughly the same radiographic density as blood within the myocardium, an enlarged cardiac shadow may represent either ventricular dilation or a pericardial effusion.

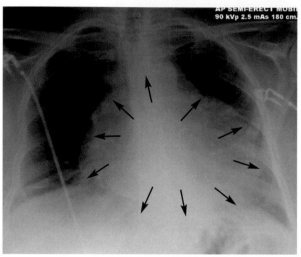

Figure 6. Chest radiographical features of a pericardial effusion.

7   **What are the features of traumatic aortic rupture on a chest radiograph (Figure 7)?**

●   Widened mediastinum.

●   Partial obliteration of the descending aorta.

●   Left apical cap.

●   Downward displacement of the left main bronchus.

●   Tracheal deviation to the right.

●   Obliteration of the aortopulmonary window.

●   Widened right paratracheal stripe.

●   Deviation of the nasogastric tube to the right.

●   Enlarged abnormal aortic contour.

●   Left haemothorax.

●   Displaced left paraspinal stripe.

●   Displaced right paraspinal stripe.

●   Fractures of the sternum, and first and second ribs.

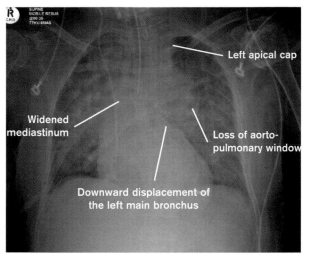

Figure 7. Chest radiographical features of traumatic aortic rupture.

8   **What are the principles of computed tomography (CT) scanning (Figure 8)?**

- Computed tomography is a non-invasive investigation where numerous X-ray beams and detectors rotate around the patient whilst the patient moves through the scanner producing a spiral path for the X-rays. This allows two-dimensional (axial, sagittal and coronal views) and three-dimensional images to be reconstructed.

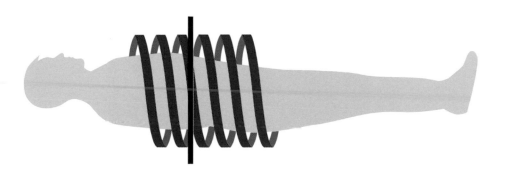

Figure 8. Principles of computed tomography, where X-ray beams rotate around the patient in a spiral path.

- Modern scanners acquire multiple slices in a single rotation allowing the whole thorax to be scanned in a few seconds.
- The degree to which the radiation is attenuated at each point is calculated and converted into a numerical value (Houndsfield units - HU) relative to the attenuation of water (which represents 0 HU).
- These numeric values are expressed graphically with the range -1000 in black and +1000 in white, with:

a)   air -1000 HU;
b)   lung -500 HU;
c)   fat -100 HU;
d)   soft tissue +20 to +80 HU;
e)   bone +1000 HU.

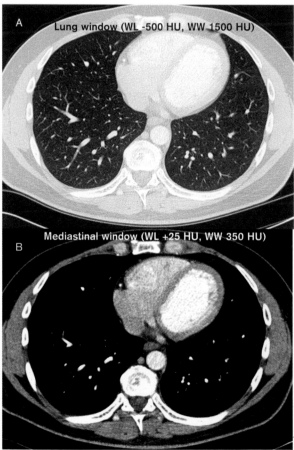

Figure 9. A) Lung and B) mediastinal windows on a CT thorax. WL = window length; WW = window width; HU = Houndsfield units.

- The window level (WL) and window width (WW) are selected around tissue of interest (Figure 9):

  a) lung windows at a WL of -500 HU and a WW of 1500 HU;
  b) mediastinal (soft tissue) windows at a WL of +25 HU and a WW of 350 HU.

- Contrast-enhanced scans are used when better delineation of vascular structures is required.

9 **What are the CT radiological features of constrictive pericarditis (Figure 10)?**

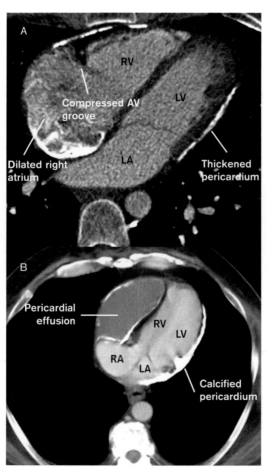

Figure 10. CT radiographical features of: A) constrictive pericarditis; and B) effusive constrictive pericarditis.

- Thickened pericardium (>4mm) with foci of calcification in 50% of patients, which most commonly occurs along the inferior diaphragmatic surface of the pericardium.
- Dilated superior and inferior venae cavae.
- Typically associated with obliteration of the pericardial space, except in cases of effusive constrictive pericarditis.

10 **What are the CT radiological features of traumatic aortic rupture (Figure 11)?**

- Aortic intimal flap.
- Contrast extravasation.
- Aortic pseudo-aneurysm.
- Peri-aortic or mediastinal haematoma.

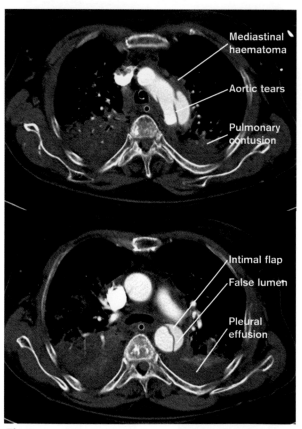

Figure 11. CT radiographical features of traumatic aortic rupture, demonstrated by aortic tears, mediastinal haematoma and a pleural effusion.

11 What are the CT radiological features of thoracic aortic aneurysms (Figures 12 and 13)?

- Dilated aortic lumen.
- Luminal thrombus.
- Atherosclerosis.

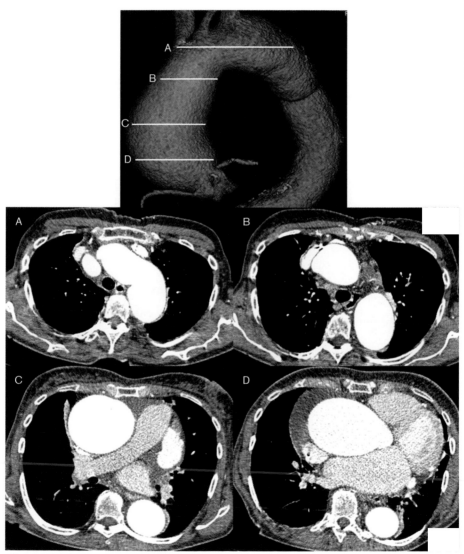

Figure 12. CT radiographical features of an ascending aortic aneurysm, demonstrated on a 3D reconstruction and serial axial images.

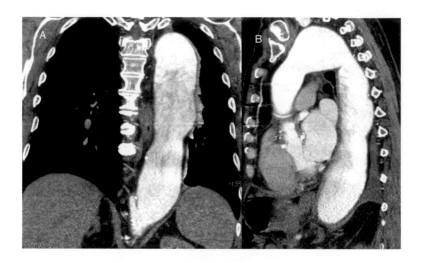

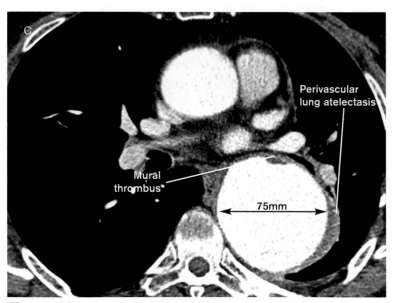

Figure 13. CT radiographical features of a descending aortic aneurysm, demonstrated by: A) coronal; B) sagittal; and C) axial images.

12 **What are the CT radiological features of thoracic aortic dissection (Figures 14, 15 and 16)?**

- Intimal flap.
- Peri-aortic haematoma.
- Left haemothorax (with Type B dissection).

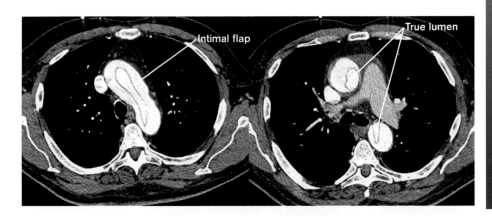

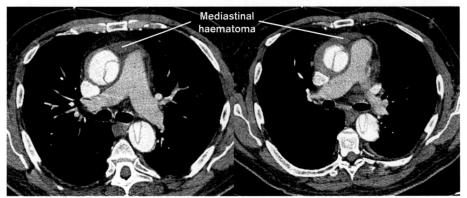

Figure 14. CT radiographical features of an acute Type A aortic dissection demonstrated on serial axial images with a mediastinal haematoma and an intimal flap separating the true and false lumens.

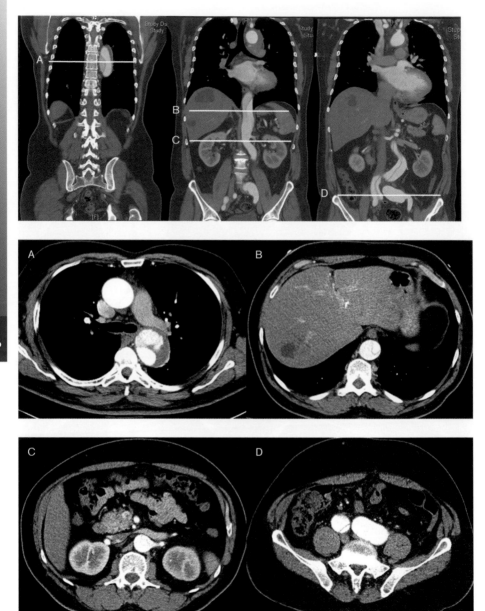

Figure 15. CT radiographical features of a Type B aortic dissection demonstrated on serial coronal and axial images.

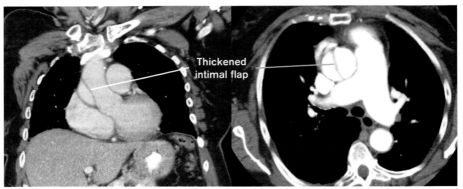

Figure 16. CT radiographical features of a chronic Type A aortic dissection demonstrated on coronal and axial images with a thickened intimal flap separating the true and false lumens.

13 What are the principles of magnetic resonance imaging (MRI)(Figure 17)?

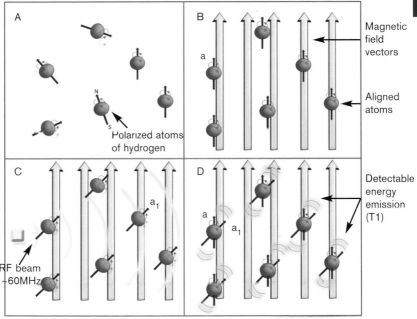

Figure 17. Principles of magnetic resonance imaging (MRI), demonstrated by: A) presence of polarized hydrogen ions in human tissue; B) alignment of the hydrogen ions by the magnetic field in a resting position (a); C) the hydrogen ions are shifted into an energized position (a1) following high-energy radiofrequency beam stimulation; D) once the beam is stopped, the hydrogen ions return to the resting position (a) and the emitted energy signal is detected by the MRI scanner.

- Normally, hydrogen atoms, which are the major component of water, spin in a random fashion.
- The magnet in the MRI scanner aligns these hydrogen atoms to spin in the same direction.
- Radio waves produced by the MRI scanner then cause the hydrogen atoms to produce signals which are detected, enabling three-dimensional images to be reconstructed.
- ECG gating allows cine images to be produced.

14 What are the indications for cardiac MRI?

- Thoracic aortic disease - for diagnosis and serial monitoring (no radiation) of aortic dissections and aneurysms (Figure 18).

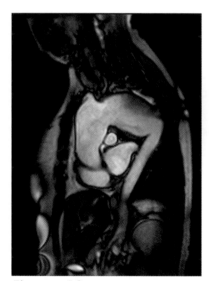 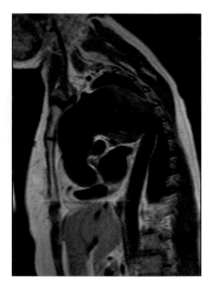

Figure 18. Sagittal magnetic resonance images demonstrating aneurysmal dilation of the ascending aorta and aortic arch.

- Ischaemic heart disease - to identify hibernating myocardium using resting, perfusion and dobutamine stress MRI.
- Cardiac tumours - to help delineate the location and spread of these lesions and thereby guide operative planning and therapeutic options.
- Constrictive pericarditis.
- Valvular and ventricular function - to quantify chamber and regurgitant volumes.

15 What are the contra-indications for MRI?

- Implanted pacemaker or defibrillator.
- Cochlear implant.
- Cerebral aneurysm clip.
- Occular metallic foreign body.
- Implanted medical device, such as a neural stimulator or drug infusion port.
- Metal shrapnel or bullet.
- Pregnant women.
- MRI is, however, safe with coronary stents, sternal wires, joint replacements and the majority of artificial heart valves.

16 What are the MRI features of viable myocardium (Figure 19)?

- Hibernating viable myocardium that is likely to recover following revascularisation can be recognised by:

   a) resting MR - end-diastolic wall thickness >6mm;

   b) contrast (gadolinium)-enhanced MR - delayed hyper-enhancement with <25% transmurality. If the delayed hyper-enhancement is >50% transmurality, it suggests that the left ventricle is unlikely to benefit from revascularisation. With 25-50% transmurality, further characterisation of viability is required by dobutamine stress MR;

   c) dobutamine stress MR - systolic wall thickening >2mm.

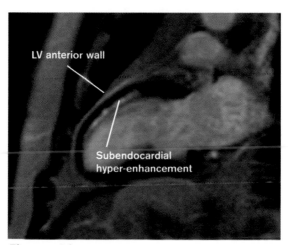

LV anterior wall

Subendocardial hyper-enhancement

Figure 19. Gadolinium-enhanced magnetic resonance imaging, demonstrating 50% transmural hyper-enhancement of the anterior left ventricular (LV) wall.

- Infarcted myocardium is characterized by the absence of living cells, with increased interstitial space between the collagen fibres. This allows accumulation of gadolinium during contrast-enhanced MRI, resulting in delayed hyper-enhancement.

17 What are the principles of positron emission tomography (PET)(Figure 20)?

- Decay of a radio-isotope causes emission of a positron (positively charged electron), which interacts with surrounding electrons to emit gamma rays that are detected by the gamma camera of the PET scanner.

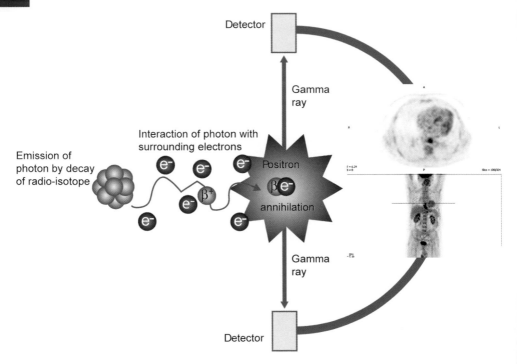

Figure 20. Principles of cardiac positron emission tomography.

- PET is better at detecting changes in physiology (metabolism) than anatomy, depicted by areas of greater uptake of the radioactive tracer (hot spot). In view of this, PET is often combined with CT as PET-CT, to identify the anatomical location of the hot spot.
- 18-fluorodeoxyglucose (^{18}FDG) is a radio-isotope marker commonly used as a surrogate of cellular metabolism, as following phosphorylation by hexokinase, ^{18}FDG becomes trapped within the cells.
- With particular respect to myocardial metabolism, during ischaemia, myocytes switch from free fatty acids to glucose as the predominant source of energy.

18 What are the indications for cardiac PET (Figure 21)?

- Myocardial perfusion - to risk stratify patients with critical coronary stenosis, using ^{13}N ammonia, ^{15}O water or ^{82}Rb (rubidium) as the radio-isotope.

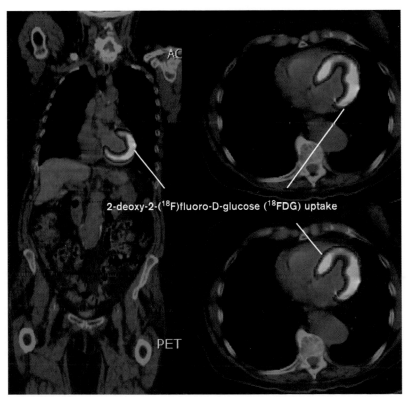

2-deoxy-2-(^{18}F)fluoro-D-glucose (^{18}FDG) uptake

Figure 21. Positron emission tomography, using ^{18}FDG uptake.

- Myocardial viability - to distinguish hibernating viable myocardium from infarcted non-viable tissue, using ^{18}FDG (metabolism) and ^{13}N ammonia (perfusion) as the radio-isotopes:

  a) hibernating myocardium is represented by normal metabolism and reduced perfusion (metabolism-perfusion mismatch);

  b) a myocardial scar (infarcted tissue) is represented by a matched reduction in metabolism and perfusion.

19 What are the principles of nuclear medicine scanning?

- Decay of radio-isotopes produces γ-rays. This is captured by external detectors, such as gamma cameras, to produce 2- or 3-dimensional images.
- Using these principles, cardiac nuclear medicine allows the assessment of:

  a) myocardial perfusion and viability;
  b) regional left ventricular contractility.

20 What are the principles of nuclear myocardial perfusion scanning (Figure 22)?

- Myocardial perfusion scanning uses the radio-isotope Thallium-201 (^{201}Th) at rest and under stress, to assess the functional importance of coronary artery disease. It is more sensitive and specific than exercise ECG at identifying coronary artery disease.
- As a potassium analogue, which is actively transported into cells via the Na-K ATPase pump, uptake of ^{201}Th into the cells is directly proportional to regional myocardial blood flow. The ^{201}Th remains in the myocyte whilst the metabolic function of the cell remains intact.
- The initial injection of ^{201}Th represents myocardial blood flow whereas re-injection of the radionucleotide marker allows assessment of redistribution, a phenomenon associated with the deranged cellular metabolism of hibernating myocardium.

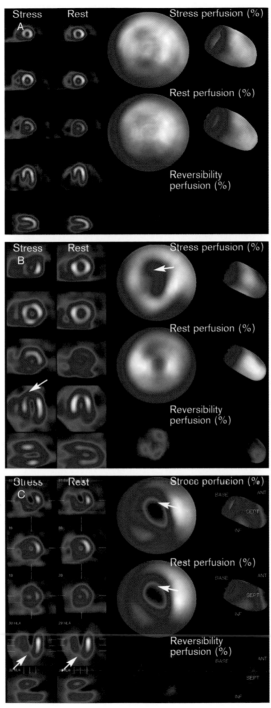

Figure 22. Myocardial perfusion scanning using Thallium-201 during stress (dobutamine 5µg/kg/min) and rest demonstrating: A) normal myocardium; B) inducible antero-apical ischaemia with a perfusion defect on the stress images (arrows) and restored perfusion on the rest images; and C) full-thickness antero-apical myocardial infarction with a fixed defect (arrows) on both the stress and rest images.

- Myocardial perfusion images are performed at rest and during stress (dobutamine, dipyridamole, adenosine or exercise) and can demonstrate a number of different conditions:

  a) normal myocardium, which is represented by normal uptake both in rest and stress images;

  b) reversible ischaemia, which is represented by a defect in the stress image that normalises after rest;

  c) a chronic scar (infarcted myocardium), which is represented by a 'fixed' defect that remains unchanged in both rest and stress images;

  d) hibernating viable myocardium, which is represented by a 'fixed' defect (in both rest and stress images) that improves on delayed imaging.

21 What are the principles of multi-gated acquisition (MUGA) scanning (Figure 23)?

- MUGA scans use the principles of cardiac nuclear medicine to provide a more accurate and reproducible cine assessment of left ventricular contractility than echocardiography.

- Following intravenous injection of a radioactive material, such as technetium-99 (^{99}Tc), which radio-labels red blood cells, gamma images are acquired, 'gated' to the patient's cardiac cycle.

- Regional wall motion abnormalities (hypokinesia, dyskinesia or akinesia) can be detected at rest and under stress (using adenosine or exercise).

- Reduced emission of gamma rays at rest usually indicate a ventricular scar following myocardial infarction, whereas defects observed during stress are indicative of areas of ischaemia.

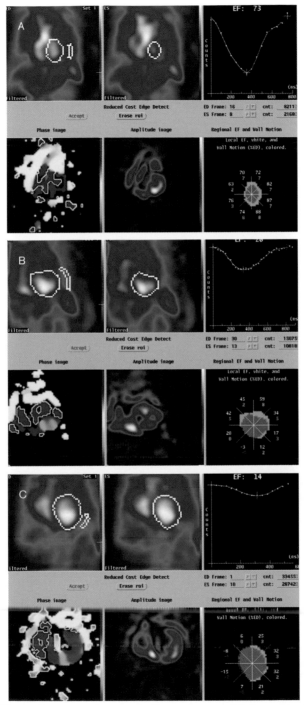

Figure 23. MUGA scan demonstrating: A) normal left ventricular function (EF 73%); B) impaired left ventricular function (EF 28%) with septal and lateral hypokinesia; and C) poor left ventricular function (EF 14%) with global hypokinesia / akinesia. EF = ejection fraction.

22 What is single photon emission computed tomography (SPECT) (Figure 24)?

- SPECT combines conventional nuclear medical techniques with 3D images provided by computed tomography. A gamma camera is rotated around the patient to allow reconstructions to determine the anatomical location of differential radionucleotide, such as 99-technetium (^{99}Tc), uptake.

- SPECT is similar to PET-CT in combining anatomical and physiological imaging but differs in that SPECT detects gamma rays directly emitted from the radionucleotide material, whereas PET detects the gamma rays produced when emitted positrons interact with surrounding electrons.

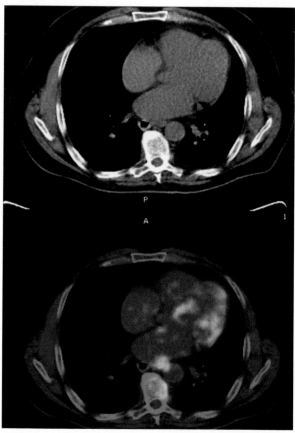

Figure 24. SPECT scan combining nuclear medicine imaging with computed tomography.

Recommended reading

1.   Kim RJ, Wu E, Rafael A, Chen EL, Parker MA, Simonetti O, Klocke FJ, Bonow RO, Judd RM. The use of contrast-enhanced magnetic resonance imaging to identify reversible myocardial dysfunction. *N Engl J Med* 2000; 343(20): 1445-53.

2.   Weinsaft JW, Klem I, Judd RM. MRI for the assessment of myocardial viability. *Cardiol Clin* 2007; 25(1): 35-56.

3.   Camici PG, Prasad SK, Rimoldi OE. Stunning, hibernation, and assessment of myocardial viability. *Circulation* 2008; 117(1): 103-14.

4.   Bengel FM, Higuchi T, Javadi MS, Lautamäki R. Cardiac positron emission tomography. *J Am Coll Cardiol* 2009; 54(1): 1-15.

Chapter 8

Cardiopulmonary bypass

1 **What are the aims of cardiopulmonary bypass (CPB)?**
- The principal aim of cardiopulmonary bypass is to facilitate cardiac and thoracic aortic procedures by excluding the heart and lungs from the circulation, whilst providing:

  a) adequate gas exchange;
  b) systemic organ perfusion;
  c) a means of controlling body temperature;
  d) salvage and safe re-transfusion of blood from the surgical field.

- As well as for cardiac surgical procedures, cardiopulmonary bypass is also used for:

  a) pulmonary embolectomy;
  b) resection of certain hepatic lesions, intracranial masses and abdominal tumours with cavo-atrial spread.

2 **Describe a cardiopulmonary bypass circuit (Figure 1)**
- Venous cannula in the right atrium, inferior and superior venae cavae or the femoral vein.
- Venous line - usually ½-inch heparin-coated tubing.
- Venous reservoir - usually a rigid high capacitance reservoir.
- Centrifugal or roller pump.
- Heat exchanger.
- Oxygenator - usually a hollow-fibre membrane oxygenator.
- Arterial filter and bubble trap.
- Arterial line - usually 3/8-inch heparin coated tubing.
- Arterial cannula - usually in the ascending aorta, femoral artery or axillary artery.
- Most bypass circuits come as sterile, pre-prepared packs, where dry and wet assembly take about 10 to 15 minutes each and the circuits can be kept on standby for up to 8 hours (wet) or 7 days (dry).

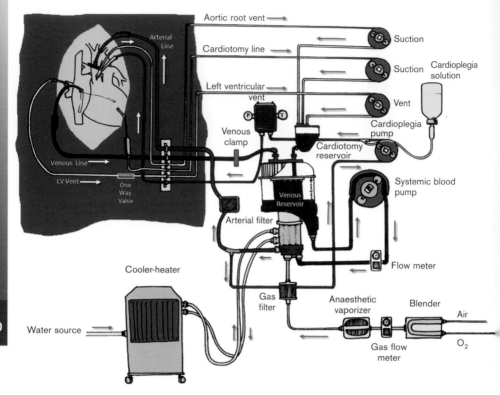

Figure 1. Cardiopulmonary bypass circuit. LV = left ventricle; P = pressure gauge; T = temperature gauge; O_2 = oxygen.

3 **Describe the principles of venous drainage (Figure 2)**
● There are several different methods of achieving venous drainage from the right atrium:

a) Ross basket, which is a perforated metal basket that lies within the right atrium, thereby avoiding any contact and potential damage with the inferior vena cava;

b) two-stage single venous cannula (34-42Fr), which is placed via the right atrial appendage and is thought to provide better venous drainage than the Ross basket, as it has openings that lie within the inferior vena cava and the body of the right atrium;

c) bicaval cannulation (24-32Fr in the superior vena cava and 28-36Fr in the inferior vena cava), either via the right atrium or directly into the cavae, with snares around the cannulas. It prevents kinking of the superior vena cava and air entrainment during mitral and tricuspid valve surgery, if a single two-stage cannula alone were used;

d) femoral venous cannula, which is placed into the right atrium under transoesophageal guidance and commonly used for minimal access cardiac surgery.

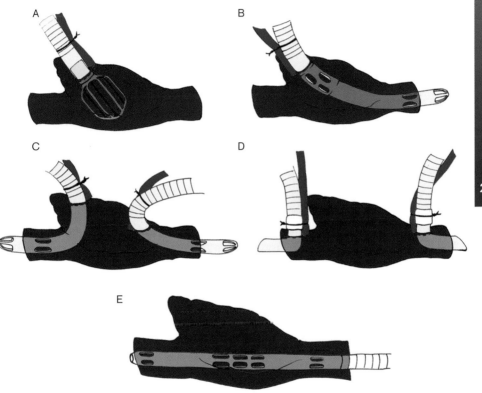

Figure 2. Venous drainage. A) Ross basket. B) Two-stage venous cannula with drainage holes in the right atrium and inferior vena cava. C) Bicaval venous drainage with cannulae passing via the right atrium. D) Bicaval venous drainage with cannulae placed directly into the inferior and superior venae cavae. E) Femoral venous cannula with drainage holes in the inferior vena cava, right atrium and superior vena cava.

- Blood leaves the right atrium using the siphon effect by gravity as the venous reservoir is 40-70cm below the level of the heart.
- The rate at which blood drains from the right atrium is determined by the:

  a) central venous pressure;
  b) height differential between the right atrium and the venous reservoir;
  c) resistance in the bypass circuit (cannulae, tubing and connectors) between the right atrium and the reservoir;
  d) absence or presence of air within the tubing.

- Venous 'chattering' is usually caused by inadequate circulating volume or an excessive siphon effect, where the venous drainage is occurring at a rate faster than the return of blood to the right atrium. It is treated by adding volume to the circuit, reducing the height differential between the right atrium and the venous reservoir or partially clamping the venous line.
- Caval snares should be released when delivering antegrade cardioplegia to ensure adequate drainage of the coronary sinus return into the right atrium.
- Complications of venous cannulation include atrial arrhythmias, atrial or caval tears and subsequent bleeding, air embolisation, catheter malposition and unexpected decannulation.

4   Describe the tubing used in cardiopulmonary bypass circuits

- Medical grade polyvinyl chloride (PVC) tubing of varying diameters is usually used as it is:

  a) flexible but resistant to kinking and collapse;
  b) non-toxic and compatible with blood;
  c) smooth, transparent and non-wettable;
  d) suitable for heat sterilisation.

- Although the tubing is heparin-bonded to reduce the inflammatory response, systemic heparinisation is still required.
- The tubing is usually connected by fluted polycarbonate connectors.
- Flow dynamics can be optimised by using wide tubing with minimal areas of turbulence. This, however, has to be balanced with the need to reduce the prime volume which is achieved with a short circuit with narrow tubing.

5 **Describe the principles of venous reservoirs (Figure 3)**

- The venous reservoir acts as:

    a) a high capacitance chamber for receiving venous return;
    b) a venous bubble trap;
    c) access to add drugs, fluids, or blood;
    d) storage for the circulating volume during deep hypothermic circulatory arrest.

- There are two main types of venous reservoir:

    a) open reservoirs (rigid, hard plastic canisters), which have a large capacity for storage of circulating volume, allow vacuum-assisted venous drainage, are easier to prime, are less expensive, can incorporate filters and allow for volume measurements and management of venous air;

A   B

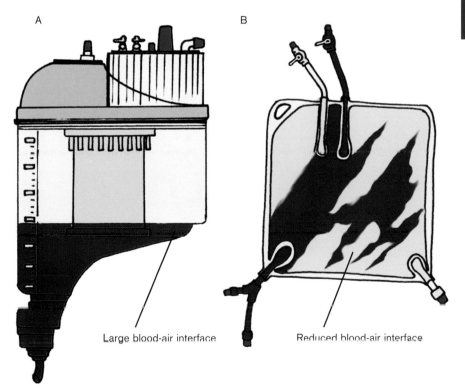

Large blood-air interface   Reduced blood-air interface

Figure 3. Venous reservoirs. **A)** Open hard reservoir. **B)** Closed soft reservoir.

b) closed reservoirs (collapsible, soft plastic bags), which are less versatile but by eliminating the blood-gas interface, are able to reduce the systemic inflammatory response and the risk of producing gas micro-emboli.

6 What are the different oxygenators available (Figure 4)?

- There are two different types of oxygenators available for use with cardiopulmonary bypass circuits:

a) membrane oxygenators, which contain sheaves of hollow fibres (120-200µm) with 0.3-0.8µm pores. They are thought to produce less particulate and gaseous micro-emboli, are less reactive to blood elements, and allow superior control of blood gases;

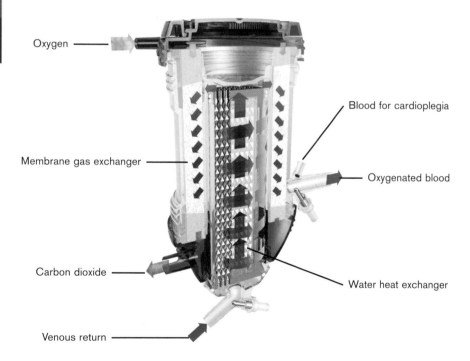

Oxygen

Blood for cardioplegia

Membrane gas exchanger

Oxygenated blood

Carbon dioxide

Water heat exchanger

Venous return

Figure 4. Combined membrane oxygenator and heat exchanger unit. Venous blood flows into the unit via the lower port. As the blood ascends, circulating water within the heat exchanger allows the temperature of the blood to be controlled. It is then oxygenated by the membrane gas exchanger, using oxygen that is infused from the upper gas port. Oxygenated blood, which has been warmed or cooled, then exits via the side port as arterial return or to be mixed with cardioplegia. *Reproduced with permission from Eurosets Medical Devices.*

b)   bubble oxygenators, which although are cheaper, produce more gaseous micro-emboli and therefore are rarely used in the Western World.

- The oxygenator also contains a flow regulator, flow meter, gas blender, oxygen analyzer, gas filter and moisture trap.
- The arterial $PaCO_2$ is controlled by gas flow, and PaO_2 by the FiO_2.

7 Describe the principles of heat exchangers

- A heat exchanger allows control of body temperature by heating and cooling blood passing through the cardiopulmonary bypass circuit.
- The heat exchanger is usually located prior to the oxygenator in the bypass circuit. This reduces the risk of producing gaseous emboli, which may occur when blood is warmed, as gases are less soluble at a higher temperature.
- The warming gradient, between the inflowing water and blood, is limited to 5°C-10°C to reduce the risk of bubble emboli.
- The blood is not heated above 40°C to reduce the risk of plasma protein denaturation.
- Blood can be cooled at approximately 1°C per minute and re-warmed at approximately 0.5°C per minute. The temperature changes more rapidly initially followed by a slower change in temperature, due to the exponential nature of the heating and cooling curves.
- Heat exchanger failure is very uncommon but may result in leakage of water into the bloodstream and subsequent haemolysis and haemoglobinuria.

8 What are the different cardiopulmonary bypass pumps available (Figure 5)?

- Roller pumps produce flow by compression of the heparin-coated bypass tubing using two rollers 180° apart. The flow rate is determined by the:

  a)   rate of rotation of the rollers;
  b)   degree of compression;
  c)   length and diameter of the tubing being compressed.

- Centrifugal pumps produce flow by using a rotating impeller. The flow rate is determined by the:

  a)   speed of rotation of the impeller;
  b)   afterload within the circuit, distal to the pump.

A   B

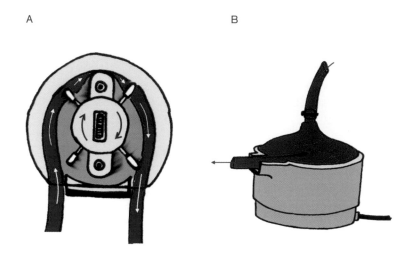

Figure 5. Cardiopulmonary bypass pumps. A) Roller pump. B) Centrifugal pump.

Table 1. Advantages and disadvantages of roller and centrifugal cardiopulmonary bypass pumps.

	Roller pumps	Centrifugal pumps
Occlusive	Nearly occlusive	Non-occlusive
Afterload dependence	Afterload independent	Afterload sensitive
Prime volume	Low	High
Cost	Low	High
Potential for pulsatile flow	Yes	No
Potential for backflow	No	Yes
Potential for massive air embolism	Yes	No
Blood trauma and haemolysis	Yes	Low
Risk of spallation and tubing rupture	Yes	Low

- Complications of cardiopulmonary bypass pumps include a runaway pump (inability to control the pump speed), flow meter damage, electrical damage and tubing rupture (with roller pumps).

9 **What filters are available within the cardiopulmonary bypass circuit?**

- Arterial line filters (40μm), which are used to reduce the cerebral embolic load.
- Leucocyte depleting filters, which remove activated neutrophils and therefore may reduce the systemic inflammatory response associated with cardiopulmonary bypass.
- Ultrafiltration and modified ultrafiltration, which remove excess fluid in patients with renal impairment and can be used to increase haematocrit levels. Cytokines generated by the systemic inflammatory response are also cleared by ultrafiltration and may have a beneficial effect by limiting subsequent tissue and end-organ injury.

10 **What are the sources of cerebral emboli during cardiopulmonary bypass?**

- Gas emboli sources include:

  a)   vents;
  b)   cardiotomy reservoir (especially with low volumes);
  c)   loose purse-string sutures (especially during augmented venous return);
  d)   priming procedures and intravenous fluids;
  e)   stopcocks, sampling and injection sites;
  f)   breaks in the perfusion circuit;
  g)   rapid warming of cold blood;
  h)   cavitation;
  i)   oxygenators;
  j)   heart and great vessels (following open heart surgery).

- Particulate emboli sources include:

  a)   thrombus formation or haemolysed red cells;
  b)   denatured proteins and cellular debris;
  c)   stored donor blood;
  d)   aortic atherosclerotic and calcific debris;
  e)   muscle, bone, fat, suture material, wax or glue aspirated via the cardiotomy suckers.

- These emboli can be detected by transcranial Doppler ultrasound or fluorescein retinal angiography.
- As the cerebral vessels are immediately upstream of the heart and the aortic cannulation site, the brain is at the greatest risk of micro-embolic injury.

11 Describe the principles of arterial cannulation

- Arterial cannulation is usually performed at the distal ascending aortic aorta.
- An epi-aortic probe should be used to detect atherosclerotic plaques, as it is more sensitive than digital palpation or trans-oesophageal echocardiography (which has a blind spot at the distal ascending aorta).
- Complications include bleeding, aortic tears, aortic dissection, air embolisation, atherosclerotic plaque disruption and embolisation, aortic back wall injury, and malposition of the cannula tip (towards the aortic valve, against the aortic wall, or in an arch vessel) (Figure 6).
- Alternative sites of cannulation include the aortic arch, innominate artery, subclavian artery, axillary artery, femoral artery and the left ventricular apex.

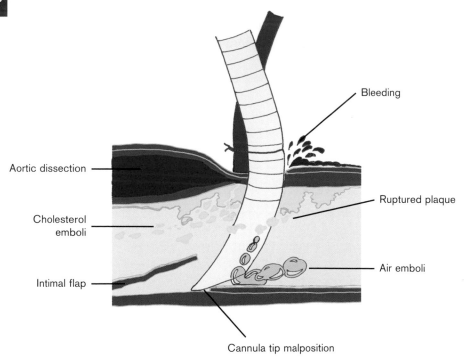

Figure 6. Complications of arterial cannulation.

● Cannulation of the femoral artery may, however, lead to:

a) limb ischaemia;
b) damage to nearby neurovascular structures;
c) disruption of debris secondary to retrograde flow;
d) organ malperfusion due to flow through the false lumen in patients with aortic dissection;
e) lower cardiopulmonary bypass flow rates, secondary to smaller calibre vessels;
f) retroperitoneal haemorrhage;
g) femoral artery stenosis or thrombosis.

12 What are the sources of blood returning to the heart during cardiopulmonary bypass?

● Right heart - from the coronary sinus, Thebesian veins and venae cavae.
● Left heart - from the aortic root (if aortic regurgitation is present) and the bronchial veins.
● Congenital anomalies - from an atrial or ventricular septal defect, patent ductus arteriosus, persistent left superior vena cava or anomalous pulmonary venous drainage.

13 Describe the principles behind venting of the heart (Figure 7)

● When the heart is not contracting, blood returning to the heart during cardiopulmonary bypass (see above) may cause:

a) cardiac rewarming;
b) ventricular distension. This may result in myofibrillar disruption and subsequent myocardial dysfunction following release of the aortic cross-clamp.

● In view of this, venting of the left ventricle is performed using a cannula in the:

a) aortic root;
b) directly through the aortic valve;
c) right superior pulmonary vein;
d) left ventricular apex;
e) main pulmonary artery.

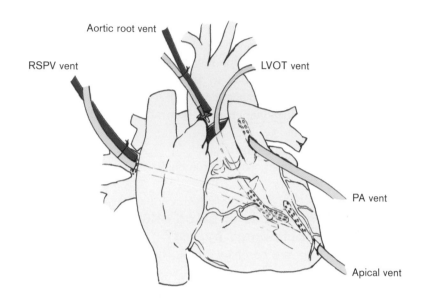

Aortic root vent

RSPV vent

LVOT vent

PA vent

Apical vent

Figure 7. Venting of the left ventricle. LVOT = left ventricular outflow tract; RSPV = right superior pulmonary vein; PA = pulmonary artery.

14 What safety devices are present on the cardiopulmonary bypass machine and circuit?

- Alarms with a cardiopulmonary bypass pump cut-off include:

  a) low venous reservoir blood level;
  b) high arterial line pressure;
  c) macrobubble detector.

- Arterial line filter.
- Back-up electrical generator supply, arterial pump head and heater-cooler device.
- One-way valved intracardiac vent lines.
- Back-up oxygen supply with filter.

15 Describe the typical constituents of priming solution

- Adult circuits require 1.5-2L of balanced electrolyte solution. Examples include:

  a) 1000mL Hartmann's solution;
  b) 500mL gelofusin;
  c) 250mL (12.5-50g) mannitol, which increases postoperative diuresis and has been shown to reduce the incidence of postoperative renal dysfunction;
  d) 10,000 U heparin;
  e) blood when the haemoglobin levels are <10g/dL.

- Before the bypass circuit is connected to the patient, the prime volume is recirculated through a micropore filter to remove any particulate debris.
- The prime volume is reduced by using as short, narrow-bore bypass tubing as possible, to decrease the haemodilution effect of the prime volume and need for blood transfusion.

16 What is the optimal haematocrit during cardiopulmonary bypass?

- The optimal haematocrit whilst on bypass is determined by the balance between using higher levels which increase oxygen delivery versus lower levels which reduce the blood viscosity and the risk of haemolysis.
- Ideally, haematocrit levels are similar to the temperature in °C, with lower levels required as the metabolic requirements are lower and the viscosity increases with hypothermia.
- As the prime volume of standard cardiopulmonary bypass circuits is approximately one third of the circulating blood volume, haemodilution occurs with a corresponding fall in the haematocrit level:

$$\text{CPB haematocrit} = \frac{\text{Blood volume}}{\text{Blood volume + prime volume}} \times \text{pre-CPB haematocrit}$$

- Oxygen delivery to the tissues during cardiopulmonary bypass can be controlled by three main factors:

  a) haematocrit;
  b) inspired oxygen concentration;
  c) cardiopulmonary bypass pump flow rate.

O_2 delivery = 10 x pump flow(L/min) x [1.34 x Hb(g/dL) x SaO_2 (%)] + [0.003 x PaO_2(mmHg)].

- The mixed venous oxygen saturations can be used to determine whether oxygen delivery is adequate and if <60%, either blood should be transfused or pump flows increased.
- Haematocrit levels are approximately three times greater than haemoglobin levels.

17 What anticoagulation regimes are used for cardiopulmonary bypass?

- The standard dose of heparin for cardiopulmonary bypass is 300-400 units (3-4mg) per kg, given intravenously; 2mg/kg is utilised for minimal extracorporeal circulation (MECC).
- After 3-4 minutes, the activated clotting time (ACT) is measured. Pump suckers can be turned on when the ACT is >400s and cardiopulmonary bypass initiated when the ACT is >480s.
- The ACT is measured every 30 minutes whilst on cardiopulmonary bypass and additional heparin boluses (5000-10,000 U) are given to maintain the ACT >480s.
- If the ACT fails to reach 480s, additional heparin should be given up to 500 U per kg. At this stage, antithrombin III deficiency should be considered, especially if the patient was receiving heparin pre-operatively, and fresh frozen plasma or recombinant antithrombin should be administered to overcome heparin resistance.
- Antithrombin is a necessary cofactor that binds circulating thrombin and heparin accelerates this reaction a thousand-fold.
- Direct thrombin inhibitors (such as argatroban, bivalirudin) may be needed if the patient is allergic or resistant to heparin. Reversal of these agents is, however, difficult.

18 What parameters are monitored during cardiopulmonary bypass?

- Patient parameters:

    a) electrocardiogram (ECG);
    b) arterial blood pressure (BP);
    c) central venous pressure (CVP);
    d) arterial oxygen saturations (SaO_2);
    e) end-tidal carbon dioxide ($ETCO_2$);
    f) peripheral and core temperature;
    g) urine output;
    h) arterial blood gases - including pH, PaO_2, $PaCO_2$, bicarbonate, lactate, base excess, potassium, glucose.

- Cardiopulmonary bypass pump parameters:

  a) blood flow rate;
  b) centrifugal or roller pump speed;
  c) arterial line pressure;
  d) arterial and venous line oxygen saturations;
  e) delivered oxygen concentration;
  f) gas flow;
  g) temperature of the pump blood;
  h) temperature of water in the heat exchanger.

19 **What is the optimal flow rate on cardiopulmonary bypass?**
- Cardiopulmonary bypass flow rates are calculated to achieve a cardiac index of 2.4L/min/m^2 at 37°C (hence 4.8L/min for an average patient with a BSA of 2m^2).
- For each 1°C reduction in temperature, the flow rate can be reduced by 7%.
- Once the optimal flow rate has been achieved, the mean arterial pressure is maintained between 55-65mmHg with the aid of vasodilators and vasoconstrictors.
- For patients with hypertension, carotid artery stenosis and renal disease, and the elderly, the mean arterial pressure needs to be maintained at a higher level, between 65-75mmHg.

20 **How is body surface area calculated?**
- Body surface area (BSA) can be calculated using the formula:

  BSA (m^2) = ([Height(cm) x Weight(kg)] / 3600)$^{1/2}$

21 **Describe the principles of anticoagulation reversal following separation of cardiopulmonary bypass**
- Protamine is a cation (derived from salmon sperm) that binds with the anion, heparin, to form stable heparin-protamine complexes.
- Protamine contains two active sites, one for neutralising heparin and one which has mild anticoagulant effects.
- For each 1mg (100U) of heparin administered initially, 1mg of protamine (maximum 3mg/kg) should be injected intravenously to reverse the anticoagulant effect.
- Heparin rebound may occur once all of the protamine is bound by circulating heparin and further tissue heparin is released maintaining

the anticoagulant effect. In this situation, a further dose of protamine (50mg) may be required.

- Once the protamine infusion has commenced, the pump suckers should be turned off.
- Protamine should be given as a slow infusion over 15 minutes to reduce the risk of protamine reactions (see below).

22 Describe the Horrow classification of protamine reactions

- Class I: hypotension caused by rapid administration of protamine. This is triggered by histamine release and can usually be treated by fluid resuscitation and vasopressors.
- Class II: anaphylactic reaction:

  a) IIa (true anaphylaxis) - hypotension, bronchospasm and angioedema, mediated by anti-protamine immunogolublin E antibody, histamine, prostaglandins and kinins. It occurs in diabetics (on protamine-zinc insulin), patients with fish allergies and those who have been exposed to protamine previously. It should be treated by immediately stopping the protamine, and administering 10mL 1:100,000 IV adrenaline, 100mg IV hydrocortisone, 10mg IV chlorphenamine (Piriton®), 100% O_2 and nebulised bronchodilators;

  b) IIb (immediate anaphylactoid) and IIc (delayed anaphylactoid) reactions are similar but less severe and are mediated by the complement pathway.

- Class III: catastrophic pulmonary vasoconstriction is caused by complement activation and the release of thromboxane A2. This results in right ventricular failure, circulatory shock and severe bronchospasm. The treatment includes immediately stopping the protamine and administering 10mL 1:100,000 IV adrenaline, milrinone, and re-institution of cardiopulmonary bypass.

23 What are the complications of cardiopulmonary bypass?

- Systemic inflammatory response induced by the contact of blood with the foreign surface of the cardiopulmonary bypass circuit, activating cytokine, kallikrein, coagulation and complement cascades. This often results in increased capillary permeability, interstitial oedema and subsequent organ dysfunction.

- Coagulopathy caused by platelet dysfunction, as well as dilution and consumption of coagulation factors and platelets.
- Haemolysis.
- Renal and splanchnic hypoperfusion.
- Cerebrovascular accident, caused by gas and particulate emboli (see earlier) and cerebral hypoperfusion.
- It has been suggested that membrane oxygenators, heparin-coated circuits, centrifugal pumps, intra-operative steroids and leucocyte depleting filters may reduce the systemic inflammatory response.

24 Describe the principles of minimal extracorporeal circulation (MECC) (Figure 8)

- In comparison to standard cardiopulmonary bypass, the principal aims of MECC are to:

  a) reduce the systemic inflammatory response by removing the venous reservoir and cardiotomy suckers, thereby reducing the blood-air interface that triggers the inflammatory cascades;

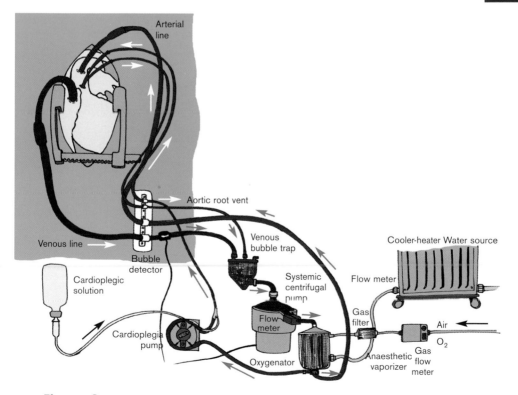

Figure 8. Minimal extracorporeal circulation (MECC) cardiopulmonary bypass circuit. O_2 = oxygen.

b) minimise haemodilution associated with cardiopulmonary bypass by reducing the prime volume by retrograde and antegrade autologous priming, where the crystalloid priming solution is 'displaced' out of the cardiopulmonary bypass circuit by the patient's own blood both in the arterial and venous lines just before the commencement of cardiopulmonary bypass.

25 Describe the principles of venous drainage in a patient with a persistent left superior vena cava (PLSVC) (Figure 9)

- When present, a PLSVC drains blood from the left subclavian and internal jugular veins via the coronary sinus into the right atrium (90%) or directly into the left atrium (10%).

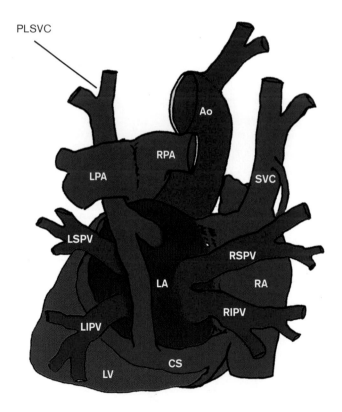

Figure 9. Persistent left superior vena cava (PLSVC). Posterior view of the heart with the PLSVC draining into the coronary sinus (CS) or the left atrium (LA). LPA = left pulmonary artery; RPA = right pulmonary artery; Ao = aorta; SVC = superior vena cava; LSPV = left superior pulmonary vein; RSPV = right superior pulmonary vein; LIPV = left inferior pulmonary vein; RIPV = right inferior pulmonary vein; RA = right atrium; LV = left ventricle.

- PLSVC occurs in 0.3-0.5% of patients and should be suspected if:

  a) the left innominate vein is small or absent;
  b) the coronary sinus is large;
  c) the right superior vena cava is small or absent.

- When undertaking cardiopulmonary bypass in the presence of a PLSVC:

  a) a single two-stage cannula can be used if the right side of the heart is not opened;
  b) if bicaval cannulation is required and a right superior vena cava is present, then the PLSVC can be snared;
  c) if bicaval cannulation is required and a right connecting innominate vein is absent, an additional coronary sinus cannula is required to prevent right atrial distension and congestion of the left cerebral hemishpere;
  d) there is systemic desaturation due to right to left shunt in cases of PLSVC to LA.

Recommended reading

1. Horrow JC. Protamine: a review of its toxicity. *Anesth Analg* 1985; 64(3): 348-61.

2. Balasundaram S, al-Halees Z, Duran CG. Persistent left superior vena cava: a simple technique for adequate drainage during cardiopulmonary bypass. *J Cardiovasc Surg (Torino)* 1991; 32(1): 59-61.

3. Murphy GS, Hessel EA 2nd, Groom RC. Optimal perfusion during cardiopulmonary bypass: an evidence-based approach. *Anesth Analg* 2009; 108(5): 1394-417.

4. Remadi JP, Rakotoarivelo Z, Marticho P, Benamar A. Prospective randomized study comparing coronary artery bypass grafting with the new mini-extracorporeal circulation Jostra System or with a standard cardiopulmonary bypass. *Am Heart J* 2006; 151(1): 198.

5. Mazzei V, Nasso G, Salamone G, Castorino F, Tommasini A, Anselmi A. Prospective randomized comparison of coronary bypass grafting with minimal extracorporeal circulation system (MECC) versus off-pump coronary surgery. *Circulation* 2007; 110(16). 1761-7.

Chapter 9

Cardiopulmonary bypass scenarios

1 **What are the important considerations when commencing cardiopulmonary bypass?**

- Cardiopulmonary bypass begins by progressively increasing the venous return to the bypass machine, whilst gradually increasing the arterial flow. At this stage, it is important to monitor several different haemodynamic parameters:

  a) decompression of the heart;
  b) venous drainage;
  c) arterial line pressures;
  d) systemic arterial and venous pressures;
  e) arterial blood oxygen concentration;
  f) venous reservoir levels.

- Once bypass has been established for 2 minutes and the above haemodynamic factors are stable, lung ventilation can be discontinued, systemic cooling commenced and the aortic cross-clamp applied, as appropriate.

2 **What are the causes of failure of the heart to arrest with antegrade cardioplegia?**

- Aortic regurgitation (check for left ventricular distension).
- Aortic cross-clamp not applied completely across the aorta.
- High-grade proximal coronary artery stenosis.
- Low potassium concentration in the cardioplegia solution.
- Poor flow through the cardioplegia line caused by kinking, clamping or the cannula trapped in the aortic cross-clamp.

3   **What are the common causes of poor venous return or an empty venous reservoir?**
- Systemic vasodilation.
- Volume loss from:

  a)   bleeding;
  b)   pooling of blood in either pleural cavity;
  c)   iatrogenic aortic dissection.

- Inadequate venous drainage, caused by:

  a)   a kinked or clamped venous line;
  b)   venous airlock;
  c)   venous cannula malposition;
  d)   obstruction to flow by caval snares;
  e)   an inferior vena caval tear caused during venous cannulation;
  f)   an inadequate height differential between the right atrium and the venous reservoir.

4   **What are the main principles for managing a large inferior vena cava (IVC) tear caused during venous cannulation?**
- Carefully advance the venous cannula into the IVC beyond the tear to obtain venous drainage along with cardiotomy suction return.
- Use a supplemental purse string to secure the venous cannula.
- Cool the patient to 18°C.
- During circulatory arrest, the IVC can be repaired by direct suture or using a bovine pericardial patch.

5   **What are the main principles of managing a massive airlock in the venous line?**
- Stop the cardiopulmonary bypass pump.
- Separate the venous cannula from the venous line.
- Manually fill the venous line with saline.
- Reconnect the venous cannula to the venous line.
- If there is a small to moderate amount of air, it can be 'chased' back into the reservoir by progressively lifting the venous line.

6   **What are the causes of raised central venous pressure whilst on cardiopulmonary bypass?**

- Poor venous drainage.
- Central venous catheter snared or abutting the superior vena cava (SVC) cannula.
- Lifted and rotated heart (e.g. when accessing the circumflex vessels during coronary artery bypass grafting).

7   **What are the main principles in managing massive arterial air embolism during cardiopulmonary bypass?**

- Stop the cardiopulmonary bypass pump and clamp both the arterial and venous lines.
- Place the patient in a steep Trendelenburg position.
- Remove the arterial cannula and aspirate any air at the site of entry.
- Remove the venous cannula.
- Place the arterial cannula via the right atrium into the superior vena cava with a snare.
- Commence temporary retrograde cerebral perfusion at 400-500mL/min for approximately 3 minutes to de-air, until bubbles stop coming out of the aorta.
- Concomitantly, mannitol and dexamethasone are given intravenously with ice packs placed around the head to aid cerebral protection.
- Antegrade circulation is then recommenced with deep hypothermia (18-20°C) for 30 minutes to increase the solubility of air.
- The perfusion pressures are kept relatively high at 70-80mmHg and 100% inspired oxygen concentration (FiO_2).
- Using transoesophageal echocardiography guidance, any residual air in the cardiac chambers and great vessels is removed.
- To de-air the vertebral arteries, intermittent occlusion of the carotid arteries is performed.
- Any sources of air ingress are also identified and corrected, including stopcocks, loose arterial connections, left ventricular vent catheters, oxygenator membrane leaks, an empty venous reservoir, loose purse-string sutures and cardioplegia infusion catheters.

8   **What are the causes of hypoxia whilst on cardiopulmonary bypass?**
- Low cardiopulmonary bypass pump flow rate.
- Low inspired oxygen concentration (FiO_2) delivered to the circuit.
- Failure of the cardiopulmonary bypass pump oxygenator.

9   **What are the main principles of managing an arterial cannula that falls out during cardiopulmonary bypass?**
- Stop the cardiopulmonary bypass pump.
- Clamp the venous line.
- Flush the arterial line with forward flow from the pump.
- Replace the arterial cannula.
- Reconnect the arterial line and the arterial cannula, ensuring the absence of air bubbles.

10 **What are the causes of a high arterial line pressure?**
- Arterial cannula abutting the arterial wall or a plaque on the arterial wall.
- Iatrogenic aortic dissection.
- Selective cannulation of an aortic arch vessel.
- Normal arterial line pressures are approximately 300mmHg.

11 **What are the causes of hypotension whilst on cardiopulmonary bypass?**
- Low cardiopulmonary bypass flow rate.
- Damped arterial line trace.
- Low systemic vascular resistance, secondary to:

    a)   sepsis;
    b)   pre-operative vasodilators;
    c)   cytokines returned to the circulation via the cardiotomy suckers from pooled blood in the pleural cavity.

- Kinked or clamped arterial cannula.
- Iatrogenic aortic dissection.
- Selective cannulation of the aortic arch vessels.

12 What are the causes of hypertension on cardiopulmonary bypass?

- High cardiopulmonary bypass pump flow rate.
- Selective cannulation of the brachiocephalic artery (with a right radial arterial line).
- Increased systemic vascular resistance (vasoconstriction), secondary to:

  a)   vasopressors;
  b)   hypothermia;
  c)   inadequate anaesthesia.

13 What are the signs of iatrogenic aortic dissection caused during aortic cannulation?

- Spreading haematoma with bleeding at a point distal to the cannulation site.
- Classically a boggy mass may be palpable in the oblique sinus which may push the heart anteriorly.
- Failure of blood to rise to the top of the arterial cannula.
- Poor swing on the arterial line following removal of the line clamp.
- High line pressures when fluid is infused via the arterial cannula.
- Profound hypotension with poor venous return.

14 What are the main principles of managing iatrogenic aortic dissection caused during aortic cannulation?

- Stop the cardiopulmonary bypass pump immediately and clamp the arterial and venous lines.
- Insert the aortic cannula into the right atrium, to rapidly infuse volume as required.
- Insert an arterial cannula into a peripheral artery or uninvolved distal aorta.
- Following deep hypothermic circulatory arrest (18°C), the ascending aorta is opened and inspected for dissection at the original site of cannulation.
- The aorta can then be repaired using a direct suture, patch or interposition graft depending on the extent of the dissection.
- It is important to recognise and treat iatrogenic aortic dissection immediately, to limit the extent of the injury and restore systemic perfusion.

- When recognised early, survival rates following iatrogenic aortic dissection are 66% to 85%, but when discovered after operation survival is approximately 50%.

15 What are the causes of oliguria on cardiopulmonary bypass?

- Pre-renal (reduced renal perfusion) secondary to:

  a)   an inadequate cardiopulmonary bypass flow rate;
  b)   hypovolaemia;
  c)   renal vasoconstriction (mediated by α-agonists);
  d)   undetected iatrogenic aortic dissection.

- Renal: pre-operative renal dysfunction.
- Post-renal: secondary to an obstructed urinary catheter (kinked, blood clot, lidocaine gel).

16 What are the causes of haematuria on cardiopulmonary bypass?

- Urinary tract trauma during catheterisation followed by systemic heparinisation for cardiopulmonary bypass.
- Haemolysis, secondary to:

  a)   cardiotomy suction;
  b)   prolonged cardiopulmonary bypass;
  c)   acquired red cell fragility (hepatic dysfunction, endocarditis);
  d)   congenital red cell anomalies (sickle cell disease, spherocytosis).

17 Describe the de-airing routine following an aortic valve replacement

- Throughout the procedure, carbon dioxide is insufflated into the surgical field. Just prior to tying down the aortotomy suture:

  a)   the patient is placed in the Trendelenburg position;
  b)   the venous line is partially occluded to fill the heart;
  c)   the heart is gently agitated whilst keeping the aortotomy open with forceps to allow release of trapped air;
  d)   the lungs are inflated to displace any air in the pulmonary veins;

e) the aortic cross-clamp is removed and the aortotomy suture line is tied;

f) the aortic root vent is turned on at 300mL/min. As the heart begins to eject, any air trapped within the left ventricle is ejected into the aorta and removed by the root vent.

- Transoesophageal echocardiography is used to aid the de-airing process.

18 **What are the important factors to consider before weaning a patient from cardiopulmonary bypass?**

- Patient factors:

a) temperature - ensure that the peripheral temperature has reached 34°C and that the central core temperature is above 36.5°C. Rewarming of the circulating blood usually commences during the last distal anastomosis (CABG) or during closure of the aortotomy (AVR) or atriotomy (MVR), with the aid of a warming blanket;

b) electrocardiogram - ensure that the:
   i) rate is above 60 bpm or consider using epicardial pacing wires;
   ii) rhythm is sinus or longstanding atrial fibrillation, otherwise consider electrical cardioversion or commencing an anti-arrhythmic agent;
   iii) ST segment is isoelectric, otherwise consider resting the heart until any ischaemic changes have resolved;

c) blood pressure - ensure that the mean arterial pressure (>60mmHg) is enough to sustain organ perfusion, otherwise consider commencing a vasopressor (such as noradrenaline).

- Surgical factors:

a) operation is complete;

b) all the surgical sites have been checked for bleeding;

c) left and right ventricular function is as expected, otherwise consider commencing inotropic support or inserting an intra-aortic balloon pump;

d) snares released in patients with bicaval cannulation;

e) decompress the pericardial and pleural cavities:
   i) suction any residual blood or topical cooling fluid;
   ii) remove any swabs;
   iii) decompress any pneumothorax.

- Anaesthetic factors:

    a)   arterial blood gases - ensure that the PaO_2 is >15kPa, $PaCO_2$ is <6kPa, base excess is <-4mmol/L and the serum potassium is <5.5mmol/L;

    b)   transoesophageal echocardiography - ensure that all intracardiac air has been removed following all open-heart cardiac surgical procedures;

    c)   ventilation - ensure that both lungs are fully expanded prior to weaning from cardiopulmonary bypass.

19 What are the steps involved in weaning a patient from cardiopulmonary bypass?

- The perfusionist gradually occludes the venous line and simultaneously reduces the pump flow, allowing the heart to gradually fill and eject independent of the cardiopulmonary bypass machine.

- Initially the volume in the venous reservoir is kept constant, but as pump flow approaches zero, volume is added or removed from the patient to produce appropriate arterial and venous pressures.
- Ideally, the patient is weaned slightly underfilled, to reduce the myocardial oxygen demands when the heart is just recovering.
- The preload can be adjusted by transfusing boluses of 50-100mL to achieve the appropriate filling pressures.
- Adequacy of filling and myocardial function is determined by a number of haemodynamic parameters that are monitored as the patient is weaned from cardiopulmonary bypass:

    a)   central venous pressure;
    b)   mean arterial pressure;
    c)   pulmonary arterial pressure;
    d)   cardiac index;
    e)   cardiac rate and rhythm;
    f)   left and right heart contractility, observed directly and echocardiographically.

- Once haemodynamic stability has been achieved and all intracardiac repairs assessed to be successful on transoesophageal echocardiography, the venous cannulae can be removed.
- Once all surgical sites have been checked for bleeding and haemostasis achieved, protamine is given. The aortic cannula is left in at this stage to allow for rapid transfusion if the patient were to develop a protamine reaction.

- Any residual blood within the cardiopulmonary bypass circuit is then washed via the cell saver and retransfused.
- The heart-lung machine can be disassembled once the sternum is closed and the patient is haemodynamically stable.

20 What are the common causes of hypotension after weaning from cardiopulmonary bypass?

- Reduced preload, secondary to:

   a)   hypovolaemia;
   b)   bleeding;
   c)   swabs compressing the heart;
   d)   'hitched up' pericardium, restricting venous return.

- Reduced ventricular contractility, secondary to:

   a)   myocardial stunning;
   b)   incomplete revascularisation;
   c)   inadequate myocardial protection;
   d)   coronary air embolism;
   e)   coronary artery bypass graft failure, secondary to anastomotic narrowing or inadequate graft length.

- Vasodilation, secondary to cardiopulmonary bypass-induced systemic inflammatory response.
- Arrhythmias, including inadequate pacing.
- Management includes treating the underlying cause, transfusing volume, achieving haemostasis, inotropic and vasopressor support, resting the heart back on cardiopulmonary bypass and inserting an intra-aortic balloon pump.

Recommended reading

1.   Lee M. *Near misses in cardiac surgery*. IUniverse, 2008.

227

Chapter 10

Adjuncts to cardiopulmonary bypass

1   What are the indications for deep hypothermic circulatory arrest?

- Surgery on the aortic arch:

  a)   aortic dissection;
  b)   arch aneurysms.

- When a bloodless field is required:

  a)   thoraco-abdominal aneurysms;
  b)   renal tumours invading the inferior vena cava and right atrium;
  c)   complex congenital cardiac surgery;
  d)   pulmonary thrombo-endarterectomy;
  e)   neurosurgery.

- When it is impossible to clamp the ascending aorta:

  a)   porcelain aorta;
  b)   distal ascending aortic aneurysms.

- To control and repair massive haemorrhage:

  a)   blood loss during resternotomy;
  b)   repair of a ruptured thoracic aorta (following dissection or trauma).

2   **What are the safe periods of circulatory arrest at the different temperatures (Table 1)?**

Temperature (°C)	Duration of safe circulatory arrest (mins)
36	1
32	5
28	10
24	20
20	30-40
16	45-60

Table 1. Duration of safe circulatory arrest.

3   **What are the effects of deep hypothermic circulatory arrest on cerebral metabolism?**

- At 20°C cerebral metabolism and oxygen consumption are approximately 20% of normothermic levels as they drop by 5% per 1°C.
- As cerebral metabolism is reduced with hypothermia, haematocrit levels can be reduced to prevent sludging of capillary beds and as reduced oxygen carrying capacity is required.
- Mortality and adverse neurologic outcomes increase after 45-60 minutes of circulatory arrest at 16°C.

4   **What are the methods of monitoring cerebral metabolism during circulatory arrest?**

- As there are no easily available direct methods of monitoring cerebral metabolism clinically, indirect methods include:

  a)   nasopharyngeal temperature;
  b)   internal jugular venous saturation >95% signifies minimal cerebral O_2 extraction and minimal cerebral activity;
  c)   electroencephalogram (EEG), although it is not always reliable to use silent EEG activity as a marker of reduced cerebral activity;
  d)   near infrared spectroscopy, which indirectly measures cerebral tissue oxygenation. There are two methods currently available,

including INVOS®, which measures changes from baseline and Foresight®, which provides the absolute value for cerebral saturation.

5 What are the complications of deep hypothermic circulatory arrest?

- Coagulopathy and platelet dysfunction.
- Systemic inflammatory response to both cardiopulmonary bypass and deep hypothermic circulatory arrest resulting in capillary leak, tissue oedema and organ dysfunction.
- Neurological injury secondary to ischaemia in watershed areas, particulate and gaseous embolism, and systemic inflammatory response.

6 What is the sequence of events for deep hypothermic circulatory arrest (DHCA) for surgery on the thoracic aorta?

- Using cardiopulmonary bypass, the patient's core (nasopharyngeal) temperature is cooled to the desired lower temperature (15-18°C), using adjuncts (see below).
- To produce a steady state of hypothermia, it is important to keep the temperature at 15-18°C for 10-15 minutes before the induction of DHCA. This ensures adequate suppression of cerebral activity and reduces the risk of cerebral rewarming occurring during the circulatory arrest time.
- The arterial line is then clamped, the circulating volume drained into the venous reservoir and the pump switched off.
- After completion of the operative procedure, the patient is placed in a deep Trendelenburg position.
- The circulation is then restarted at a slow rate (~500mL/min) in an antegrade direction, using the side arm of the ascending aortic interposition graft if appropriate.
- De-airing can also be facilitated by retrograde cerebral perfusion to flush out particulate and gaseous debris through the anastomotic line as well as using an aortic root vent.
- After cardiopulmonary bypass is re-established, a period of cold reperfusion for approximately 10 minutes is maintained at 15-18°C before steady active rewarming (0.2-0.5°C/min).
- It is important to avoid cerebral hyperthermia or aggressive rewarming, which may result in neurological injury during reperfusion.

7   **What adjuncts are used to minimise cerebral injury during deep hypothermic circulatory arrest?**
*   Ice packs around the head to ensure uniform cooling and prevent rewarming during the circulatory arrest period.
*   Pharmacological methods to reduce cerebral oedema include 100mg dexamethasone and 1mg/kg mannitol, but their efficacy is still debated.
*   Thiopentone is often not used as the large doses required to suppress cerebral metabolism have negative inotropic side effects.
*   Antegrade or retrograde cerebral perfusion (see below).
*   Normoglycaemia, as hyperglycaemia can contribute to brain injury.

8   **How is antegrade cerebral perfusion performed?**
*   A typical set-up would involve (Figure 1):

    a)   cannulating the right axillary artery (using an 18Fr cannula) either directly or indirectly with an 8mm Gortex graft attached to the artery;
    b)   clamping the brachiocephalic artery at its origin to ensure antegrade flow from the right axillary artery into the right common carotid artery and cerebral circulation;
    c)   clamping the left common carotid artery and left subclavian artery.

*   Alternatively, the brachiocephalic artery and left common carotid artery can be cannulated directly from the arch using 18Fr and 14Fr cannulae, respectively, with the left subclavian artery snared without a cannula.
*   The circulation is then perfused with:

    a)   cold blood between 10-18°C;
    b)   a flow rate of 10mL/kg/min (i.e. 700-900mL/min);
    c)   perfusion pressures restricted to 30-70mm Hg.

*   If the perfusion pressures are too high, there is a risk of dislodging atheromatous emboli, causing air embolism or developing cerebral oedema.
*   A complete Circle of Willis is important to ensure total cerebral perfusion.
*   The extent to which safe deep hypothermic circulatory arrest times may be potentially extended with antegrade cerebral perfusion remains unestablished.

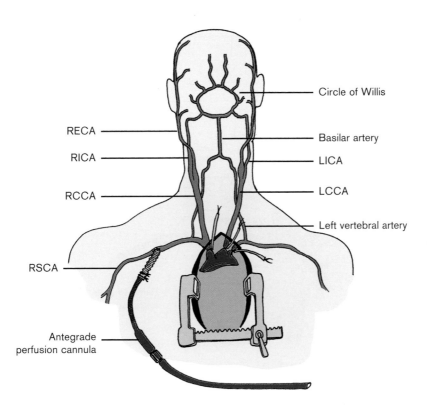

Figure 1. Antegrade cerebral perfusion. RECA = right external carotid artery; RCCA = right common carotid artery; RICA = right internal carotid artery; RSCA = right subclavian artery; LCCA = left common carotid artery; LICA = left internal carotid artery.

9 **How is retrograde cerebral perfusion performed?**

● A typical set-up would involve (Figure 2):

a) cannulating the superior vena cava (24Fr cannula) attached to the arterial line via a Y-connector with the downstream limb of the arterial line clamped;

b) a snare placed around the superior vena cava cannula superior to the origin of the azygos vein to reduce run-off.

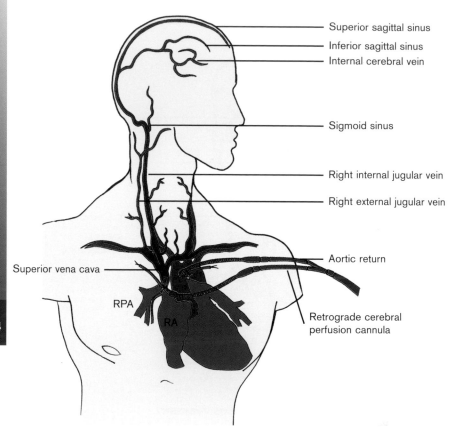

Figure 2. Retrograde cerebral perfusion. RPA = right pulmonary artery; RA = right atrium.

- The circulation is then perfused with:

  a)   cold blood between 10-18°C;
  b)   a flow rate of 250-400mL/min;
  c)   perfusion pressures restricted to 25-40mm Hg.

- Historically, retrograde cerebral perfusion was developed to manage massive air embolism.
- The effectiveness of retrograde cerebral perfusion in protecting the brain is not clear but it may enhance cerebral cooling and wash out particulate and gaseous emboli from the cerebral circulation. During retrograde cerebral perfusion, however, dark de-oxygenated blood usually returns into the aortic arch, indicating cerebral oxygen uptake may be taking place.

10 What strategies exist in the management of acid-base metabolism during deep hypothermic circulatory arrest?

- As the temperature decreases, there is increased solubility of a given gas (Boyles' law) resulting in more CO_2 in solution but less in gaseous form, thereby producing a reduced $PaCO_2$ and an increased pH (i.e. more alkalotic).
- During hypothermia, there are two methodologies to maintain acid-base homeostasis:

  a) pH-stat - adding CO_2 to keep the $PaCO_2$ at 5kPa and pH at 7.4, which are normal levels in arterial blood at 37°C;
  b) alpha-stat - not adding CO_2, thereby allowing the pH and $PaCO_2$ to drift as dictated by the solubility at a given temperature, producing alkalotic blood during the cooling process.

- One strategy is to use:

  a) pH-stat on cooling; this enhances cerebral perfusion by maintaining $PaCO_2$ and facilitates cooling;
  b) alpha-stat on re-warming to reduce the micro-embolic load on the cerebral circulation.

11 What are the advantages and disadvantages of alpha-stat and pH-stat methodology?

- pH-stat methodology has the advantage of a more rapid and homogenous cooling but an increased risk of cerebral embolism.
- Alpha-stat methodology has the advantage of reducing the risk of cerebral embolism and the alkalosis produced may also be beneficial in terms of reducing cerebral and myocardial metabolism.
- Several prospective, randomised studies have shown the benefit of alpha-stat methodology by reducing the number of postoperative cerebral events.
- pH-stat methodology is often used in paediatric cardiac surgery.

12 How is the haematocrit managed during deep hypothermic circulatory arrest?

- As temperature decreases:

  a)   the metabolic rate decreases thereby reducing the oxygen requirement of the tissues;
  b)   blood viscosity increases resulting in an increased risk of sludging if the haematocrit remains >35%.

- In view of this, as the temperature decreases, the haematocrit is proportionally reduced to match the temperature in degrees centigrade, i.e. at temperatures of 20°C the haematocrit is maintained at about 20%.

13 What are the complications of blood transfusion?

- Historically, approximately 60% of patients undergoing cardiac surgery received blood transfusion, but this is associated with:

  a)   transmission of blood-borne pathogens - HIV, hepatitis B / C;
  b)   transfusion reactions - haemolytic, allergic, febrile;
  c)   cost;
  d)   increased bacterial infections;
  e)   reduced immune function.

- In view of this, it is important to avoid blood transfusion if possible with the usual triggers for blood transfusion being a haemoglobin of <8g/dL, with <10g/dL used in elderly and high-risk patients.

14 What are the different options available for blood conservation?

- Pharmacological:

  a)   aprotinin (although concerns have been raised about its use; see below);
  b)   tranexamic acid;
  c)   epsilon-aminocaproic acid;
  d)   recombinant erythropoietin.

- Autologous pre-donation.
- Intra-operative cell salvage.
- Auto-transfusion of washed shed postoperative mediastinal fluid.

15 What is the standard dosing regime for aprotinin (see Chapter 3)?

- Standard Hammersmith regime:

  a) loading dose 2 million units (= 280mg) IV;
  b) pump prime 2 million units (= 280mg);
  c) continuous infusion 0.5 million units (= 70mg) per hour.

- The dose should be adjusted with the patient's body weight and renal function (as aprotinin is excreted by the renal tubules).

16 What are the clinical effects of aprotinin following cardiac surgery?

- The IMAGE trial showed that aprotinin:

  a) reduces postoperative mediastinal blood loss;
  b) reduces the need for postoperative blood transfusions;
  c) reduces the need for postoperative platelets and blood product requirements;
  d) reduces the resternotomy for bleeding rate.

17 What are the side effects of aprotinin?

- Thrombotic risk - anecdotal reports of thrombosis associated with heart surgery.
- Graft patency - data from the IMAGE trial suggested that aprotinin reduces graft patency in coronary arteries with poor run-off.
- Hypersensitivity - usually within 6 months of first exposure.
- Mortality - data from the BART trial suggested that aprotinin used in cardiac surgical patients is associated with an increased incidence of mortality, renal impairment, heart failure and myocardial infarction. In view of this, aprotinin use has been suspended in cardiac surgical patients pending further studies.

18 What are the clinical effects of tranexamic acid following cardiac surgery?

- Tranexamic acid has been shown to reduce postoperative mediastinal blood losses, blood product transfusion and resternotomy for bleeding rate but is thought to be less effective than aprotinin.

19 What is autologous pre-donation?

- Autologous pre-donation is defined as blood venesected either several weeks pre-operatively or immediately prior to commencing cardiopulmonary bypass and then transfused postoperatively.
- Although it has been shown to reduce transfusion requirements, the fact that most cardiac surgical patients have one of the contra-indications (anaemia, unstable angina, aortic stenosis, heart failure) means that it is rarely used in current cardiac surgical practice.

20 What are the principles of intra-operative cell salvage?

- All fluid (heparinised and non-heparinised) not returned to the bypass circuit can be scavenged by a cell saver system.
- The fluid is washed, filtered and centrifuged to produce concentrated red blood cells with a haemoglobin of 20g/dL or a haematocrit of 60% (Figure 3).
- The washing process eliminates platelets and plasma proteins, including clotting factors and fibrinogen degradation products.
- Several studies have shown that the use of cell salvage reduces postoperative blood transfusion requirements and is cost effective.

21 What are the principles of autotransfusion of washed shed postoperative mediastinal fluid?

- Shed blood collected via the pleural and pericardial drains postoperatively can be re-infused after processing through a cell salvage system.
- Although the washing process eliminates platelets and clotting factors, studies have shown this system to reduce postoperative transfusion requirements.
- As a minimum, 500mL of drainage is required to produce a meaningful volume after washing. It is not used after all cardiac surgical cases due to cost-effectiveness.

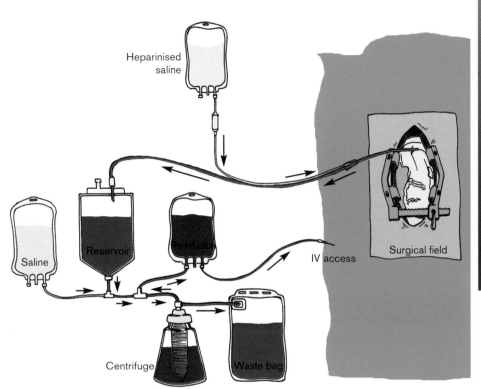

Heparinised saline

Saline

Reservoir

Re-infusion

IV access

Surgical field

239

Centrifuge

Waste bag

Figure 3. Intra-operative cell salvage. Blood and other fluids drained from the chest cavity through the sucker are continuously flushed with normal saline and heparin. The heparinised diluted blood is collected into a reservoir and subsequently washed with non-heparinised normal saline before entering the centrifuge where red cells are differentiated and filtered to be collected into a re-infusion bag. Saline solution, plasma, platelets and leucocytes are discarded into a waste bag. The concentrated red cells can then be re-transfused into the patient.

22 What are the techniques of blood conservation available for Jehovah's Witness patients undergoing cardiac surgery?

- Pre-operatively:

  a) erythropoietin;

  b) stop all antiplatelets (aspirin, clopidogrel) and anticoagulants (warfarin, heparin) for 7 days if clinically possible.

- Intra-operatively:

  a) pharmacological adjuncts - aprotinin or tranexamic acid;

  b) meticulous haemostasis;

  c) continuous cell salvage circuit;

  d) consider 'off-pump' or minimal extracorporeal circulation (MECC) with a low prime volume;

  e) consider fibrin glue.

- Postoperatively:

  a) autotransfusion of washed shed postoperative mediastinal fluid;

  b) low threshold for resternotomy for bleeding.

Recommended reading

1. Murkin JM, Martzke JS, Buchan AM, Bentley C, Wong CJ. A randomized study of the influence of perfusion technique and pH management strategy in 316 patients undergoing coronary artery bypass surgery. II. Neurologic and cognitive outcomes. *J Thorac Cardiovasc Surg* 1995; 110(2): 349-62.

2. Treasure T. The safe duration of total circulatory arrest with profound hypothermia. *Ann R Coll Surg Engl* 1984; 66(4): 235-40.

3. Alderman EL, Levy JH, Rich JB, Nili M, Vidne B, Schaff H, Uretzky G, Pettersson G, Thiis JJ, Hantler CB, Chaitman B, Nadel A. Analyses of coronary graft patency after aprotinin use: results from the International Multicenter Aprotinin Graft Patency Experience (IMAGE) trial. *J Thorac Cardiovasc Surg* 1998; 116(5): 716-30.

4. Fergusson DA, Hébert PC, Mazer CD, Fremes S, MacAdams C, Murkin JM, Teoh K, Duke PC, Arellano R, Blajchman MA, Bussières JS, Côté D, Karski J, Martineau R, Robblee JA, Rodger M, Wells G, Clinch J, Pretorius R; BART Investigators. A comparison of aprotinin and lysine analogues in high-risk cardiac surgery. *N Engl J Med* 2008; 358(22): 2319-31.

5.   McGill N, O'Shaughnessy D, Pickering R, Herbertson M, Gill R. Mechanical methods of reducing blood transfusion in cardiac surgery: randomised controlled trial. *BMJ* 2002; 324(7349): 1299.

6.   Klein AA, Nashef SA, Sharples L, Bottrill F, Dyer M, Armstrong J, Vuylsteke A. A randomized controlled trial of cell salvage in routine cardiac surgery. *Anesth Analg* 2008; 107(5): 1487-95.

7.   Society of Thoracic Surgeons Blood Conservation Guideline Task Force, Ferraris VA, Ferraris SP, Saha SP, Hessel EA 2nd, Haan CK, Royston BD, Bridges CR, Higgins RS, Despotis G, Brown JR; Society of Cardiovascular Anesthesiologists Special Task Force on Blood Transfusion, Spiess BD, Shore-Lesserson L, Stafford-Smith M, Mazer CD, Bennett-Guerrero E, Hill SE, Body S. Perioperative blood transfusion and blood conservation in cardiac surgery: the Society of Thoracic Surgeons and The Society of Cardiovascular Anesthesiologists clinical practice guideline. *Ann Thorac Surg* 2007; 83(5 Suppl): S27-86.

8.   Apostolakis E, Akinosoglou K. The methodologies of hypothermic circulatory arrest and of antegrade and retrograde cerebral perfusion for aortic arch surgery. *Ann Thorac Cardiovasc Surg* 2008; 14(3): 138-48.

9.   Svensson LG, Nadolny EM, Penney DL, Jacobson J, Kimmel WA, Entrup MH, D'Agostino RS. Prospective randomized neurocognitive and S-100 study of hypothermic circulatory arrest, retrograde brain perfusion, and antegrade brain perfusion for aortic arch operations. *Ann Thorac Surg* 2001; 71(6): 1905-12.

Chapter 11

Myocardial protection

1 **What are the principles of myocardial protection during cardiac surgery?**

- Using cardiopulmonary bypass and cross-clamping of the aorta, the coronary arteries are deprived of oxygenated blood. During this ischaemic time, damage to the myocardium needs to be minimised, hence the concept of myocardial protection.

- Several different methods of myocardial protection can be used to reduce myocardial O_2 demands:

  a) unloading the heart (cardiopulmonary bypass);
  b) stopping the heart (cardioplegic diastolic arrest);
  c) cooling the heart (hypothermia).

- By arresting the heart, O_2 demands are reduced by 90% (Table 1; Figure 1).

Table 1. Cardiac metabolic demands.	
Cardiac metabolic demands	
Beating loaded heart	10ml O_2 per 100mg myocardium per minute
Unloaded heart (cardiopulmonary bypass)	6ml O_2 per 100mg myocardium per minute
Arrested heart (cardioplegia)	1ml O_2 per 100mg myocardium per minute

- Hypothermia further reduces the myocardial oxygen consumption and metabolic rate by a factor of 7% for every 1°C decrease in temperature.

- Using 'off-pump' coronary artery bypass surgery removes the ischaemic insult of aortic cross-clamping but has ischaemic issues of its own (see below).

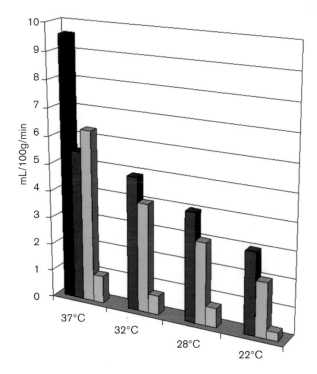

Figure 1. Myocardial oxygen demand (mVO_2) at different states of ventricular work. The graph demonstrates a significant reduction in myocardial oxygen consumption in the arrested heart and additionally with hypothermia.

2 What are the effects of cooling on the myocardium?
- Cooling the heart results in:

a) decreased metabolic rate;
b) decreased enzyme function;
c) decreased membrane stability;

d)   increased calcium sequestration;
e)   increased glucose utilization;
f)   decreased ATP generation;
g)   decreased tissue oxygen uptake;
h)   decreased osmotic homeostasis;
i)   increased hyperviscosity with rouleaux formation.

- The reduction in myocardial metabolism attributable to hypothermia is much less compared to that caused by diastolic arrest.

3   What is ischaemia-reperfusion injury?

- Ischaemia-reperfusion injury represents damage to tissues following restoration of blood supply after a period of ischaemia.
- The reperfusion triggers an inflammatory response inducing tissue damage secondary to oxygen-free radicals, calcium influx, leucocytes, lactate accumulation and high-energy phosphate depletion.
- Oxygen-free radicals cause tissue damage by inducing interstitial and intracellular oedema, endothelial injury and increased microvascular permeability.
- Ischaemia-reperfusion injury of the heart may result in cardiac arrhythmias, myocardial stunning and myocyte cell death.

245

4   What are the options for myocardial protection during cardiac surgery?

- Cardioplegic arrest.
- Aortic cross-clamping with electrically-induced fibrillation.
- Hypothermic arrest with fibrillation (where the aorta remains unclamped).
- 'Off-pump' coronary artery surgery.
- Pre-operative and peri-operative measures to optimize the balance between the myocardial oxygen supply and demand are also important, including:

a)   administering supplemental oxygen;
b)   minimizing tachycardia (beta blockers) and hypotension;
c)   when indicated, using an intra-aortic balloon pump;
d)   giving pre-operative nitrates.

5 **What are the different routes for delivering cardioplegia?**

● Antegrade cardioplegia delivered via the aortic root (standard method) proximal to the aortic cross-clamp at a pressure of 60-100mmHg at 250mL/min usually results in arrest within 30-60s. Delivery may be unpredictable due to coronary artery disease and should not be used in the presence of severe aortic regurgitation, to avoid ventricular damage by mechanical dilation (Figure 2).

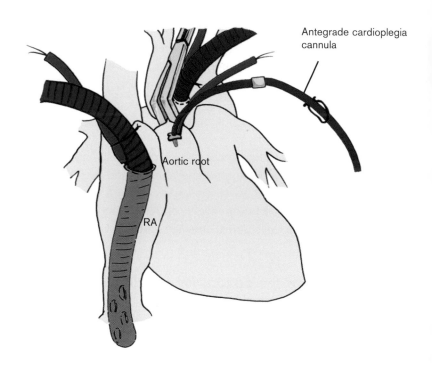

Antegrade cardioplegia cannula

Aortic root

RA

Figure 2. Antegrade cardioplegia delivered via a cannula placed in the ascending aorta. RA = right atrium.

● Antegrade cardioplegia delivered directly into the coronary ostia, such as during aortic valve and root procedures (Figure 3).

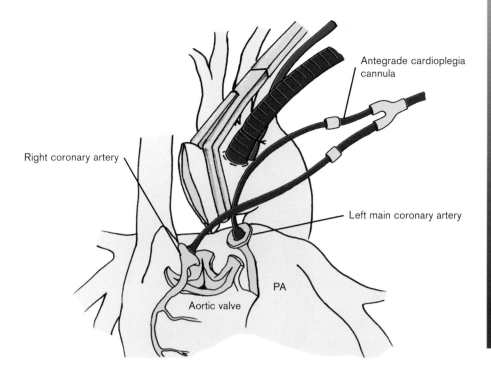

Antegrade cardioplegia
cannula

Right coronary artery

Left main coronary artery

PA

Aortic valve

Figure 3. Antegrade cardioplegia delivered directly into the coronary ostia. The aortic root has been excised, aortic valve exposed and coronary ostia mobilized as buttons. PA = pulmonary artery.

- Retrograde cardioplegia delivered via the coronary sinus at a pressure of 30-50mmHg at 150mL/min usually results in arrest over 2-4 minutes (Figure 4).
- An alternative method of delivering retrograde cardioplegia is independent cannulation of the SVC and IVC, which are then isolated with tapes. Cardioplegia is then delivered directly into the right atrium. This is a useful technique when these cannulae are already in position during mitral surgery. It also ensures that cardioplegia is delivered via both the Thebesian veins and coronary sinus, and avoids the pitfalls of incorrect cannula position within the coronary sinus and/or variations in coronary venous anatomy.

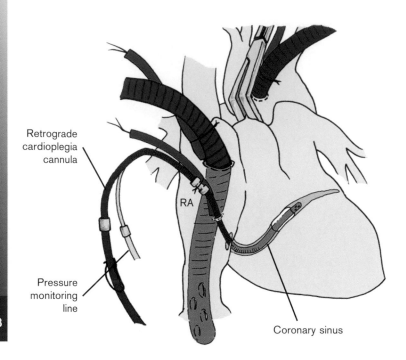

Retrograde
cardioplegia
cannula

RA

Pressure
monitoring
line

Coronary sinus

Figure 4. Retrograde cardioplegia. RA = right atrium.

- Cardioplegia is delivered through a separate roller pump with a bubble trap and microfilter.

6 How is a retrograde cardioplegia cannula inserted?

- A 1cm^2 purse-string is placed ~4cm inferior to the right atrial appendage.
- Following institution of cardiopulmonary bypass, the right atrium is filled with blood (via the bypass machine) to avoid entrapment of air.
- The tip of the retrograde cardioplegia cannula is curved to 120° and passed over the inferior vena cava cannula.
- The left hand of the operating surgeon is used to guide the retrograde cannula past the Thebesian valve into the coronary sinus within the atrioventricular groove.
- The position of the retrograde cannula can be checked by:

  a)   palpation of the cannula within the coronary sinus;

b) manometry with the coronary sinus pressure ~20-30mmHg;
c) aspirating dark venous blood (as the myocardium has a high oxygen uptake).

- Complications include malposition and rupture or tearing of the coronary sinus.

7 What are the advantages and disadvantages of using retrograde cardioplegia?

- Advantages:

a) it is useful in patients with severe aortic regurgitation, significant coronary arterial occlusive disease or severe coronary ostial stenosis;
b) retrograde cardioplegia can also be given without interrupting the flow of the operation.

- Disadvantages:

a) it has less predictable distribution than antegrade cardioplegia;
b) there are concerns regarding protection of the right ventricle when using retrograde cardioplegia alone.

8 What are the different cardioplegia solutions available?

- Crystalloid cardioplegia, usually given cold (4-10°C).
- Blood cardioplegia, which can be given hypothermic or normothermic.
- Although crystalloid and blood cardioplegia have equal efficacy in patients with normal ventricles, some studies have shown the benefit of blood cardioplegia in patients with unstable angina or left ventricular dysfunction.

9 How does cardioplegia cause cardiac arrest?

- Cardioplegic solutions induce diastolic arrest by altering the resting potential (-90mV) and ionic gradients (Na, K, Ca, Cl) in the myocyte with two main mechanisms of action:

a) extracellular solutions (such as St. Thomas' solution), which prevent cardiomyocyte repolarisation by increasing the potassium concentration in the extracellular fluid;

b)   intracellular solutions (such as Bredtschneider's solution), which block depolarisation by lowering extracellular sodium concentrations.

10 What are the main components of cardioplegia solution?

- Crystalloid cardioplegia (St. Thomas' solution) contains:

    a)   sodium - 110mmol/L;
    b)   potassium - 16mmol/L;
    c)   calcium - 1.2mmol/L;
    d)   magnesium - 16mmol/L;
    e)   chloride - 160mmol/L.

- Blood cardioplegia contains blood and St. Thomas' solution at a ratio of 4:1, procaine (membrane stabilizer), glutamate, aspartate, oxygen-free radical scavengers and adenosine.
- Magnesium blocks phosphorylase activity of myosin, delays calcium flux and inhibits excitation-contraction coupling.

11 What are the advantages of blood cardioplegia over crystalloid cardioplegia?

- Blood:

    a)   provides oxygen and nutrients;
    b)   provides a buffering capacity;
    c)   minimises intracellular oedema due to its oncotic proteins;
    d)   distributes cardioplegia more evenly thereby inducing a faster onset of arrest;
    e)   scavenges oxygen-free radicals as it contains superoxide dismutase, catalase, glutathione and vitamins C and E.

12 What are the principles of terminal warm blood cardioplegia ('hot-shot')?

- A 'hot shot' represents a dose of warm cardioplegia given immediately before removing the aortic cross-clamp.
- Warm cardioplegia:

    a)   allows washout of the products of anaerobic metabolism, such as lactic acid;

b) provides substrate resuscitation of ischaemic myocytes with oxygen and ATP.

- It has been shown to improve myocardial metabolism and contractility once ventricular contractions resume.

13 **What myocardial protection strategies are available for patients undergoing redo cardiac surgery with a patent left internal mammary artery (LIMA)?**

- LIMA balloon (positioned pre-operatively under fluoroscopic guidance), which can be occluded when giving cardioplegia.
- Dissect out the LIMA and temporarily occlude when giving cardioplegia.
- Moderate hypothermic fibrillatory arrest (without occluding the LIMA).
- Cooling (28°C) with either continuous retrograde cardioplegia or intermittent antegrade cold blood cardioplegia without isolation of the LIMA.

14 **What is the sequence of events when using the cross-clamp fibrillation technique?**

- Establish cardiopulmonary bypass with mild hypothermia (32-34°C).
- Decompress the left ventricle.
- Induce ventricular fibrillation using an electric fibrillator.
- Apply the aortic cross-clamp during minimal flow on cardiopulmonary bypass.
- Perform the distal anastomosis.
- Remove the aortic cross-clamp.
- DC cardiovert into sinus rhythm (if necessary).
- Perform the proximal anastomosis.
- Repeat the sequence with the next distal anastomosis.

15 **What are the principles of cross-clamp fibrillation?**

- The heart is electrically fibrillated prior to aortic cross-clamping thereby inducing global ischaemia with fibrillation followed by anoxic arrest.
- Some degree of myocardial protection is afforded by unloading the heart (cardiopulmonary bypass), reducing myocardial work (fibrillation) and ischaemic pre-conditioning (see below).
- The left ventricle is decompressed before placing the aortic cross-clamp in order to prevent myocardial distension, subendocardial ischaemia and myofibrillar disruption.

- Mild hypothermia (32-34°C) increases permissible global ischaemia to approximately 15 minutes and dampens the amplitude of the fibrillation.
- Lower temperatures, however, cannot be used as it is difficult to defibrillate below 30°C.

16 What are the advantages and disadvantages of cross-clamp fibrillation?

- Advantages: simple, inexpensive, shorter aortic cross-clamp and cardiopulmonary bypass times, and facilitates identification and differentiation of coronary arteries from veins.
- Disadvantages: aortic trauma and thrombo-embolism from repeated aortic cross-clamping (especially in arteriopaths).
- Several prospective trials have shown the efficacy of cross-clamp fibrillation is similar to cold blood cardioplegia as regards postoperative enzyme release and left ventricular function.

17 What is ischaemic pre-conditioning?

- Repeated brief insults of sub-lethal ischaemia followed by reperfusion protects the myocardium during subsequent prolonged episodes of ischaemia by preserving myocardial ATP, thereby resulting in improved recovery of contractile function after reperfusion.
- The 'first window' of improved recovery immediately follows the ischaemic insult and lasts about 12 hours, with the 'second window' of recovery occurring 24-36 hours after the ischaemic insult.
- Ischaemic pre-conditioning occurs through adenosine receptors.
- The cross-clamp fibrillation technique with sequential graft construction allows gradually increased areas of myocardium to be reperfused, using ischaemic pre-conditioning.

18 What techniques are available for myocardial protection during 'off-pump' coronary artery bypass surgery?

- Intracoronary shunts.
- Ischaemic pre-conditioning.
- Constructing the left internal mammary artery to left anterior descending artery anastomosis as the first graft.

Recommended reading

1. Buckberg GD, Brazier JR, Nelson RL, Goldstein SM, McConnell DH, Cooper N. Studies of the effects of hypothermia on regional myocardial blood flow and metabolism during cardiopulmonary bypass. I. The adequately perfused beating, fibrillating, and arrested heart. *J Thorac Cardiovasc Surg* 1977; 73(1): 87-94.

2. Teoh KH, Christakis GT, Weisel RD, Fremes SE, Mickle DA, Romaschin AD, Harding RS, Ivanov J, Madonik MM, Ross IM. Accelerated myocardial metabolic recovery with terminal warm blood cardioplegia. *J Thorac Cardiovasc Surg* 1986; 91(6): 888-95.

3. Buckberg GD. Normothermic blood cardioplegia. Alternative or adjunct? *J Thorac Cardiovasc Surg* 1994; 107(3): 860-7.

4. Teoh LK, Grant R, Hulf JA, Pugsley WB, Yellon DM. A comparison between ischemic preconditioning, intermittent cross-clamp fibrillation and cold crystalloid cardioplegia for myocardial protection during coronary artery bypass graft surgery. *Cardiovasc Surg* 2002; 10: 251-5.

Chapter 12

Aortic valve disease

1 **What is the natural history of untreated aortic stenosis (AS)(Figure 1)?**

- Asymptomatic patients have a long latent period before the onset of symptoms and the majority of these patients are not at risk of sudden death.

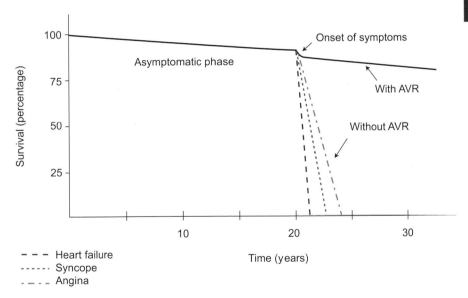

Figure 1. Graph demonstrating good survival whilst patients are asymptomatic, but a rapid decline in mean survival following the onset of symptoms. AVR = aortic valve replacement.

- Following the onset of symptoms, however, patients with AS have a markedly reduced mean survival:

  a) angina - 5 years;
  b) syncope - 3 years;
  c) dyspnoea - 2 years.

- In patients with AS, sudden death is rare within 3 months of symptom onset.

2   What is the pathophysiology of aortic stenosis?

- Aortic stenosis induces a progressive pressure overload on the left ventricle. This generates increasing intra-ventricular pressures, producing an aortic transvalvular gradient, where the left ventricular systolic pressure is greater than the aortic systolic pressure.
- Left ventricular hypertrophy occurs as a compensatory mechanism in an attempt to reduce wall stress, as per Laplace's law (Figure 2):

$$WS = \frac{P \times r}{2 \times Th}$$

where WS = wall stress, P = LVEDP, r = LV cavity radius, Th = LV wall thickness.

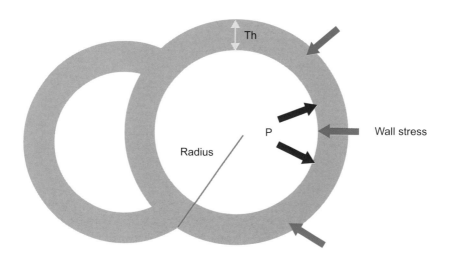

Figure 2. Laplace's law demonstrating the inter-relationship between wall stress, radius, pressure and thickness. Th = wall thickness; P = LVEDP.

- There is, however, a cost to these compensatory mechanisms:

    a) reduced left ventricular compliance, as left ventricular hypertrophy produces a thick-walled non-compliant chamber which impairs the ability of the left ventricle to fill adequately under normal pressures (diastolic dysfunction). This is associated with increased left ventricular end-diastolic pressures (LVEDP), where the left ventricle is more dependent upon diastolic filling (atrial contraction), hence often decompensates with atrial fibrillation;

    b) increased myocardial oxygen requirements to meet increased metabolic demands;

    c) reduced coronary blood flow secondary to raised LVEDP, hence patients may experience angina even with normal coronary arteries.

- Eventually left ventricular systolic dysfunction occurs when increasing pressure overload overwhelms left ventricular contractile reserve resulting in left ventricular dilation and subsequent left ventricular failure.

257

3   **How is the severity of aortic stenosis quantified?**
- According to the American Heart Association (AHA) guidelines, there are three main criteria (Table 1).

Table 1. AHA guidelines for the severity of aortic stenosis.

	Mild	Moderate	Severe
Aortic valve area (cm²)	1.5-2.5	1.0-1.5	<1.0
Mean pressure gradient (mmHg)	15-25	25-40	>40
Peak velocity (m/s)	<3.0	3.0-4.0	>4.0

- Although commonly used in clinical practice, the peak aortic gradient is not included in the AHA criteria for the severity of AS, because the peak gradient varies with other clinical factors such as volume status and left ventricular function.
- Aortic valve area (AVA) can be calculated by:

    a) planimetry using short axis aortic valve 2D echocardiography;

b) Continuity equation (Figure 3):

$$AVA = \frac{Area_{LVOT} \times VTI_{LVOT}}{VTI_{AoV}}$$

where LVOT = left ventricular outflow tract, VTI = velocity time intergral, AoV = aortic valve;

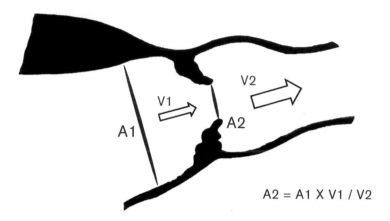

$$A2 = A1 \times V1 / V2$$

Figure 3. Continuity equation demonstrating that the total flow (area x velocity) of blood that passes through the LVOT is the same as the total flow of blood passing through the aortic valve. A1 = LVOT area; V1 = LVOT flow velocity; A2 = aortic valve area; V2 = intra-aortic flow velocity.

c) Gorlin equation:

$$AVA = \frac{CO}{44.3 \times HR \times LVET \times \sqrt{mean\ gradient}}$$

where CO = cardiac output, HR = heart rate, LVET = left ventricular ejection time.

- Information regarding the degree of leaflet movement, valve morphology, underlying aetiology of AS and changes in left ventricular function and size are also important when assessing the severity of AS.

4   What are the causes of aortic stenosis?

- The commonest causes of AS worldwide are:

a) rheumatic fever, which produces commissural fusion with leaflet thickening and fibrosis, resulting in a triangular aortic valve orifice (Figure 4);

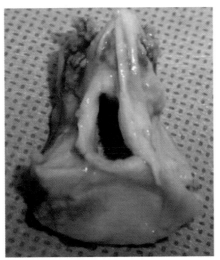

Figure 4. Rheumatic aortic valve disease.

b) calcific degeneration, which begins at the base of the cusps and progresses toward the leaflet edges with the commissures remaining open;

c) bicuspid aortic valve, where the cusps are prone to earlier progressive thickening and calcification with age (Figure 5).

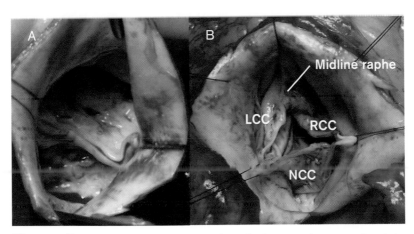

Figure 5. Bicuspid aortic stenosis. A) Cusps of approximately equal size and no midline raphe (Sievers type 0). B) Midline raphe caused by partial fusion of the right and left coronary cusps (Sievers type 1). NCC = non-coronary cusp; RCC = right coronary cusp; LCC = left coronary cusp.

- In the developed world, the percentages change depending upon age:

  a) <70 years old: bicuspid 50%, rheumatic fever 25%, calcific degeneration 18%;

  b) >70 years old: calcific degeneration 48%, rheumatic fever 23%, bicuspid 21%.

5 Describe the pathological findings of calcific degeneration (Figure 6)

- Masses of lipocalcification lying on the aortic side of the valve consisting of:

  a) inflammatory cell infiltrate (macrophages, T lymphocytes);
  b) lipids (low-density lipoprotein, lipoprotein A);
  c) microscopic calcification;
  d) proteins.

- The macrophages produce proteins, such as osteopontin, which cause calcification of the inflammatory mass.

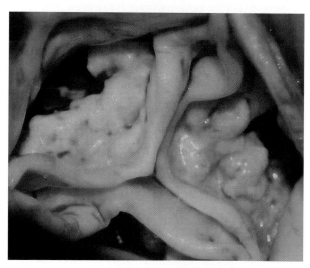

Figure 6. Calcific degeneration of the aortic valve.

6 **What are the symptoms of aortic stenosis?**

- Aortic stenosis is a progressive disease and, therefore, patients can remain asymptomatic for many years.
- Angina pectoris caused by increased myocardial O_2 demand secondary to increased left ventricular cavity pressure, left ventricular ejection time and muscle mass. Fifty percent of patients with AS also have co-existing coronary artery disease.
- Syncope or presyncope usually occurs following exertion where the cardiac output is fixed, resulting in arterial hypotension and reduced cerebral perfusion.
- Dyspnoea and congestive heart failure due to raised left ventricular end-diastolic pressure with outflow obstruction resulting in back pressure onto the lungs.

7 **What are the signs of aortic stenosis?**

- Pulsus tardus (slow-rising pulse).
- Pulsus parvus (small amplitude pulse).
- Apical impulse sustained but not displaced, reflecting prolonged left ventricular ejection.
- Single second heart sound (HS) as the A2 component is diminished due to calcification and stiffening of the aortic valve.
- Paradoxical splitting of the second HS due to prolonged left ventricular ejection with severe AS, resulting in a delayed A2 component.
- Fourth HS and pre-systolic thrust generated from atrial contraction into a hypertrophied and non-compliant left ventricle.
- Crescendo-decrescendo systolic murmur caused by turbulent flow across the narrowed aortic valve. It is best heard over the ascending aorta in the right second intercostal space radiating to the carotids. The murmur begins after isovolumetric contraction (0.06s after the first HS) and ends before the second HS; therefore, the murmur of AS is not pan-systolic. In comparison, the pan-systolic murmur of mitral regurgitation begins immediately after the first HS and extends into the second HS. Late peaking of the AS murmur indicates severity rather than intensity of the murmur, which depends on the transaortic volume flow rate (e.g. low cardiac output), transmission of the murmur through the chest wall (e.g. obesity, emphysema) and orientation of the turbulent jet as well as the severity of AS.

8 **What are the indications for valve replacement in patients with aortic stenosis?**

AHA guidelines

- Class I:

    a)   severe AS with symptoms (dyspnoea, angina, syncope);
    b)   severe AS in a patient undergoing cardiac surgery (CABG, mitral valve, thoracic aorta);
    c)   severe AS with left ventricular systolic dysfunction (ejection fraction [EF] <50%).

- Class IIa:

    a)   moderate AS in a patient undergoing cardiac surgery (CABG, mitral valve, thoracic aorta).

- Class IIb:

    a)   severe AS with an abnormal response to exercise (<20mmHg rise in systolic blood pressure);
    b)   severe AS with rapid progression of the stenosis;
    c)   extremely severe AS (mean gradient >60mmHg, peak velocity >5m/s, aortic valve area <0.6cm^2);
    d)   mild AS in a patient undergoing CABG and with rapid progression of the stenosis.

9 **When should patients undergoing CABG have an aortic valve replacement for aortic stenosis?**

AHA guidelines

- Class I: patients with severe AS.
- Class IIa: patients with moderate AS.
- Class IIb: patients with mild AS with moderate to severe calcification or rapid progression of the stenosis.
- It is also important to consider the degree of aortic valve calcification, leaflet movement, left ventricular function (as this may generate a low gradient due to low flow), patient's wishes, patient's age, hypercalcaemia, renal failure and risk of redo aortic valve replacement with patent coronary artery bypass grafts.

10 What is low-flow, low-gradient aortic stenosis and how is it managed?

- Low-flow, low-gradient AS is defined as patients with a low ejection fraction of <40%, a mean pressure gradient of <30mmHg or peak aortic velocity of <3.5m/s and a calculated aortic valve area of <1.0cm^2.
- Dobutamine stress echocardiography, where 5-20µg/kg/min of dobutamine is administered in increments of 5µg every 5 minutes, is used to distinguish:

  a) patients with severe AS but a low gradient (~30mmHg) due to low cardiac output with poor left ventricular function, who would benefit from aortic valve replacement (AVR) (operative mortality 5%);
  b) patients with mild or moderate AS with low flow due to primary contractile dysfunction, who would not benefit from AVR (operative mortality 32%) (Table 2).

263

Table 2. Results of dobutamine stress echocardiography to distinguish severe AS from primary contractile dysfunction.

	Stroke volume	Peak pressure gradient	Aortic valve area
Severe AS	↑	↑	↔
Primary contractile dysfunction	↑	↔	↑ (by >0.2cm^2 or to 1.2cm^2)

- If the stroke volume fails to rise, each case is decided on an individual patient basis.
- Information regarding the degree of leaflet calcification, valve morphology, and leaflet motion on echocardiography and fluoroscopy is also used in the decision making process.

11 How is a patient with asymptomatic aortic stenosis managed?

- Firstly, it is important to ensure the patient does not have any symptoms by detailed questioning and then proceed to an exercise test to determine whether the patient is truly asymptomatic.

- Look for evidence of other AHA criteria for aortic valve replacement surgery:

  a) left ventricular dysfunction;
  b) extremely severe AS;
  c) rapid progression of the stenosis;
  d) if the patient is undergoing other cardiac surgery (CABG, mitral valve, thoracic aorta).

- If the patient is truly asymptomatic and there are no other criteria for surgery, the patient should be followed up with serial echocardiograms and clinic monitoring depending on the severity of the aortic stenosis:

  a) mild - every 5 years;
  b) moderate - every 3 years;
  c) severe - every year.

12 What is the natural history of patients with untreated aortic regurgitation (AR)?

- 6% of asymptomatic patients with good left ventricular function either become symptomatic or develop left ventricular dysfunction per year.
- 25% of asymptomatic patients with left ventricular dysfunction develop symptoms per year.
- Symptomatic patients have a 10% mortality per year.

13 How is aortic regurgitation quantified?

- According to the AHA guidelines, there are five main criteria (Table 3).

Table 3. AHA guidelines for the severity of aortic regurgitation.			
	Mild	Moderate	Severe
Jet width (% LVOT diameter)	<25	25-65	>65
Vena contracta (cm)	<0.3	0.3-0.6	>0.6
Regurgitant volume (mL)	<30	30-60	>60
Regurgitant fraction (%)	<30	30-50	>50
Effective regurgitant orifice area (cm^2)	<0.1	0.1-0.3	>0.3

- Additional criteria used to quantify AR, which are not in the AHA guidelines, are shown below in Table 4.

Table 4. Additional criteria used to quantify the severity of aortic regurgitation.			
	Mild	**Moderate**	**Severe**
Deceleration rate (m/s²)	<2.0	2.0-3.0	>3.0
Pressure half-time (ms)	>400	300-400	<300

- Information regarding the aortic root and ascending aorta dimensions, valve morphology, flow reversal in the descending aorta, changes in left ventricular function and size, and other valvular lesions are also important when assessing AR.

14 What are the causes of aortic regurgitation?

- The aetiology of AR can be sub-divided according to the anatomical location of the disease process:

   a)   leaflet - calcific degeneration, rheumatic fever, bicuspid aortic valve, infective endocarditis;
   b)   annulus, aortic root or ascending aorta - aneurysm, dissection.

- The commonest causes of acute AR include aortic dissection, infective endocarditis and trauma.

15 What are the symptoms of aortic regurgitation?

- Aortic regurgitation is a gradually progressive disease and therefore patients can remain asymptomatic for many years.
- Dyspnoea, orthopnoea and paroxysmal nocturnal dyspnoea due to raised left ventricular end-diastolic pressure, resulting in back pressure onto the lungs.
- Fatigue.
- Congestive cardiac failure and pulmonary oedema when left ventricular compensatory mechanisms are overwhelmed.

16 What are the signs of aortic regurgitation?

- A widened pulse pressure occurs due to augmentation of the total cardiac output resulting in distension of the peripheral arterial system followed by quick collapse secondary to regurgitant flow through the aortic valve. Clinically, this manifests itself through several eponymous signs:

a)   Duroziez's sign - to-and-fro (systolic and diastolic) murmur audible over the femoral artery when compressed with a stethoscope;

b)   Quinke's sign - pulsation in the capillary membranes of the fingertips;

c)   Traube's sign - pistol-shot sound audible over the femoral artery;

d)   De Musset's sign - head bobbing with a collapsing pulse;

e)   Corrigan's pulse - water-hammer collapsing pulse;

f)   Mueller's sign - pulsation of the uvula;

g)   Hill's sign - systolic blood pressure in the leg greater than the systolic pressure in the arm by at least 20mmHg.

- Apical impulse is hyperdynamic and displaced inferolaterally.
- 3rd HS loudest at the apex with the patient lying on their left side using the bell of the stethoscope.
- Decrescendo diastolic murmur heard best at the left sternal edge with the patient sitting forward in expiration.
- Systolic flow murmur related to the ejection of a large stroke volume.
- Austin Flint low-pitched diastolic murmur occurs due to the Bernoulli effect of turbulence on the mitral valve. It is best heard at the apex of the heart with the patient lying on their left side using the bell of the stethoscope.

17 What are the indications for valve replacement in patients with aortic regurgitation?

AHA guidelines

- Class I:

a)   severe AR with symptoms (dyspnoea);

b)   severe AR in patients undergoing cardiac surgery (CABG, mitral valve, thoracic aorta);

c)   severe AR with left ventricular systolic dysfunction (EF <50%).

- Class IIa:

a)   severe AR with left ventricular dilation (end-systolic diameter >55mm and end-diastolic diameter >75mm);

- Class IIb:

  a) severe AR with an abnormal response to exercise (<20mmHg rise in systolic blood pressure);
  b) severe AR with rapid progression of the regurgitation;
  c) severe AR with left ventricular dilation (end-systolic diameter >50mm and end-diastolic diameter >70mm);
  d) moderate AR in patients undergoing cardiac surgery (CABG, mitral valve, thoracic aorta).

18 How is a patient with asymptomatic aortic regurgitation managed?

- Firstly, it is important to ensure the patient does not have any symptoms by detailed questioning and then proceed to an exercise test to determine whether the patient is truly asymptomatic.
- Look for evidence of other AHA criteria for aortic valve replacement surgery:

  a) left ventricular dysfunction;
  b) rapid progression of the regurgitation;
  c) if the patient is undergoing other cardiac surgery (CABG, mitral valve, thoracic aorta).

- If the patient is truly asymptomatic and there are no other criteria for surgery, the patient should be followed up with serial echocardiograms and clinic monitoring depending on the severity of the aortic regurgitation:

  a) mild - every 5 years;
  b) moderate - every 3 years;
  c) severe - every year.

19 When should patients undergoing aortic valve replacement (AVR) with coronary artery disease undergo concomitant bypass grafting?

AHA guidelines

- Class I - coronary stenosis >70%.
- Class IIa - coronary stenosis between 50-70%.

20 Which patients should have aortic valve replacement on an in-hospital urgent basis rather than being placed on a routine elective waiting list?

- Patients with pulmonary oedema and congestive cardiac failure, secondary to decompensated AS or AR.
- Patients with recurrent syncopal episodes with AS.
- Patients with symptoms, such as chest pain or dyspnoea, at rest.

21 What structures are at risk during aortic valve surgery (Figure 7)?

- Anterior mitral valve leaflet (beneath the non-coronary and left coronary cusps).
- Membranous septum (beneath the non-coronary and right coronary cusps).
- Bundle of His (beneath the commissure between the non-coronary and right coronary cusps).
- Left and right coronary ostia.

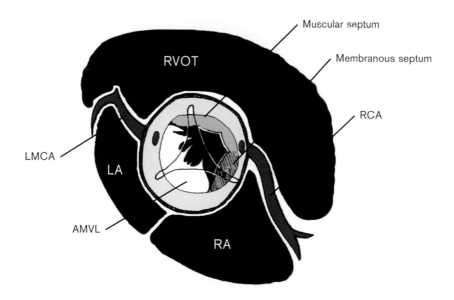

Figure 7. Surgical anatomy and inter-relationships of the aortic valve. RVOT = right ventricular outflow tract; RA = right atrium; LA = left atrium; RCA = right coronary artery; LMCA = left main coronary artery; AMVL = anterior mitral valve leaflet.

22 What are the surgical approaches to the aortic valve?

- Oblique aortotomy (J-shaped).
- Transverse aortotomy.
- Greater curve aortotomy, which can be combined with an aortoplasty to reduce the size of a moderately enlarged ascending aorta.

23 What are the different methods of implanting an aortic valve prosthesis?

- Interrupted sutures technique, which is slower, but has the theoretical reduced risk of a paravalvular leak (Figure 8). It is generally used in patients with friable tissues secondary to endocarditis, often combined with pledgets:

  a) everting sutures place the prosthetic valve in an intra-annular position thereby reducing the relative effective orifice area (EOA) of the annulus allowing a smaller valve to be implanted;
  b) non-everting sutures place the prosthetic valve in a supra-annular position, thereby increasing the effective orifice area of the annulus, allowing a larger valve to be implanted, relative to the everting suture technique.

- Semi-continuous technique, which is faster, but has a theoretical increased risk of a paravalvular leak. By the nature of this technique the sutures are placed using everting sutures but the valve can be positioned into a supra-annular or intra-annular position.

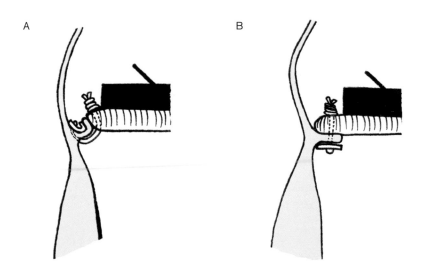

A   B

Figure 8. A) Everting and B) non-everting sutures for aortic valve replacement.

24 What is the definition of patient prosthesis mismatch (PPM)?

- PPM is defined as the EOA of an implanted prosthetic valve being too small relative to the patient's body surface area.
- It is sub-classified by a prosthetic valve EOAI (EOA indexed):

a)   mild - >0.85cm^2/m^2;
b)   moderate - 0.65-0.85cm^2/m^2 ;
c)   severe - <0.65cm^2/m^2.

- Although PPM leads to persistently high transvalvular pressure gradients, reduced left ventricular mass regression, reduced symptom improvement and reduced exercise tolerance, there is controversy regarding the effects of PPM on short and long-term mortality.

25 What surgical options are available in patients with a small aortic root?

A small aortic root results in the inability to implant an aortic valve prosthesis suitable for the patient's size and activity. In view of this several surgical options need to be considered:

- Implanting an aortic valve prosthesis with an improved effective orifice area:

a)   supra-annular (such as Carbomedics Top Hat®, Medtronic SAV);
b)   improved haemodynamics (such as the St Jude Regent®);
c)   small sewing ring (such as the CE Perimount Magna®);
d)   stentless (such as the Elan™ bioprosthesis).

- Aortic root enlargement with a bovine pericardial patch.
- Aortic annular enlargement:

a)   Nicks' annuloplasty (Figure 9);
b)   Manougian's annuloplasty (Figure 10);
c)   Konno.

- Aortic root replacement.
- Apico-aortic valved conduit (composite graft from the left ventricular apex to the descending aorta).

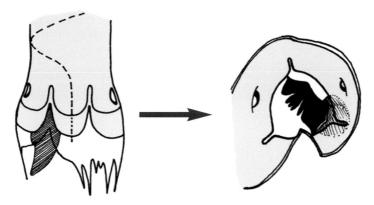

Figure 9. Nick's aortic annuloplasty with the incision passing through the non-coronary sinus.

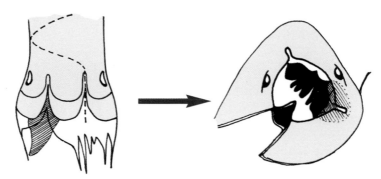

271

Figure 10. Manougian's aortic annuloplasty with the incision passing through the commissure between the left and non-coronary sinuses.

26 How are patients followed up after an aortic valve replacement?

- Ideally all patients have an echocardiogram pre-discharge to look for valve function, paravalvular leak, left ventricular function, pericardial effusion and damage to nearby structures. Furthermore, it serves as a baseline for further surveillance.
- Routine postoperative follow-up comprises of a 6-8 week appointment, a 6 month appointment and then annual out patient visits.
- Mechanical valve patients do not require routine echocardiography follow-up unless the patient develops new symptoms or a murmur.
- Bioprosthesis valve patients, however, require an annual echocardiogram follow-up after 5 years to identify any evidence of structural valve deterioration.

27 What are the approximate peak aortic gradients (mmHg) through prosthetic valves (Table 5)?

Table 5. Peak aortic gradients (mmHg) through prosthetic valves.					
Valve size (mm)	19	21	23	25	27
Carbomedics Top Hat® (M)	30	20	18	16	10
St Jude Regent® (M)	21	16	13	12	8
Edwards Perimount® (B)	28	24	20	18	18

M = mechanical prosthesis; B = biological prosthesis

28 What are the approximate effective orifice areas (EOA cm²) of prosthetic valves (Table 6)?

Table 6. Effective orifice areas (cm²) of prosthetic valves.					
Valve size (mm)	19	21	23	25	27
Carbomedics Top Hat® (M)	1.0	1.5	1.6	2.0	2.4
St Jude Regent® (M)	1.7	2.0	2.5	2.6	3.5
Edwards Perimount® (B)	1.2	1.8	2.0	2.1	2.4

M = mechanical prosthesis; B = biological prosthesis

29 What were the results of the two main randomised controlled trials looking at mechanical and bioprosthetic valve replacements?

Veterans Affairs Trial

- This trial looked at 575 men, who underwent valve replacement (384 aortic valve replacements, 181 mitral valve replacements) between 1987-1992, with a 15-year follow-up.
- Patients who underwent mechanical AVR (Bjork-Shiley®) had a better long-term survival than those with bioprosthetic AVR (Hancock®).
- Patients who underwent mechanical AVR had a lower re-operation at 15 years than those with bioprosthetic AVR (3% vs. 29%).
- There was no evidence of structural valve degeneration of the mechanical prostheses (Bjork-Shiley®).

- In young patients (aged less than 65 years old), structural valve deterioration occurred approximately 7-8 years following bioprosthetic AVR.
- Bioprosthetic valves were associated with less bleeding but the same thrombo-embolism rates as mechanical valves.

Edinburgh Heart Valve Trial

- This trial looked at 541 men and women, who underwent valve replacement (211 aortic valve replacements, 261 mitral valve replacements) between 1975 - 1979, with a 20-year follow-up.
- There was no survival difference between patients who underwent mechanical AVR (Bjork-Shiley®) and bioprosthetic AVR (Hancock®/ Carpentier Edwards porcine).
- Re-operation rates were greater following bioprosthetic AVR than mechanical AVR.
- Thrombo-embolism and prosthetic valve endocarditis rates were the same for both valves.
- Bleeding rates were greater following mechanical AVR than bioprosthetic AVR.

30 When should allografts, autografts and stentless aortic valves be used?

- Aortic valve homografts (allografts) are used for patients with an aortic root abscess or a small aortic root.
- Pulmonary autografts (Ross operation) are used in children but in the absence of connective tissue disorders.
- Stentless aortic valves are usually used depending on surgeon choice, as there is a perceived benefit in avoiding patient prosthesis mismatch. The long-term benefits of this, however, have not been confirmed in the three randomised controlled trials that have been conducted.

31 What is the freedom from structural valve deterioration (Figure 11) for the different aortic valve prostheses?

- For patients greater than 70 years old, the freedom from structural valve deterioration at 15 years is:

    a) mechanical prosthesis - 97%;
    b) aortic valve homograft - 85%;
    c) bovine pericardial valve - 85%;
    d) porcine bioprosthesis - 80%;
    e) stentless bioprosthesis - 80%;
    f) pulmonary autograft (Ross) - 74% for the aortic valve, 80% for the pulmonary valve.

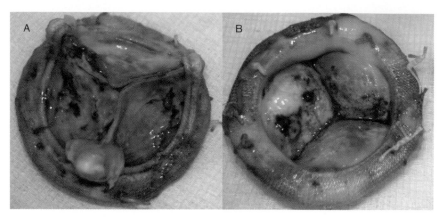

Figure 11. Structural valve deterioration, demonstrated by thickening and calcification of the bovine pericardial leaflets. A) Aortic side. B) Left ventricular side.

- Structural valve deterioration (SVD) in bioprosthetic valves is greater in the younger population due to increased haemodynamic demands. SVD at 10 years is:

  a) 40% in patients aged 0-40 years;
  b) 30% in patients aged 40-69 years;
  c) 10% in patients aged >70 years.

- Structural valve deterioration and calcification occur at the areas of greatest stress, such as commissures and zones of flexion.

32 What is the significance of a patient with a bicuspid aortic valve?

- It is the commonest congenital cardiac condition, occurring in 1-2% of the population, with an autosomal dominant inheritance pattern.
- Patients with a bicuspid aortic valve are more likely to have:

  a) a short left main stem coronary artery;
  b) a left dominant coronary artery circulation;
  c) an anomalous position of the coronary ostia;
  d) aortopathy resulting in dissection or aneurysm;
  e) coarctation of the aorta;
  f) earlier onset of aortic stenosis.

- Histological analysis of the aorta in patients with a bicuspid aortic valve reveals cystic medial necrosis, reduced fibrillin-1 production and elastin fragmentation.

33 What factors should be considered when choosing between a mechanical and bioprosthetic aortic valve (Figures 12-14)?

- Prosthesis type does not influence survival, thrombo-embolism or infective endocarditis rates.
- Bleeding is more frequent with mechanical valves.
- SVD is more common with bioprosthetic valves.
- Mechanical valves are the preferred choice if:

   a)   the patient is already on warfarin with another mechanical valve;

   b)   the patient is young (age <60) and does not want another operation.

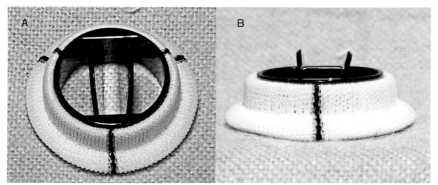

Figure 12. Bileaflet mechanical aortic valve from: A) top view; and B) side view.

- Bioprosthetic valves are the preferred choice if:

   a)   the patient is aged >65;

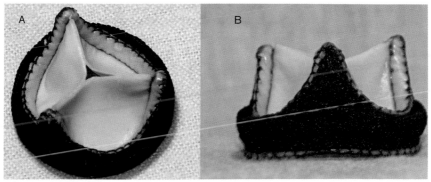

Figure 13. Bovine pericardial bioprosthetic aortic valve from: A) top view; and B) side view.

b)   the patient wants to avoid warfarin (patient preference, contra-indication to warfarin, woman of child-bearing age, young patient with active lifestyle, recent GI bleed, awaiting future operation for malignancy, etc).

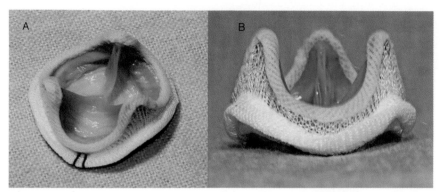

Figure 14. Porcine bioprosthetic aortic valve from: A) top view; and B) side view.

276

34 What valve should be used in patients with renal failure on haemodialysis?

- The AHA guidelines in 1998 suggested using a mechanical prosthesis; however, the AHA guidelines in 2006 made no recommendation.
- It has been suggested that most modern bioprosthetic valves will last longer than these patients with end-stage renal failure, hence by implanting a bioprosthetic valve, it is possible to avoid the use of long-term anticoagulation in these difficult cases.

35 How is a patient with a thrombosed aortic valve managed?

AHA guidelines

- Patients with NYHA III-IV symptoms or a large thrombus burden should undergo an emergency operation.
- Patients with NYHA I-II symptoms or a small clot burden should undergo fibrinolysis.

36 **What factors should be considered when choosing which aortic valve prosthesis to implant in women of child-bearing age?**

- Bioprosthetic valves degenerate quicker in younger patients and this process can be accelerated by pregnancy.
- Mechanical valves obligate the need for anticoagulation and this may cause problems with warfarin during pregnancy.
- A pulmonary autograft or aortic homograft can be used but would involve complex subsequent redo surgery.
- One strategy would be to consider a bioprosthesis until the patient has completed her family and then replace it with a mechanical valve when the bioprosthesis degenerates.

37 **What are the important factors to consider in a pregnant patient with a mechanical valve *in situ*?**

- It is critical to explain the risks and benefits of all the options to the patient and her partner.
- As warfarin crosses the placenta, there is an increased risk of abortion, prematurity and stillbirth.
- Warfarin is also associated with a risk of embryopathy (in 5-10% of patients but is lower if the dose is <5mg/day). It is thought to probably be safe to use warfarin during weeks 1-6 and during the second and third trimesters.
- Heparin, however, does not cross the placenta and therefore does not cause embryopathy but may induce bleeding at the uteroplacental junction.
- One strategy in the management of a pregnant patient with a mechanical valve *in situ* includes:

  a) warfarin during weeks 1-6;
  b) unfractionated heparin during weeks 6-12;
  c) warfarin during weeks 12-36;
  d) unfractionated heparin from week 36;
  e) stop heparin before delivery;
  f) restart unfractionated heparin 4-6 hours post-placental separation once bleeding is controlled.

38 Describe the options available for minimally invasive aortic valve replacement

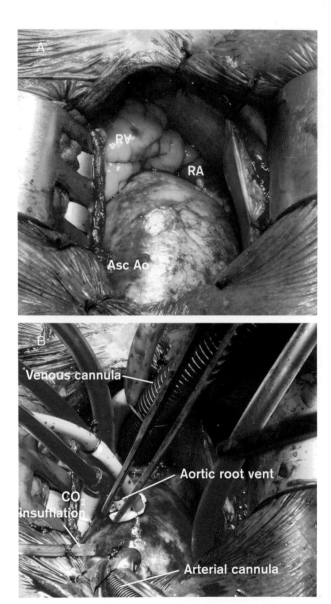

Figure 15. A) Cardiac structures exposed following an upper hemisternotomy. B) Set-up for an aortic valve replacement through an upper hemi-sternotomy prior to aortotomy. RA = right atrium; RV = right ventricle; Asc Ao = ascending aorta.

- Hemisternotomy (Figure 15) - performed with a J-shaped incision from the suprasternal notch to the 4th intercostal space on the right.
- Transcatheter aortic valve implantation (TAVI):

  a) transapical route - via a small left anterior thoracotomy, which allows the aortic valve to be approached in an antegrade direction (see below);
  b) transfemoral route - via the femoral artery, which allows the aortic valve to be approached in a retrograde direction.

39 Describe the steps involved in a transapical transcatheter aortic valve implantation (Figure 16)

- General anaesthesia.
- A temporary right ventricular pacing wire is inserted via the left femoral vein.
- A pig-tail catheter is inserted into the aortic root via the right femoral artery and is used for contrast injection and pressure measurements.
- A small (approximately 5cm) left anterior thoracotomy is performed, usually made in the 6th intercostal space but echocardiography is used to locate the left ventricular apex.
- The pericardium is incised anterior to the left phrenic nerve to gain access to the left ventricular apex.
- A pledgeted 2/0 Prolene® purse string is placed at the apex of the left ventricle.
- Using a stab incision, a balloon dilator is passed through the apex and positioned across the aortic valve using fluoroscopic guidance.
- Using rapid ventricular pacing (200 bpm) to reduce cardiac output across the aortic valve, the balloon is dilated to 45 atmospheres for 5 seconds.
- The preloaded crimped stented valve is then passed through the left ventricular apex and again positioned across the aortic valve using fluoroscopic guidance.
- Again using rapid ventricular pacing (200 bpm), the balloon inside the valve is dilated to 45 atmospheres for 5 seconds.
- Transoesophageal echocardiography is used to check positioning of the implanted aortic valve prosthesis and for the presence of any paravalvular regurgitation.

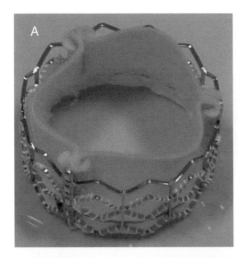
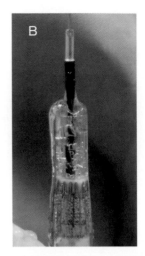

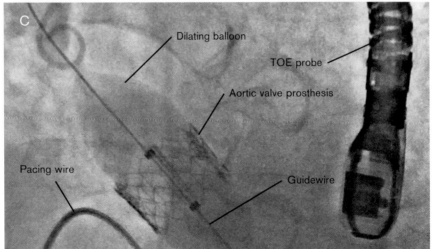

Figure 16. Transcatheter aortic valve implantation. A) Transcatheter aortic valve prosthesis, consisting of bovine pericardial leaflets attached to a balloon-expandable stainless steel stent. B) Crimped transcatheter aortic valve prosthesis mounted on a balloon catheter. C) Fluoroscopy image demonstrating expansion of the catheter balloon and deployment of the prosthesis across the aortic valve.

Recommended reading

1.   Bonow RO, Carabello BA, Kanu C, de Leon AC Jr, Faxon DP, Freed MD, Gaasch WH, Lytle BW, Nishimura RA, O'Gara PT, O'Rourke RA, Otto CM, Shah PM, Shanewise JS, Smith SC Jr, Jacobs AK, Adams CD, Anderson JL, Antman EM, Faxon DP, Fuster V, Halperin JL, Hiratzka LF, Hunt SA, Lytle BW, Nishimura R, Page RL,

Riegel B. ACC/AHA 2006 Guidelines for the management of patients with valvular heart disease. *Circulation* 2006; 114; e84-e231.

2. Oxenham H, Bloomfield P, Wheatley DJ, Lee RJ, Cunningham J, Prescott RJ, Miller HC. Twenty-year comparison of a Bjork-Shiley mechanical heart valve with porcine bioprostheses. *Heart* 2003; 89(7): 715-21.

3. Hammermeister K, Sethi GK, Henderson WG, Grover FL, Oprian C, Rahimtoola SH. Outcomes 15 years after valve replacement with a mechanical versus a bioprosthetic valve: final report of the Veterans Affairs randomized trial. *J Am Coll Cardiol* 2000; 36(4): 1152-8.

4. Pibarot P, Dumesnil JG. Prosthesis-patient mismatch: definition, clinical impact, and prevention. *Heart* 2006; 92(8): 1022-9.

5. Nicks R, Cartmill T, Bernstein L. Hypoplasia of the aortic root. The problem of aortic valve replacement. *Thorax* 1970; 25: 339-46.

6. Manouguian S, Seybold-Epting W. Patch enlargement of the aortic valve ring by extending the aortic incision into the anterior mitral leaflet. *J Thorac Cardiovasc Surg* 1979; 78: 402-12.

7. Monin JL, Quéré JP, Monchi M, Petit H, Baleynaud S, Chauvel C, Pop C, Ohlmann P, Lelguen C, Dehant P, Tribouilloy C, Guéret P. Low-gradient aortic stenosis: operative risk stratification and predictors for long-term outcome: a multicenter study using dobutamine stress hemodynamics. *Circulation* 2003; 108(3): 319-24.

Chapter 13

Mitral valve disease

1   What is the natural history of mitral regurgitation (MR)?

- Asymptomatic patients can have a long latent period before the onset of symptoms as chronic MR is well tolerated if left ventricular function is well preserved.
- Deterioration in left ventricular function, however, is masked by the unloading effect of a leaking valve resulting in a pseudo-normal left ventricular ejection fraction (EF).
- Poor prognostic features of MR include:

  a)   symptoms for >1 year;
  b)   atrial fibrillation;
  c)   age >60 yr;
  d)   EF <50%;
  e)   left ventricular end-diastolic volume >100mL/m^2, left ventricular end-systolic volume >60mL/m^2;
  f)   left ventricular end-systolic diameter >5cm, left ventricular end-diastolic diameter >7cm.

2   What is the pathophysiology of mitral regurgitation?

- Chronic left ventricular volume overload associated with MR leads to eccentric hypertrophy of the left ventricle.
- Stroke volume is initially maintained by the Frank-Starling mechanism.
- Eventually left ventricular contractile function declines producing increased left ventricular end-systolic volume, raised left ventricular filling pressures, and raised left atrial and pulmonary venous pressures, finally resulting in pulmonary oedema and congestive heart failure.
- Once the left ventricular ejection fraction falls below approximately 60%, left ventricular systolic dysfunction is almost certainly present as some of the ejected volume flows into the left atrium (afterload-reducing effect of MR).

3   How is mitral regurgitation classified?

- According to Carpentier's functional classification (Figure 1):

   a)   Type I: normal leaflet motion, e.g. annular dilation, leaflet perforation;

   b)   Type II: excess leaflet motion, e.g. myxomatous degeneration, chordal rupture;

   c)   Type III: restricted leaflet motion:

       i)   IIIa: restricted opening, e.g. rheumatic fever;

       ii)   IIIb: restricted closure, e.g. ischaemic cardiomyopathy.

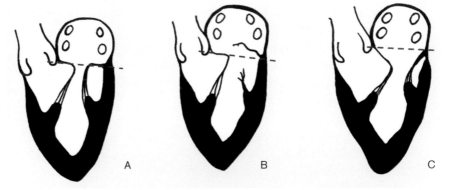

Figure 1. Carpentier's functional classification of mitral regurgitation. A) Type I - normal leaflet motion usually producing central regurgitation. B) Type II - excessive leaflet motion above the annular plane usually producing eccentric regurgitation. C) Type III - restricted leaflet motion below the annular plane usually producing eccentric regurgitation.

4   What are the causes of chronic mitral regurgitation?

- Myxomatous degeneration (Type II).
- Rheumatic fever (Type IIIa).
- Ischaemic cardiomyopathy (mainly Type IIIb and Type I, see below).

5   What are the causes of acute mitral regurgitation?

- Chordal rupture (Type II).
- Infective endocarditis (Type I).
- Papillary muscle rupture (following myocardial infarction, Type II)(Figure 2).

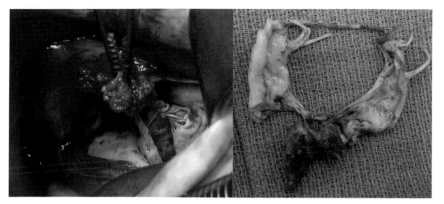

Figure 2. Papillary muscle rupture following acute myocardial infarction.

6   What is the aetiology of ischaemic mitral regurgitation?

- Acute ischaemic MR is usually caused by infarcted, ruptured or non-ruptured papillary muscle (Type II).
- Chronic ischaemic MR is caused by a combination of restricted movement of P2 and P3 scallops of the posterior mitral valve (MV) leaflet due to left ventricular dilation displacing the papillary muscles (Type IIIb) and functional dilation of the MV annulus (Type I).
- In addition, reduced contraction of the MV annulus and reduced ventricular closing forces on the MV due to poor LV function contribute to ischaemic MR.

7   What are the symptoms of mitral regurgitation?

- Mitral regurgitation is a progressive disease and hence patients can be asymptomatic for many years.
- Fatigue and weakness related to low cardiac output.
- Dyspnoea, orthopnoea and paroxysmal nocturnal dyspnoea.
- Eventually patients may develop pulmonary hypertension and right heart failure.

8   What are the signs of mitral regurgitation?

- Displaced volume-loaded apex beat.
- Apical thrill.
- 3rd heart sound.
- Apical pansystolic murmur - radiating to the axilla (the intensity of the murmur does not necessarily correlate with the severity of MR).

- Apical diastolic flow murmur (due to increased flow across the MV in diastole).
- Right ventricular heave and an increased pulmonary component of the 2nd heart sound (if pulmonary hypertension is present).

9 How is mitral regurgitation quantified echocardio-graphically?

- According to the American Heart Association (AHA) guidelines, there are five main criteria (Table 1).

Table 1. AHA guidelines for the severity of mitral regurgitation.			
	Mild	Moderate	Severe
Jet area (% LA area)	<20%	20-40%	>40%
Vena contracta (cm)	<0.3	0.3-0.7	>0.7
Regurgitant volume (mL)	<30	30-60	>60
Regurgitant fraction (%)	<30	30-50	>50
Effective regurgitant orifice area (cm^2)	<0.2	0.2-0.4	>0.4

- Information regarding the left atrial size, valve morphology, flow reversal in the pulmonary veins, the underlying aetiology of MR, and changes in left ventricular function and size are also important when assessing the severity of MR.
- For ischaemic MR, regurgitant volume >30mL and an effective regurgitant orifice area >0.2cm^2 are considered severe.
- Vena contracta refers to the narrowest part of the regurgitant jet just after the valve orifice.

10 What are the indications for mitral valve surgery in patients with mitral regurgitation?

AHA guidelines

- Class I: severe MR with symptoms (NYHA II-IV) or left ventricular changes (end-systolic diameter >40mm or EF <60%).
- Class IIa: severe MR in an asymptomatic patient with good LV function and size, where the likelihood of repair in the operating centre is >90%.

- Class IIa: severe MR with AF or pulmonary hypertension (>50mmHg at rest or 60mmHg with exercise).
- Class IIb: severe MR, poor left ventricular function (EF <30%) and symptoms (NYHA III-IV) despite maximal anti-failure medical therapy and biventricular pacing.

11 When should transoesophageal echocardiography (TOE) be performed in patients with severe mitral regurgitation?

AHA guidelines

- Class I: intra-operative TOE, pre-bypass to assess the feasibility of repair and post-bypass to assess the success of the repair.
- Class IIa: pre-operative TOE to guide whether asymptomatic patients have a >90% chance of repair (see AHA guidelines on MR).

12 What is mitral valve prolapse due to Barlow's disease?

- Mitral valve prolapse is defined as >2mm billowing of the anterior or posterior mitral valve leaflet beyond the annular plane into the left atrium with or without MR.
- It can be familial or non-familial and may be associated with Marfan syndrome.
- Histological analysis reveals marked myxomatous proliferation of acid mucopolysaccharides within the zona spongiosa of the mitral valve leaflets, resulting in thinning and elongation of the chordae tendinae.
- Patients with mitral valve prolapse can be asymptomatic or present with severe MR or arrhythmias (atrial fibrillation or ventricular tachycardia).
- Surgery is indicated as per AHA guidelines for non-ischaemic MR.

13 What is the natural history of mitral stenosis (MS)?

- Patients usually become symptomatic on exertion when the mitral valve area (MVA) becomes <2.5cm^2 and symptomatic at rest when the MVA becomes <1.5cm^2.
- The natural progression of MS causes the mitral valve area to reduce by 0.1-0.3cm^2 per year.
- The progression from onset of rheumatic fever to onset of signs of MS takes 10-20 years.
- The progression from signs of MS to mild symptoms of MS takes 10-20 years.

- The progression from mild symptoms of MS to decompensation (often precipitated by AF) takes 10-20 years.
- The 10-year survival is 80% (in patients with NYHA I/II symptoms) and 10-15% (in patients with NYHA III/IV symptoms).
- In patients with pulmonary hypertension (>50mmHg), the mean survival is 3 years.

14 What is the pathophysiology of mitral stenosis?

- Restricted left ventricular inflow results in increased left atrial pressure; back pressure on the pulmonary circulation causes dyspnoea and eventually pulmonary hypertension, right ventricular failure and subsequent left ventricular failure.
- Pulmonary hypertension occurs secondary to compensatory vasoconstriction and hypertrophy of the pulmonary arterioles.
- The patient's haemodynamic state is worsened by tachycardia or atrial fibrillation which reduces the diastolic filling period.

288

15 What are the causes of mitral stenosis?

- The majority of cases are caused by rheumatic fever (Lancefield group A β-haemolytic *Streptococcus*)(Figure 3).
- Very rare causes include a congenital parachute mitral valve, endocardial fibroelastosis and carcinoid syndrome.
- The pathophysiology of MS can also be caused by cor triatriatum, left atrial myxoma and pulmonary vein stenosis.

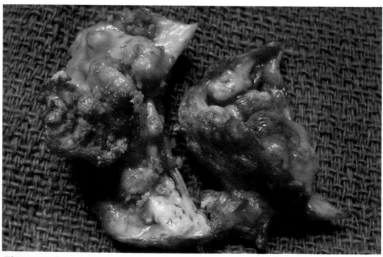

Figure 3. Rheumatic mitral stenosis.

16 What are the symptoms of mitral stenosis?

- Mitral stenosis has a long latent period and therefore can be asymptomatic for many years.
- Fatigue.
- Dyspnoea, orthopnoea and paroxysmal nocturnal dyspnoea.
- Left atrial distension resulting in:

  a) atrial fibrillation and subsequent thrombo-embolic events;
  b) left recurrent laryngeal nerve compression presenting with hoarseness (Ortner's syndrome);
  c) oesophageal compression producing dysphagia;
  d) rarely, left main bronchus compression causing left lung collapse.

- Pulmonary hypertension and right heart failure which present as:

  a) peripheral oedema and ascites;
  b) haemoptysis due to distension and rupture of bronchial veins.

17 What are the signs of mitral stenosis?

- Low volume pulse.
- Irregular pulse.
- Tapping non-displaced apex beat.
- Opening snap.
- Loud S1 heart sound.
- Mid-diastolic rumbling murmur loudest at the apex.
- Pulmonary hypertension:

  a) mitral facies;
  b) central cyanosis;
  c) loud P2 heart sound;
  d) tricuspid regurgitation - pan-systolic murmur at the right sternal edge;
  e) pulmonary regurgitation - Graham Steel early diastolic murmur on inspiration.

18 How is mitral stenosis quantified?

- According to the American Heart Association (AHA) guidelines, there are three main criteria:

	Mild	Moderate	Severe
Table 2. AHA guidelines for the severity of mitral stenosis.			
Mitral valve area (cm^2)	>1.5	1.0-1.5	<1.0
Mean pressure gradient (mmHg)	<5	5-10	>10
Pulmonary artery systolic pressure (mmHg)	<30	30-50	>50

- The mitral valve area (MVA) can be calculated by:

a) planimetry: short axis mitral valve on 2D echocardiography;

b) pressure half-time (PHT) equation: $MVA = \dfrac{220}{PHT}$

where MVA = mitral valve area, PHT = pressure half-time;

c) continuity equation: $MVA = \dfrac{Area_{LVOT} \times VTI_{LVOT}}{VTI_{MV}}$

where LVOT = left ventricular outflow tract, VTI = velocity time integral, MV = mitral valve;

d) Gorlin equation: $MVA = \dfrac{CO}{38 \times HR \times DFP \times \sqrt{mean\ gradient}}$

where CO = cardiac output, HR = heart rate, DFP = diastolic filling period.

- Information regarding the left atrial size, valve morphology, presence of left atrial thrombus, underlying aetiology of MS, and changes in left ventricular function and size are also important when assessing the severity of mitral stenosis.

19 What are the indications for mitral valve surgery in patients with mitral stenosis?

AHA guidelines

- Class I: moderate-severe MS with symptoms (NYHA III-IV) where percutaneous mitral balloon valvuloplasty (PMBV) is not suitable (see below).

- Class IIa: severe MS with severe pulmonary hypertension (>50mmHg) or symptoms (NYHA I-II) where PMBV is not suitable.
- Class IIb: moderate-severe MS with recurrent embolic events on anticoagulation.

20 What are the determinants of the Wilkins mitral stenosis score (Figure 4)?

- Leaflet mobility, leaflet thickening, leaflet calcification and subvalvular thickening.
- Each scores between 0-4, with a maximum score of 16.
- A Wilkins score >9 suggests the lesion is unlikely to be amenable to PMBV.

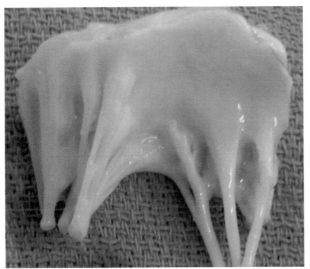

Figure 4. Thickening of the mitral valve leaflet and sub-valvular apparatus, associated with mitral stenosis.

21 What are the indications for percutaneous mitral balloon valvuloplasty (PMBV) in patients with mitral stenosis?

AHA guidelines

- Class I: moderate-severe MS with either symptoms (NYHA II-IV) or pulmonary hypertension (>50mmHg at rest or 60mmHg on exercise).

- Class IIa: moderate-severe MS with symptoms (NYHA III-IV) in patients with a non-pliable valve or in patients who are at a high surgical risk of death.

  PMBV should be only performed in patients with favourable valve morphology (Wilkins score of 8 or less) and no contraindications (left atrial thrombus, moderate-severe MR).

22 How is percutaneous mitral balloon valvuloplasty (PMBV) performed?

- Using local anaesthetic and sedation, a valvuloplasty balloon is passed via the femoral vein into the right atrium, across the intra-atrial septum, into the left atrium, across the mitral valve and inflated (Figure 5).
- Results are best when the leaflets are thin, mobile, not calcified, in the younger age group and where the subvalvular chordae have not fused/calcified.

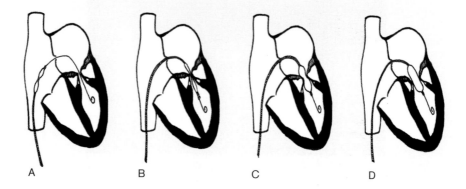

A   B   C   D

Figure 5. Percutaneous trans-septal mitral balloon valvuloplasty. The femoral vein is accessed using 9-11Fr sheaths. A) The coiled tip guide wire is then advanced into the left ventricle, via the right atrium, interatrial septum, left atrium and mitral valve. B) A valvuloplasty balloon (Jomiva™, Numed, Hopkinton, New York, USA or Inoue-Balloon™, Toray International America Inc., Houston, USA) is advanced into the mitral valve orifice using transoesophageal echocardiography and fluoroscopy guidance. C) The balloon is then progressively inflated with controlled hydraulic pressure, until a satisfactory diameter is reached. D) Following completion, the balloon is deflated and the mitral valve function is assessed.

- PMBV typically increases the mitral valve area from 1 to 2cm^2.
- Complications include mortality 1%, cardiac perforation 1%, stroke 2% and severe MR 3%.

23 How is a closed mitral valvotomy performed?

- Following a left posterolateral thoracotomy, the pericardium is opened anterior to the phrenic nerve. An index finger is then inserted into the left atrium and a Tubbs dilator is passed via the apex through the left ventricle, using purse strings to reduce blood loss and air embolism. The dilator is then guided manually through the mitral valve orifice and opened along the natural inter-commissural line. The resulting dilation is assessed manually and by transoesophageal echocardiography (Figure 6).

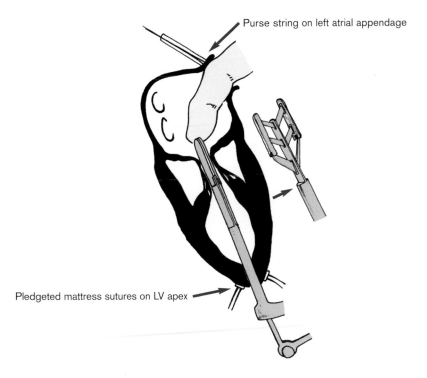

Purse string on left atrial appendage

Pledgeted mattress sutures on LV apex

Figure 6. Closed mitral valvotomy.

24 What are the surgical approaches to the mitral valve (Figure 7)?

- Standard left atriotomy:

    a)   the pericardial reflections around the inferior and superior pulmonary veins are mobilised;

    b)   Waterson's interatrial groove is developed thereby reflecting the right atrium back over the left atrium;

    c)   an incision is then made in the left atrium anterior and medial to the right superior pulmonary vein and continued inferiorly.

- Bi-atrial trans-septal incision, where an oblique incision from the right atrial free wall through the right atrial appendage and down to the left atrial roof, is joined by a second incision (dashed red line) through the fossa ovalis, medial to the crista terminalis, from the Eustachian valve to the edge of the superior limbus. The sino-atrial nodal artery is at risk during this incision.

- Superior roof incision, where an incision is made across the right atrial free wall and continued between the superior vena cava and the right atrial appendage. From there, it is extended across the interatrial septum and the roof of the left atrium passing behind the aortic root towards the commissure between the left coronary cusp and the non-coronary cusp. There is a risk of damage to the left main coronary artery, non-coronary sinus of the aorta and superior vena cava.

- Bi-atrial (Dubost) incision, where a vertical incision is made between the right superior and inferior pulmonary veins, which extends across

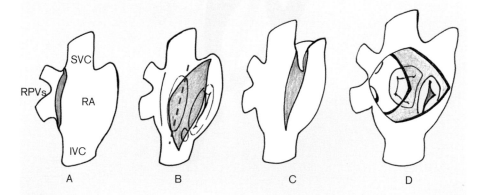

Figure 7. Surgical approaches to the mitral valve. A) Standard left atriotomy. B) Bi-atrial vertical trans-septal incision. C) Superior roof incision. D) Bi-atrial Dubost incision. SVC = superior vena cava; IVC = inferior vena cava; RA = right atrium; RPVs = right pulmonary veins.

the left atrium, right atrium and interatrial septum. It allows good access but can be difficult to close.
- Right anterolateral thoracotomy, which is used for minimal access or redo surgery.

25 How is the mitral valve assessed intra-operatively?
- The valve is inspected using nerve hooks to measure the degree of motion of each scallop (P1, P2, P3, A1, A2, A3) of both leaflets compared against a reference point (usually P1 or the anterolateral commissure).
- The valve competency can be checked before repair by distending the left ventricle with cold saline and identifying the aetiology and location of the regurgitation jet.
- Competence of the valve following repair is assessed by:

  a) static testing under direct vision by distending the left ventricle with cold saline;
  b) TOE with an appropriately filled left ventricle off cardiopulmonary bypass support.

26 What structures are at risk during mitral valve surgery (Figure 8)?

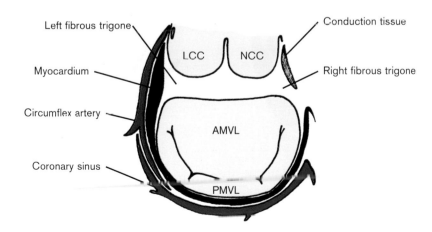

Figure 8. Anatomical relations of the mitral valve. AMVL = anterior mitral valve leaflet; PMVL = posterior mitral valve leaflet; LCC = left coronary cusp of the aortic valve; NCC = non-coronary cusp of the aortic valve.

- Circumflex coronary artery.
- Coronary sinus.
- Aortic valve (left and non-coronary cusps).
- Atrioventricular node and conducting bundles.

27 What is systolic anterior motion (SAM) of the mitral valve?

- Systolic anterior motion occurs when the tips of the mitral valve leaflets are displaced anteriorly into the left ventricular outflow tract. This results in a Venturi effect pulling on the mitral valve leaflets causing MR and left ventricular outflow tract obstruction. In comparison, during diastole the left ventricular outflow diameter is normal (Figure 9).
- SAM is more common in patients with hypertrophic obstructive cardiomyopathy (HOCM) and small elderly women with asymmetric septal hypertrophy.

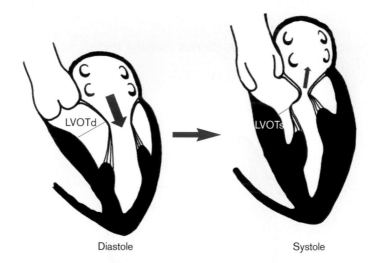

Diastole   Systole

Figure 9. Systolic anterior motion (SAM) of the mitral valve. LVOTd = left ventricular outflow tract in diastole; LVOTs = left ventricular outflow tract in systole.

28 How is systolic anterior motion (SAM) of the mitral valve prevented?

- The risk of SAM can be reduced by avoiding excess anterior mitral valve leaflet tissue or excess height of the posterior mitral valve leaflet

(>1.5cm), as this will cause the line of leaflet coaptation to be displaced anteriorly into the left ventricular outflow tract.

- SAM is exacerbated by hypovolaemia, excess inotropes and tachycardia.

29 How is systolic anterior motion (SAM) post-mitral valve repair treated?

- Conservative - ensure adequate volume status, increase afterload, reduce tachycardia, reduce inotropes.
- Surgical (Figure 10) - remove the annuloplasty ring then consider:

    a)   sliding annuloplasty to reduce the height of the posterior mitral valve leaflet;

    b)   implanting an incomplete mitral annuloplasty ring (e.g. Cosgrove® or Duran®);

    c)   increasing the size, particularly the anteroposterior (AP) diameter, of the mitral annuloplasty ring;

    d)   implanting a low profile prosthetic mitral valve (e.g. St Jude® mechanical prosthesis).

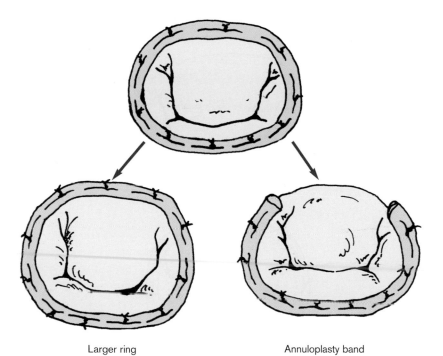

Larger ring   Annuloplasty band

Figure 10. Surgical management of systolic anterior motion (SAM) of the mitral valve includes implanting a larger annuloplasty ring or implanting an annuloplasty band.

30 What are the surgical treatment options for diseases of the mitral valve?

- Posterior MVL prolapse (Figures 11 and 12A): quadrangular or triangular resection, sliding annuloplasty, artificial chord implantation.

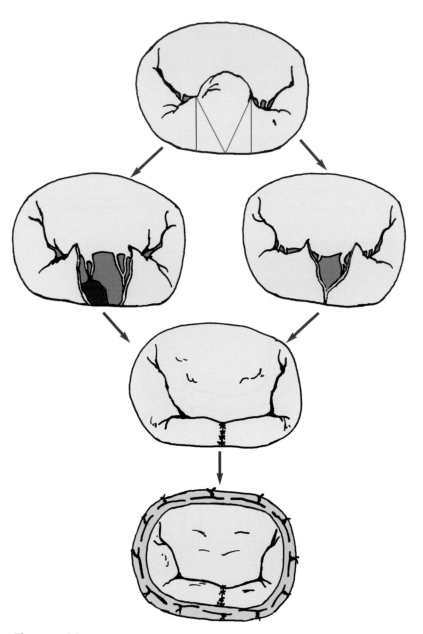

Figure 11. Surgical options for prolapse of the P2 segment of the posterior mitral valve leaflet include quadrangular resection (left image) or triangular resection (right image). This is followed by reattaching the P1 and P3 segments and implantation of an annuloplasty ring.

- Anterior MVL prolapse (Figure 12B): triangular resection, artificial chord implantation.
- Bileaflet MV prolapse: leaflet resection, artificial chord implantation, Alfieri stitch, MV replacement.
- Partial papillary muscle rupture: reimplantation of the papillary muscle.
- Complete papillary muscle rupture: MV replacement.

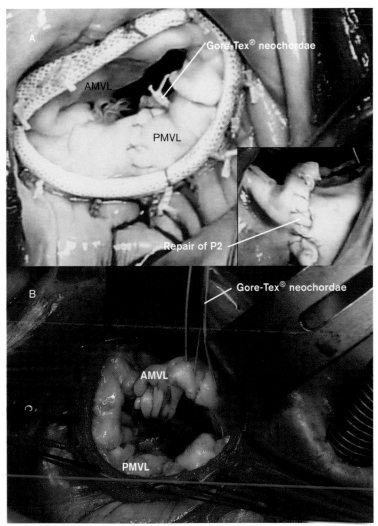

Figure 12. Operative images following mitral valve repair. A) Posterior mitral valve leaflet prolapse treated by triangular resection of the P2 segment, implantation of Gore-Tex® neochordae and ring annuloplasty. B) Anterior mitral valve leaflet prolapse treated by implantation of Gore-Tex® neochordae and ring annuloplasty. AMVL = anterior mitral valve leaflet; PMVL = posterior mitral valve leaflet.

- Leaflet perforation: bovine pericardial patch.
- Annular dilation: complete flexible annuloplasty ring (e.g. Physio®)
- Ischaemic MR: McCarthy-Adams IMR® ring, downsizing annuloplasty, MV replacement.
- Rheumatic MS: MV replacement.

31 When is a sliding annuloplasty used in addition to a simple quadrangular resection (Figure 13)?

- Following excessive posterior mitral valve leaflet resection.
- To reduce the risk of SAM (where the posterior mitral valve leaflet height is greater than 1.5cm or there is a long anterior mitral valve leaflet).

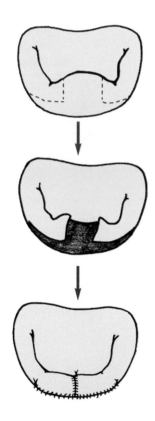

Figure 13. Posterior mitral valve leaflet repair with quadrangular resection and sliding annuloplasty. Quadrangular resection of the P2 segment is followed by partially detaching the P1 and P3 segments from the posterior mitral valve annulus. The repair is completed by reattaching the P1 and P3 segments to each other and then to the posterior annulus, thereby decreasing the height of the posterior leaflet. The repair procedure is completed with implantation of an annuloplasty ring.

32 What are the benefits of a mitral annuloplasty ring?

- Corrects annular dilation.
- Prevents further annular dilation.
- Increases leaflet coaptation.
- Reinforces annular suture lines.

33 What are the features of each of the different mitral valve ring prostheses (Figure 14)?

- Carpentier-McCarthy-Adams IMR ETlogix Annuloplasty Ring® - for ischaemic MR.
- Cosgrove-Edwards Annuloplasty System® (incomplete, flexible) - when concerned about SAM (with excess anterior mitral valve leaflet height in comparison to the intercommissural distance, as an incomplete ring does not fix the anterior mitral valve leaflet).

A   B

C   D

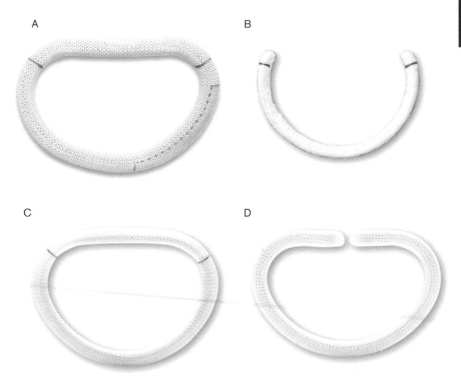

Figure 14. Mitral valve annuloplasty rings (Edwards Lifesciences, Irvine, USA). A) Carpentier-McCarthy-Adams IMR ETlogix Annuloplasty Ring®. B) Cosgrove-Edwards Annuloplasty System®. C) Carpentier-Edwards Physio Annuloplasty Ring®. D) Carpentier-Edwards Classic Annuloplasty Ring®.

- Carpentier-Edwards Physio Annuloplasty Ring® (complete, semi-flexible) - frequently used annuloplasty ring.
- Carpentier ring® (rigid, complete) - where the AP diameter can be adjusted for a bespoke ring shape.

34 What are the advantages of repairing the mitral valve rather than replacing it?

- As compared with mitral valve replacement, mitral valve repair is associated with greater freedom from mortality (operative and long-term), structural valve deterioration, re-operation, infective endocarditis, thrombo-embolism and haemorrhage.
- As more of the sub-valvular apparatus is preserved, mitral valve repair is better at maintaining left ventricular geometry and hence is associated with less left ventricular dysfunction compared with mitral valve replacement.

35 Describe the therapeutic options for ischaemic mitral regurgitation

- Coronary artery bypass grafting.
- Implantation of a mitral valve annuloplasty ring (McCarthy-Adams IMR ring®), which is specifically designed with a reduced anterior-posterior diameter and a concavity in the region of the P2/P3 scallops.
- Downsizing annuloplasty of the mitral valve.
- Mitral valve replacement.

36 What is the freedom from re-intervention for patients older than 70 years for the different mitral valve prostheses and repair techniques available?

- Repair of anterior mitral valve leaflet - 78% at 10 years.
- Repair of posterior mitral valve leaflet - 98% at 10 years.
- Open mitral valve commissurotomy - 80% at 10 years.
- Closed mitral valve commissurotomy - 70% at 10 years.
- Percutaneous mitral balloon valvuloplasty - 80% at 10 years.
- Porcine bioprosthesis - 75% at 10 years.
- Bovine pericardial bioprosthesis - 80% at 10 years.
- Mechanical prosthesis - 98% at 10 years.

37 How is atrioventricular disruption following mitral valve replacement treated?

- Put the patient back on cardiopulmonary bypass.
- Remove the prosthetic valve.
- Implant a bovine pericardial patch across the atrioventricular groove.
- Implant a smaller prosthetic valve with a low profile.
- Avoid lifting the heart with the prosthesis *in situ*.

Recommended reading

1. Bonow RO, Carabello BA, Kanu C, de Leon AC Jr, Faxon DP, Freed MD, Gaasch WH, Lytle BW, Nishimura RA, O'Gara PT, O'Rourke RA, Otto CM, Shah PM, Shanewise JS, Smith SC Jr, Jacobs AK, Adams CD, Anderson JL, Antman EM, Faxon DP, Fuster V, Halperin JL, Hiratzka LF, Hunt SA, Lytle BW, Nishimura R, Page RL, Riegel B. ACC/AHA 2006 Guidelines for the management of patients with valvular heart disease. *Circulation* 2006; 114; e84-e231.

2. Levine RA, Schwammenthal E. Ischemic mitral regurgitation on the threshold of a solution: from paradoxes to unifying concepts. *Circulation* 2005; 112(5): 745-58.

3. Oliveira JM, Antunes MJ. Mitral valve repair: better than replacement. *Heart* 2006; 92(2): 275-81.

4. Wilkins GT, Weyman AE, Abascal VM, Block PC, Palacios IF. Percutaneous balloon dilatation of the mitral valve: an analysis of echocardiographic variables related to outcome and the mechanism of dilatation. *Br Heart J* 1988; 60(4): 299-308.

5. Moorjani N, Viola N, Janusauskas V, Livesey S. Adjusting the length of artificial polytetrafluoroethylene chordae in mitral valve repair by a single loop technique. *J Thorac Cardiovasc Surg* 2009; 138(6): 1441-2

Chapter 14

Tricuspid valve disease

1   What are the causes of tricuspid regurgitation (TR)?

- Normal leaflet motion - annular dilation (secondary to pulmonary hypertension, right ventricular failure, mitral valve disease), infective endocarditis.
- Excessive leaflet motion - myxomatous degeneration.
- Restricted leaflet motion - rheumatic fever, Ebstein's anomaly.

2   What is Ebstein's anomaly?

- It is defined as dysplasia of the tricuspid valve leaflets (Figure 1) resulting in:

  a)   fused, perforated or absent leaflets with abnormal chordae;

  b)   apical displacement of the septal leaflet into the body of the right ventricle;

  c)   a thin atrialised portion of the right ventricle;

  d)   severe right ventricular dysfunction and dilation;

  e)   tricuspid regurgitation;

  f)   right ventricular outflow tract obstruction caused by the displaced leaflets.

- Ebstein's anomaly is also associated with rhythm disturbances, including supraventricular tachycardia, ventricular tachycardia and Wolff-Parkinson-White syndrome.

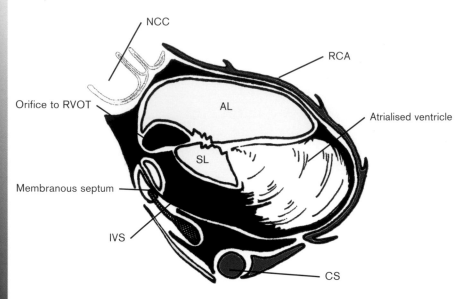

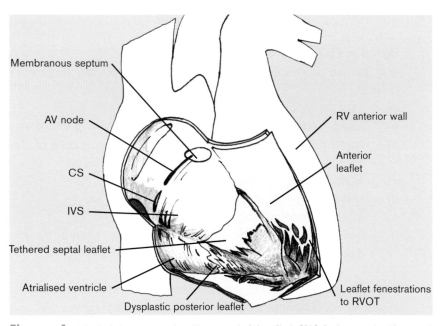

Figure 1. Ebstein's anomaly. The septal leaflet (SL) is hypoplastic and plastered to the interventricular septum (IVS), and the posterior leaflet is absent. A large segment of atrialised ventricle occupies the posterior aspect of the inlet of the right ventricle. A small opening towards the right ventricular outflow tract (RVOT) is seen beneath the anterior leaflet. NCC = non-coronary cusp of the aortic valve; RCA = right coronary artery; CS = coronary sinus; IVS = interventricular septum; AL = anterior leaflet of the tricuspid valve; SL = septal leaflet of the tricuspid valve; RVOT = right ventricular outflow tract; RV = right ventricle; AV node = atrioventricular node.

3 **What are the symptoms of tricuspid regurgitation?**
- Dyspnoea and fatigue due to reduced cardiac output.
- Peripheral oedema and ascites due to back pressure on the systemic venous circulation.

4 **What are the signs of tricuspid regurgitation?**
- Increased jugular venous pressure with a prominent V wave.
- Peripheral oedema and ascites.
- Pan-systolic murmur prominent at the left sternal edge, increased with inspiration.
- 3rd heart sound (gallop rhythm).
- Right ventricular heave.
- Jaundice secondary to hepatic congestion in severe TR.

5 **How is tricuspid regurgitation quantified by echocardiography?**

- According to the American Heart Association (AHA) guidelines, the main criteria is a vena contracta (narrowest part of regurgitant jet) width >0.7cm for severe TR.
- Severe TR is also associated with systolic flow reversal in the hepatic veins.
- Additional methods used to quantify tricuspid regurgitation include using colour-flow Doppler to measure the size of the regurgitant jet in relation to the right atrium, PISA (proximal isovelocity area) radius and right atrial size.

6 **What are the causes of tricuspid stenosis (TS)?**
- Rheumatic fever.
- Carcinoid heart disease.
- Congenital tricuspid stenosis.

7 **What are the symptoms of tricuspid stenosis?**
- Dyspnoea and fatigue due to reduced cardiac output.
- Peripheral oedema and ascites due to back pressure on the systemic venous circulation.

8　**What are the signs of tricuspid stenosis?**
- Increased jugular venous pressure with a prominent A wave.
- Peripheral oedema and ascites.
- Tricuspid opening snap.
- Diastolic rumbling murmur prominent at the left sternal edge, increased with inspiration.
- Split 1st heart sound.

9　**How is tricuspid stenosis quantified by echocardiography?**
- According to the AHA guidelines, the main criteria is a tricuspid valve area (TVA) <1cm^2 for severe TS.
- The TVA can be calculated by the continuity equation or planimetry.
- The mean tricuspid diastolic pressure gradient can also be used to quantify tricuspid stenosis.

10　**What are the indications for tricuspid valve surgery in the absence of mitral valve disease?**

AHA guidelines

- Class IIa - severe TR in symptomatic patients.
- Other considerations include tricuspid valve annulus size (>40mm), right ventricular function and size, pulmonary hypertension (>50mmHg at rest, 60mmHg on exercise), right atrial size and the presence of atrial fibrillation.

11　**What are the indications for tricuspid valve repair in patients undergoing mitral valve surgery?**

AHA guidelines

- Class I: severe TR.
- Class IIb: less than severe TR with pulmonary hypertension or a dilated tricuspid valve annulus (>40mm).

12 What are the surgical options for tricuspid valve annular dilation?

- Bicuspidisation/plication of the tricuspid valve - a running suture along the posterior TV annulus to shorten or eliminate the posterior leaflet resulting in a bicuspid valve.
- De Vega annuloplasty (Figure 2) - two arms of a running suture weaving along the TV annulus from the anteroseptal to posteroseptal commissures. The first arm of the weaved suture is started at the anteroseptal commissure, superficially and close to the annulus, to avoid the non-coronary cusp of the aortic valve. This is then continued clockwise to the posteroseptal commissure. The suture is then weaved back counter-clockwise and secured with Teflon® pledgets at both ends (Figure 2A). The stitch is tightened over an appropriately sized Hegar dilator (Figure 2B).
- Ring annuloplasty (Figures 3 and 4) - using interrupted mattress sutures, an appropriately sized tricuspid valve ring is implanted into the tricuspid valve annulus.
- During tricuspid valve surgery it is important to avoid the atrioventricular node and Bundle of His, which are located in the triangle of Koch.

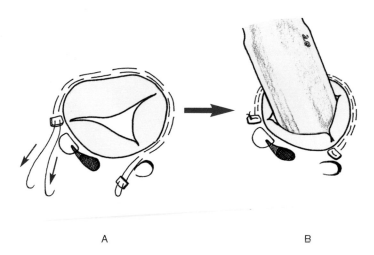

A   B

Figure 2. De Vega tricuspid valve annuloplasty.

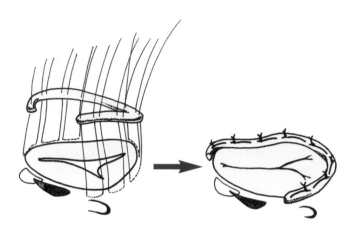

Figure 3. Tricuspid valve ring annuloplasty.

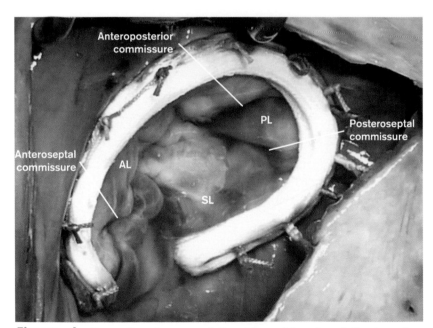

Figure 4. Operative image of the tricuspid valve following ring annuloplasty. AL = anterior leaflet of the tricuspid valve; SL = septal leaflet of the tricuspid valve; PL = posterior leaflet of the tricuspid valve.

13 What structures are at risk during tricuspid valve surgery (Figure 5)?

- Atrioventricular node (at the centre of the triangle of Koch) and Bundle of His (at the apex of the triangle of Koch).
- Aortic valve (non-coronary cusp).
- Coronary sinus.
- Right coronary artery.
- Atrioventricular nodal artery.

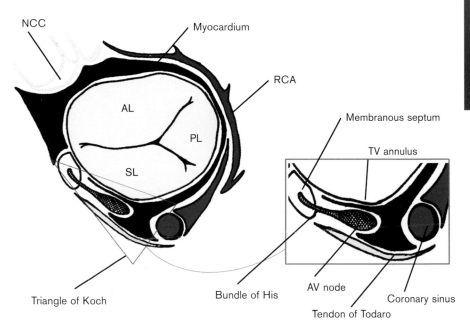

Figure 5. Anatomical relations of the tricuspid valve. NCC = non-coronary cusp of the aortic valve; RCA = right coronary artery; AL = anterior leaflet of the tricuspid valve; SL = septal leaflet of the tricuspid valve; PL = posterior leaflet of the tricuspid valve; TV annulus = tricuspid valve annulus; AV node = atrioventricular node.

14 How is the tricuspid valve annulus sized for ring annuloplasty (Figure 6)?

- Annuloplasty sizers, which measure the anterior leaflet of the tricuspid valve.
- Alternatively, fixed sizes of 30-32mm for women and 32-34mm for men are used.

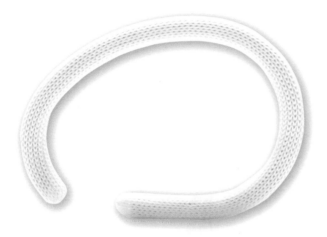

Figure 6. Tricuspid valve annuloplasty ring (Edwards Lifesciences, Irvine, USA). The gap in the ring avoids suturing the conducting system at the apex of the Triangle of Koch.

Recommended reading

1. Bonow RO, Carabello BA, Kanu C, de Leon AC Jr, Faxon DP, Freed MD, Gaasch WH, Lytle BW, Nishimura RA, O'Gara PT, O'Rourke RA, Otto CM, Shah PM, Shanewise JS, Smith SC Jr, Jacobs AK, Adams CD, Anderson JL, Antman EM, Faxon DP, Fuster V, Halperin JL, Hiratzka LF, Hunt SA, Lytle BW, Nishimura R, Page RL, Riegel B. ACC/AHA 2006 Guidelines for the management of patients with valvular heart disease. *Circulation* 2006; 114; e84-e231.

2. Anyanwu AC, Chikwe J, Adams DH. Tricuspid valve repair for treatment and prevention of secondary tricuspid regurgitation in patients undergoing mitral valve surgery. *Curr Cardiol Rep* 2008; 10(2): 110-7.

Chapter 15

Infective endocarditis

1 What is the risk of infective endocarditis?

- Native valve endocarditis has an incidence of 2-4 cases per 100,000 persons per year.
- The risk of prosthetic valve endocarditis is 0.5-1% per year following valve surgery.
- Infective endocarditis usually affects the left-sided valves (mitral valve more common than the aortic valve) with 5% of cases involving the tricuspid valve and the pulmonary valve rarely being affected.

2 What is the pathogenesis of infective endocarditis?

- Normal cardiac endothelium is resistant to infection.
- Even with transient bacteraemia, normal immune mechanisms including thrombocidins (microbicidal proteins released by platelets) prevent endocarditis.
- Risk factors for native valve endocarditis include:

  a) endothelial disruption;
  b) valvular lesions such as aortic stenosis or mitral regurgitation resulting in non-laminar flow.

- These risk factors induce platelet-fibrin thrombus formation with subsequent bacterial colonisation resulting in vegetation formation and spread into the surrounding tissues or embolisation.

3 What are the clinical features of infective endocarditis?

- Clinical features of infection - fever, night sweats, rigors, weight loss, malaise, anaemia, and clubbing and splenomegaly if chronic.
- Clinical features of immune complex deposition are:

  a) Roth spots - retinal boat-shaped haemorrhage with a pale centre;
  b) splinter haemorrhages - thin reddish-brown lines in the nailbed;

c)   Osler's nodes - painful pulp infarcts on fingers, toes, palms or soles;
d)   Janeway lesions - painless flat palmar or plantar erythema;
e)   vasculitis (brain, skin, kidney) and arthralgia.

- Clinical features of the cardiac lesion - new or changing murmur, heart block, heart failure, pyopericardium.
- Clinical features of emboli (cerebral, retinal, splenic, mesenteric, renal or lower limb), resulting in organ infarct or abscess, especially with fungal endocarditis (due to friable emboli).

4   **What are the commonest organisms in patients with native valve infective endocarditis?**

- *Streptococcus* (45%) - *viridans* (including *milleri*, *oralis*, *mitis*, *mutans*, *salivarius*) or *bovis*.
- *Staphylococcus aureus* or *epidermidis* (35%).
- *Enterococcus faecalis* (10%).
- Diptheroid bacilli and micro-aerophilic *Streptococci*.
- HACEK organisms (see below).
- Anaerobic gram negative bacilli - *Fusobacterium*, *Bacteroides*, *Streptobacillus moniliformis*, *Propionibacterium acnes*, *Listeria monocytogenes*, *Brucella abortus*, *Legionella*.
- *Coxiella burnetii* (Q fever).
- *Chlamydia psittaci* or *trachomatis*.
- Fungal - *Candida*, *Aspergillus*, *Histoplasma*.

5   **What are the HACEK organisms?**

- A group of gram negative fastidious bacilli that require prolonged culture in 10% CO_2:

a)   *Haemophilus* species (including *aphrophilus* but not *influenzae*);
b)   *Actinobacillus actinomycetemcomitans*;
c)   *Cardiobacterium hominis*;
d)   *Eikenella corrodens*;
e)   *Kingella kingae*.

6   **What are the commonest organisms in patients with early (<2 months) prosthetic valve infective endocarditis?**

● *Staphylococcus aureus* and *epidermidis* (45-50%).
● Gram negative bacilli.
● Fungi.
● *Streptococcus* and *Enterococcus* (<10%).

7   **What are the commonest organisms in patients with late (>2 months) prosthetic valve infective endocarditis?**

● *Streptococcus viridans* (45%).
● *Staphylococcus aureus* and *epidermidis* (35%).
● *Enterococcus faecalis* (10%).

8   **Which antibiotics should be used for the common organisms in infective endocarditis?**

● If the organism is unknown benzylpenicillin and gentamicin should be used (to cover the main organisms, especially *Streptococcus*) or vancomycin and gentamicin (if *Staphylococcus* is suspected).
● *Streptococcus viridans* - benzylpenicillin and gentamicin.
● *Staphylococcus aureus* - vancomycin and gentamicin.
● *Enterococcus* - amoxycillin and gentamicin.
● HACEK (often beta-lactam resistant) - ceftriaxone.

9   **What are the causes of culture-negative infective endocarditis?**

● Prior antibiotic therapy.
● Slow-growing or fastidious organisms (HACEK, nutritionally variant *Streptococci*, *Brucella*, *Legionella*, *Corynebacterium*, *Listeria*, *Bartonella*).
● Fungal endocarditis.
● Obligate intracellular parasites (*Coxiella burnetii*, *Chlamydiae*).
● Non-infective endocarditis (marantic endocarditis) - see below.

315

10 What are the causes of non-infective (marantic) endocarditis?

- Mucinous adenocarcinoma (pancreas, lung, upper gastrointestinal tract).
- Other malignant disease - lymphoma, bladder carcinoma.
- Anti-phospholipid syndrome (Hughes' syndrome).
- Acute rheumatic fever (Lancefield group A β-haemolytic *Streptococcus*).
- Libman-Sacks endocarditis (systemic lupus erythematosus, scleroderma).

11 What are the causes of persistent or recurrent fever in patients with suspected infective endocarditis whilst on antibiotic treatment?

- Wrong antibiotic.
- Wrong diagnosis.
- Spread of infection - paravalvular or intracardiac abscess, metastatic infection or mycotic aneurysm.
- Secondary infection, e.g. hospital-acquired chest infection, venous line infection.
- Antibiotic hypersensitivity (usually penicillin).

12 What are Duke's major criteria for infective endocarditis?

- Three positive blood cultures (12 hours apart) showing typical organisms - *Streptococcus viridans* or *bovis*, *Staphylococcus aureus*, *Enterococci*, HACEK.
- Evidence of endocardial infection - vegetation, abscess, prosthetic valve dehiscence, new regurgitation.

13 What are Duke's minor criteria for infective endocarditis?

- Predisposing factors (e.g. cardiac lesion, intravenous drug abuser).
- Fever >38°C.
- Embolic or vascular phenomena (e.g. splinter haemorrhages, vasculitis).
- Immunological phenomena (e.g. Osler's nodes, Roth spots).
- Serology consistent with infective endocarditis.
- Blood cultures compatible with but not typical for endocarditis.

- Other echocardiographic findings consistent with infective endocarditis and not covered by major criteria.

14 What is the significance of Duke's criteria?

- Definite endocarditis (specificity 99%, sensitivity >80%):

  a) clinical diagnosis is made by:
  - i)   two major criteria;
  - ii) one major and three minor criteria;
  - iii) five minor criteria;
  - iv) pathological diagnosis by histological evidence of active infective endocarditis (from surgical specimen or post mortem).

- Possible endocarditis - findings consistent with infective endocarditis but do not satisfy the requirements of definite infective endocarditis.
- Rejected diagnosis of endocarditis:

  a) firm alternative diagnosis;
  b) resolution of manifestations within 4 days of antibiotic treatment;
  c) no evidence of infective endocarditis at surgery or post mortem after therapy for >4 days.

15 What are the indications for surgery in patients with native valve endocarditis (Figure 1)?

AHA guidelines

- Class I:

  a) valvular regurgitation or stenosis leading to heart failure;
  b) aortic or mitral regurgitation with raised left ventricular end-diastolic pressure, left atrial pressure or moderate pulmonary hypertension;
  c) infective endocarditis caused by fungal or highly resistant organisms;
  d) local invasion resulting in heart block, annular or aortic abscess, fistula or leaflet perforation.

- Class IIa: recurrent emboli with persistent vegetation despite antibiotics.
- Class IIb: mobile vegetation >10mm.

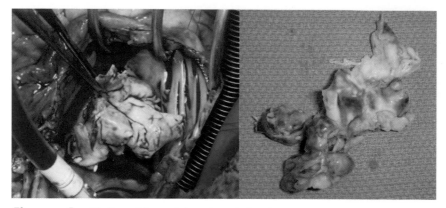

Figure 1. Native tricuspid valve infective endocarditis. A) Large vegetation attached to the septal and anterior tricuspid valve leaflets. B) Excised vegetation and valve leaflets.

16 What are the indications for surgery in patients with prosthetic valve endocarditis (Figure 2)?

AHA guidelines

- Class I: heart failure, valve dehiscence, worsening regurgitation or obstruction, or local invasion.
- Class IIa: persistent bacteraemia or recurrent emboli despite antibiotic therapy, or relapsing infection.
- Class III (contra-indication): uncomplicated prosthetic valve endocarditis with a sensitive organism.

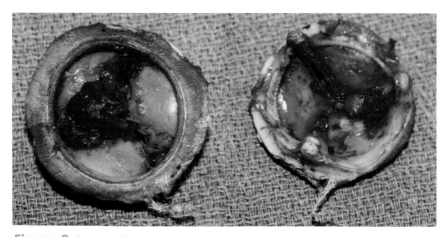

Figure 2. Prosthetic aortic valve endocarditis. The valve is seen from left ventricular (left) and aortic (right) views with vegetations present on both the inflow and outflow aspects of the valve.

318

17 What are the principles of surgery for infective endocarditis?

- Debridement of infected tissues.
- Closure of cardiac defects.
- Valve repair or replacement (repair is the preferred option in mitral and tricuspid valve endocarditis, especially if <50% of the valve is affected).
- Aortic homografts are useful in patients with aortic root abscesses.
- In intravenous drug abuse patients with tricuspid valve endocarditis, it may be necessary to perform tricuspid valvectomy without replacement to reduce the risk of recurrence but only in the absence of significant pulmonary hypertension.

18 What are the treatment options for aortic peri-annular abscesses?

- Bovine pericardial patch.
- Aortic valve homograft.

19 What is the operative mortality and long-term survival of patients undergoing surgery for infective endocarditis?

- Operative mortality - native valve endocarditis 5-10%, prosthetic valve endocarditis 10-20%.
- 5-year survival - native valve endocarditis 80%, prosthetic valve endocarditis 60%.

20 What are the antibiotic prophylaxis regimes for patients with prosthetic cardiac valves used prior to dental procedures?

- Standard - amoxycillin (3g oral 1 hr pre-operatively or 2g IV 30 min pre-operatively).
- Standard (patients with penicillin allergy) - clindamycin (600mg oral 1 hr pre-operatively).
- Patients with previous infective endocarditis - amoxycillin (2g IV 30 min pre-operatively) and gentamicin (120mg IV 30 min pre-operatively).
- Patients with previous infective endocarditis and penicillin allergy - vancomycin (1g IV 1 hr pre-operatively) and gentamicin (120mg IV 30 min pre-operatively).
- Recently, NICE (National Institute for Health and Clinical Excellence) guidelines have suggested that prophylactic antibiotics are not

required for all patients with prosthetic valves undergoing dental procedures. These guidelines, however, are very controversial and many surgeons still advocate the use of antimicrobial prophylaxis in these patients.

Recommended reading

1.   Bonow RO, Carabello BA, Kanu C, de Leon AC Jr, Faxon DP, Freed MD, Gaasch WH, Lytle BW, Nishimura RA, O'Gara PT, O'Rourke RA, Otto CM, Shah PM, Shanewise JS, Smith SC Jr, Jacobs AK, Adams CD, Anderson JL, Antman EM, Faxon DP, Fuster V, Halperin JL, Hiratzka LF, Hunt SA, Lytle BW, Nishimura R, Page RL, Riegel B. ACC/AHA 2006 Guidelines for the management of patients with valvular heart disease. *Circulation* 2006; 114; e84-e231.

2.   Durack DT, Lukes AS, Bright DK. New criteria for diagnosis of infective endocarditis: utilization of specific echocardiographic findings: Duke Endocarditis Service. *Am J Med* 1994; 96: 200-9.

3.   Wilson W, Taubert KA, Gewitz M, Lockhart PB, Baddour LM, Levison M, Bolger A, Cabell CH, Takahashi M, Baltimore RS, Newburger JW, Strom BL, Tani LY, Gerber M, Bonow RO, Pallasch T, Shulman ST, Rowley AH, Burns JC, Ferrieri P, Gardner T, Goff D, Durack DT. Prevention of infective endocarditis: guidelines from the American Heart Association. *J Am Dent Assoc* 2007; 138(6): 739-45, 747-60.

4.   Shanson D. New British and American guidelines for the antibiotic prophylaxis of infective endocarditis: do the changes make sense? A critical review. *Curr Opin Infect Dis* 2008; 21(2): 191-9.

Chapter 16

Thoracic aortic disease

1   **What are the normal dimensions of the thoracic aorta (Figure 1)?**

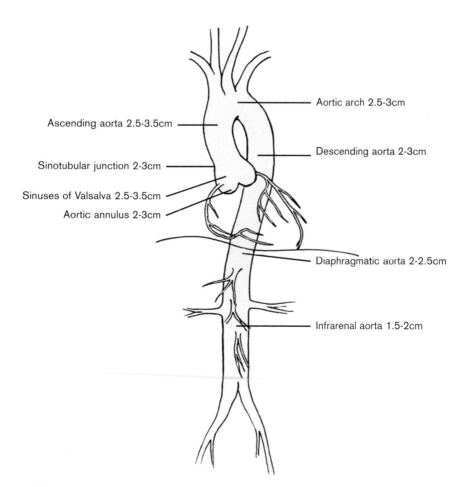

Ascending aorta 2.5-3.5cm

Sinotubular junction 2-3cm

Sinuses of Valsalva 2.5-3.5cm

Aortic annulus 2-3cm

Aortic arch 2.5-3cm

Descending aorta 2-3cm

Diaphragmatic aorta 2-2.5cm

Infrarenal aorta 1.5-2cm

Figure 1. Normal dimensions of the thoracic aorta.

- An aneurysm is defined as permanent localised dilation of an artery (≥150% diameter of the normal calibre).

2 Describe the anatomical layers of the thoracic aorta (Figure 2)

- The intima (inner layer of the aorta) consists of endothelial cells, a subendothelial layer of connective tissue and an elastic membrane.
- The media (middle layer of the aorta) consists of elastin, collagen, smooth muscle cells and ground matrix.
- The adventitia (strong outer covering of the aorta) consists of connective tissue, collagen and elastic fibres.

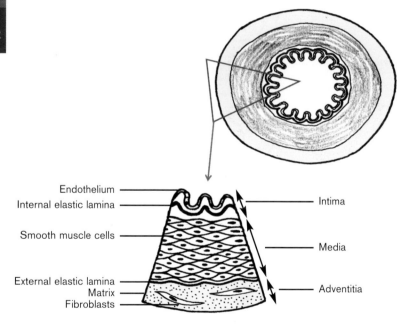

Figure 2. Histological layers of the thoracic aorta.

3 **How are aortic aneurysms classified (Figure 3)?**
- Pathology:

  a) true aneurysm, which is caused by outpouching of all three layers of the vessel wall (Figure 3A);

  b) false aneurysm (pseudoaneurysm), which consists of thrombus contained by adventitia and surrounding tissues (Figure 3B).

- Shape - saccular (Figure 3C) or fusiform (Figure 3D).
- Aetiology - atherosclerotic, dissecting or mycotic.
- Location - ascending, arch or descending (Figure 4).

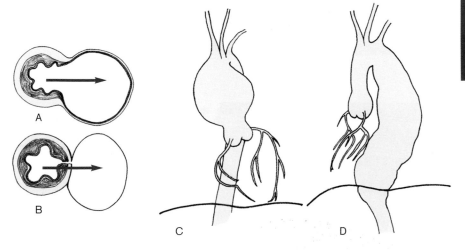

Figure 3. Thoracic aortic aneurysms. A) True aneurysm showing dilation of vessel wall involving all three arterial layers. B) False aneurysm, following rupture of the arterial wall, with the haematoma and blood still in continuity with the arterial lumen and contained within the adventitia and surrounding tissues. C) Saccular aneurysm of the ascending aorta. D) Fusiform aneurysm involving the descending thoracic aorta.

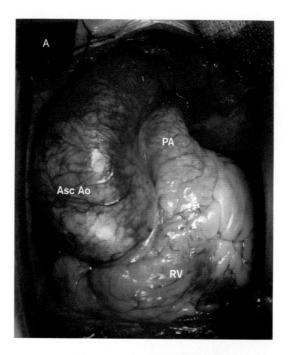

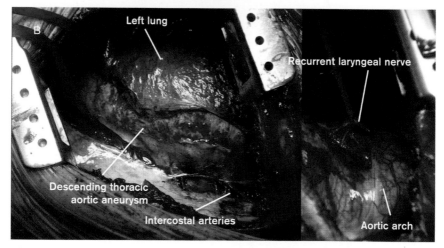

Figure 4. A) Ascending aortic aneurysm. Asc Ao = ascending aorta; PA = pulmonary artery; RV = right ventricle. B) Descending thoracic aortic aneurysm, viewed through a double left thoracotomy, with the majority of the aneurysm lying beneath the adherent left lung. The intercostal arteries can be seen branching posteriorly (left panel, lower thoracotomy) with the left recurrent laryngeal nerve passing over the aortic arch (right panel, upper thoracotomy).

4   **Describe Crawford's classification of thoraco-abdominal aortic aneurysms (Figure 5)**

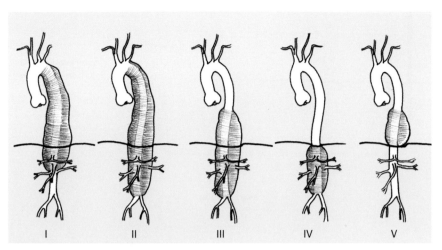

Figure 5. Crawford's classification of thoraco-abdominal aortic aneurysms.

- I: most of the descending thoracic aorta (just beyond the left subclavian artery to the suprarenal abdominal aorta).
- II: just beyond the left subclavian artery to the infrarenal abdominal aorta.
- III: lower descending aorta (below the 6th rib) into the abdomen.
- IV: below the diaphragm, i.e. an abdominal aortic aneurysm.
- V: mid-descending thoracic aorta to above the diaphragm (new addition to the classification).

5   **What is the natural history of thoracic aortic aneurysms?**

- Surgically untreated thoracic aortic aneurysms carry the risk of rupture, dissection and death.
- Expansion of thoracic aneurysms occurs at a faster rate in larger aneurysms (0.2cm per year in aneurysms <5cm compared to 0.8cm per year in aneurysms >5cm), as per Laplace's Law.
- The risk of rupture increases as the size of the aneurysm increases (0.3% per year for aneurysms 4-5cm compared to 3.6% for aneurysms >6cm).
- The median size for rupture is 6cm for ascending and 7cm for descending thoracic aortic aneurysms (Figure 6).

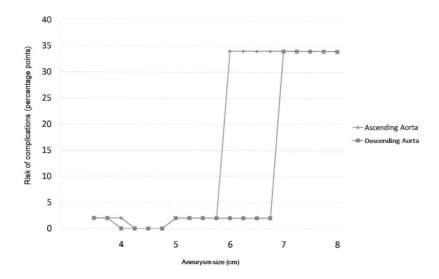

Figure 6. Graph demonstrating the risk of rupture significantly increases when ascending and descending aortic diameters are larger than 6 and 7cm, respectively.

- The mean time from onset of symptoms to rupture of the aneurysm is 2 years.
- The 5-year survival of surgically untreated (symptomatic and asymptomatic) thoracic aortic aneurysms is 39% and thoracoabdominal aneurysms, 23%.

6 What is the pathophysiology of aortic aneurysm formation?

- The media of the aorta normally contains elastin, collagen, smooth muscle cells and ground matrix.
- Aneurysms form after loss of smooth muscle cells and fragmentation of elastin fibres (a process known as cystic medial degeneration), which results in loss of elasticity and tensile strength of the media.
- The aorta normally expands and recoils with systole and diastole but dilates when elastic recoil is lost.

7 What are the predisposing factors for a thoracic aortic aneurysm?

- A: age, atherosclerosis.

- B: bicuspid aortic valve (associated with fibrillin deficiency), blood pressure (hypertension).
- C: connective tissue disorders (Marfan syndrome, Ehlers-Danlos syndrome).
- D: dissection, degenerative (cystic medial degeneration).
- E: trauma, aortitis, infection, syphilis.

8 **What are the independent risk factors for rupture of an aortic aneurysm?**
- Aortic diameter.
- Pain or other symptoms of expansion.
- Age.
- Chronic obstructive pulmonary disease (COPD).
- Smoking.

9 **What is Marfan syndrome (Figure 7)?**
- Marfan syndrome is an autosomal dominant condition associated with mutation of the fibrillin gene on chromosome 15.
- As there are many different genetic mutations, it results in many different phenotypes.

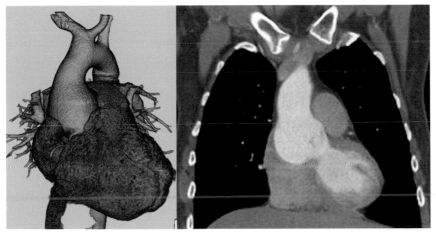

Figure 7. Computed tomography scan demonstrating a classical 'onion-shaped' aortic root aneurysm associated with Marfan syndrome.

- The diagnosis of Marfan syndrome is based on two or more of the following clinical features:

  a) tall thin patient - arm span greater than height;
  b) arachnodactyly - long tapered fingers;
  c) high arched palate;
  d) scoliosis, pectus excavatum or protusio acetabulae;
  e) hypermobility of joints with skin laxity;
  f) spontaneous pneumothorax with apical bullae;
  g) eye signs - ectopia lentis (upward dislocation of lens), myopia, retinal detachment;
  h) floppy mitral valve resulting in mitral regurgitation and chordal rupture;
  i) aortopathy with weakened aortic wall which dilates even in normotensive patients. This is caused by cystic medial necrosis and may result in a thoracic aortic aneurysm or dissection.

10 What is Ehlers-Danlos syndrome?

- Ehlers-Danlos syndrome is an autosomal dominant condition.
- Type IV Ehlers-Danlos syndrome results in a structural defect of Type III collagen and subsequent aortopathy.
- It is less common than Marfan syndrome.

11 What are the clinical features of patients with thoracic aortic aneurysms?

- Asymptomatic - incidental finding on imaging.
- Pain - anterior chest pain or back pain (typically intrascapular), with sudden onset of the pain suggesting dissection or impending rupture.
- Compression of nearby structures resulting in hoarseness (recurrent laryngeal nerve), dysphagia (oesophagus) and stridor or dyspnoea (trachea).
- Fistula resulting in haematemesis (oesophagus) or haemoptysis (lung, bronchi).

12 What are the indications for intervention on thoracic aortic aneurysms?

- Size:

  a) ascending aortic aneurysms >5.5cm;
  b) ascending aortic aneurysms >4.5cm for patients undergoing AVR or CABG;
  c) ascending aortic aneurysms 4.0-5.0cm (or when the ratio of the maximal ascending or aortic root area (πr^2) in cm^2 divided

by the patient's height in metres exceeds 10) for patients with Marfan syndrome or other connective tissue disorders;
d) aortic arch aneurysms >5.5cm;
e) descending aortic aneurysms >5.5cm;
f) thoraco-abdominal aneurysms >6.0cm.

- Symptoms of expansion, compression or fistula formation - chest pain, back pain, dyspnoea, dysphagia, hoarseness, haematemesis or haemoptysis.
- Rapid rate of expansion >1cm/year.
- Recurrent emboli (especially cerebral emboli from the aortic arch).

13 What are the indications for an aortic root replacement?

- Annulo-aortic ectasia - dilation of the aortic root, using similar size criteria for the ascending aorta (see above).
- Aneurysm of the sinus of Valsalva (which occurs most frequently in the non-coronary sinus, then the right coronary sinus and least often in the left coronary sinus). In these patients, it may be possible to perform a selective sinus replacement, instead of a complete aortic root replacement.
- Aortic root abscess.
- Stanford Type A thoracic aortic dissection extending into the aortic root.
- Small aortic root if root-sparing techniques are not possible.

14 What are the principles of surgery when operating on aortic aneurysms?

- The aim of surgery is to prevent rupture, dissection, local compression and fistula formation.
- Surgery should be offered when the combined risk of operative mortality and permanent neurological deficit is less than the combined risk of rupture and dissection.
- Operative mortality is 2-5% for aortic root or ascending aortic surgery, 5-10% for aortic arch surgery and 10-20% for thoraco-abdominal aortic surgery.
- Risk of neurological injury: 5-10% stroke; 5-10% paraplegia (for descending aortic replacement).

15 What is the 5-year survival following surgery for thoracic aortic aneurysms?

- Ascending aortic aneurysm - 82%.
- Aortic arch aneurysm - 70%.
- Descending aortic aneurysm - 65%.

- Thoraco-abdominal aortic aneurysm - 65%.
- As part of the long-term follow-up after thoracic aortic surgery, these patients need beta-blockade and annual radiological scanning (CT or MRI) to assess the residual native aorta.

16 What are the operative choices for an aortic root replacement (Figure 8)?

- If the aortic root is dilated but the aortic valve is structurally normal, a valve-sparing procedure should be considered (e.g David or Yacoub procedure):

    a) David reimplantation procedure: the commissural pillars are re-implanted within a Dacron® interposition tube graft and the coronary buttons are re-anastomosed. The sutures are passed from the left ventricular outflow tract from inside to out of the graft, thereby stabilising the aortic annulus. The Dacron® tube diameter is equal to the average length of the free margins of three leaflets (Figure 8A);

    b) Yacoub remodelling procedure: the ascending aorta and sinuses are replaced with a Dacron® interposition tube graft that is scalloped to incorporate the aortic valve commissural pillars. The coronary buttons are then re-implanted. As the aortic valve annulus is not stabilised, this technique is not suitable for patients with connective tissue disorders or where the aortic valve annulus is dilated >30mm (Figure 8B).

- If the aortic root is dilated and the aortic valve diseased (e.g. stenotic), an aortic root and valve replacement is performed:

    a) classic Bentall procedure (inclusion technique): a valved conduit is placed within the aneurysmal aortic root and flow to the coronary button is provided by holes within the prosthesis. This procedure is rarely used now (Figure 9A);

    b) modified Bentall procedure: the aneurysmal aortic root is excised and replaced by a valved conduit (such as a Carboseal® mechanical prosthesis or BioValsalva™ bioprosthesis) with re-implantation of the coronary buttons (Figure 9B).

- A Cabrol procedure may be used to avoid tension on the coronary reimplantation by using a prosthetic interposition graft (8mm Dacron® tube), such as when the coronary ostia are laterally displaced by a large aneurysm (Figure 9C).
- Homograft aortic root replacement: a cadaveric human aortic root is implanted followed by re-anastomosis of the coronary buttons. It is

A

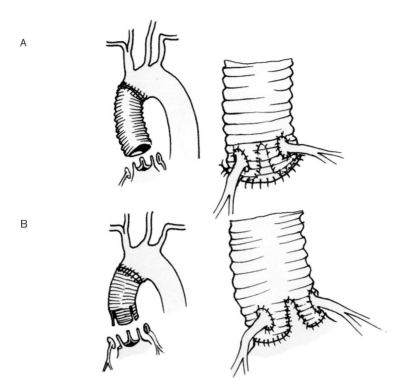

B

C

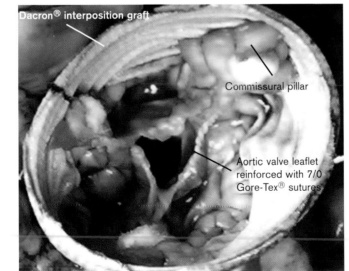

Dacron® interposition graft

Commissural pillar

Aortic valve leaflet
reinforced with 7/0
Gore-Tex® sutures

Figure 8. Valve-sparing aortic root surgery. A) David
procedure. B) Yacoub procedure. C) Operative image
demonstrating the David procedure with re-implantation
of the aortic valve commissural pillars inside the Dacron®
interposition graft. The free edges of the aortic valve
leaflets have also been reinforced with 7/0 Gore-Tex®
sutures.

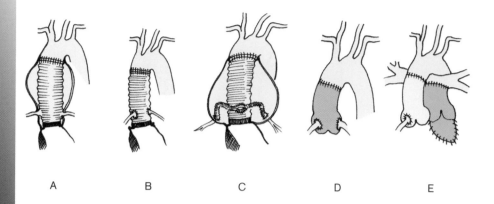

A   B   C   D   E

Figure 9. Aortic root surgery. A) Classic Bentall procedure. B) Modified Bentall procedure. C) Cabrol procedure. D) Aortic homograft implantation. E) Ross procedure.

often used in patients with an aortic root abscess following infective endocarditis of the aortic valve (Figure 9D).

- Ross procedure: the aortic root is replaced with the patient's own pulmonary trunk, which itself is replaced with a pulmonary homograft (Figure 9E).

17 What are the surgical options for the treatment of ascending aortic aneurysms (Figure 10)?

- Ascending aortic replacement: a Dacron® interposition graft is implanted just distal to the sinotubular junction and proximal to the origin of the innominate artery.
- Reduction aortoplasty: the ascending aorta is incised along its greater curve, with or without excision of a section of the aortic wall, followed by a two-layered everting overlapping closure, supported by Teflon® strips.
- Supporting aortoplasty: a mesh of Gore-Tex® or Prolene® is wrapped around the ascending aorta and secured with adventitial stitches to avoid migration over the coronary ostia or the origin of the innominate artery.

18 What is acute aortic syndrome (Figure 11)?

- It is defined as a group of life-threatening thoracic aortic pathologies that includes aortic dissection, penetrating aortic ulcer, intramural haematoma and leaking aortic aneurysm.

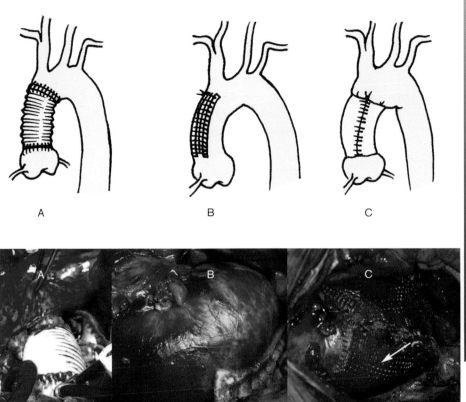

Figure 10. Surgical options for the treatment of ascending aortic aneurysms. A) Ascending aortic replacement. B) Reduction aortoplasty. C) Supporting aortoplasty using a Prolene mesh® (arrow).

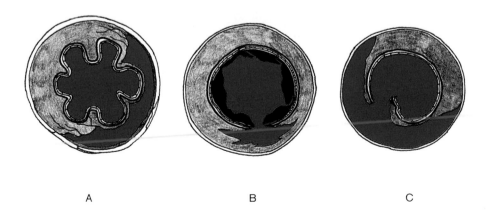

Figure 11. Acute aortic syndrome. A) Intramural haematoma. B) Penetrating aortic ulcer. C) Aortic dissection.

333

- Management of patients with acute aortic syndrome should be similar to those with acute thoracic aortic dissection:

  a) ascending aorta - surgery;
  b) descending aorta - medical management but stenting or surgery should be considered in patients with impending rupture, unremitting pain or organ malperfusion.

19 What is an intramural haematoma of the aorta (Figure 12)?

- It is defined as blood within the aortic media without the presence of an intimal tear.
- Aetiology:

  a) rupture of the vasa vasorum of the media;
  b) haemorrhage within an atherosclerotic plaque;
  c) progression from a penetrating aortic ulcer.

- It may resolve spontaneously or progress and increase in size.
- Unlike dissections, intramural haematomas occur closer to the adventitia and hence are at a greater risk of rupture than dissections.

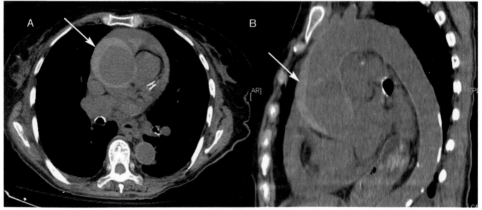

Figure 12. Intramural haematoma (arrows) of the ascending aorta demonstrated on A) axial and B) sagittal computed tomography scans.

20 What are penetrating aortic ulcers (Figure 13)?

- They are defined as focal intimal defects occurring at the site of atherosclerotic plaques.
- Progressive intimal erosion eventually results in pulsatile blood entering the media and hence penetrating ulcers may lead to intra-mural haematomas, dissection, and rupture, as well as pseudo-aneurysm and aneurysm formation.
- Surgery is indicated for patients with:

  a)   descending aortic ulcers with a diameter >20mm and depth >10mm;

  b)   ascending aortic ulcers.

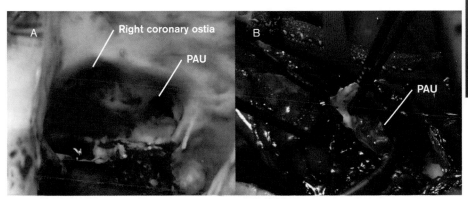

Figure 13. Penetrating aortic ulcers (PAU) observed in the A) right coronary sinus of the aortic root and B) lesser curve of the aortic arch.

21 How are thoracic aortic dissections classified (Figure 14)?

- Aortic dissection is defined as an intimal tear resulting in a split in the aortic wall between the internal and external elastic laminae within the media.
- Timing:

  a)   acute (<14 days);

  b)   sub-acute (14 days - 2 months);

  c)   chronic (>2 months).

- Location:

  a) Stanford classification:
    i) Type A: ascending aorta involved;
    ii) Type B: ascending aorta not involved;
  b) DeBakey classification:
    i) Type I: whole aorta involved;
    ii) Type II: only ascending aorta involved;
    iii) Type IIIa: only descending aorta involved;
    iv) Type IIIb: descending and abdominal aorta involved.

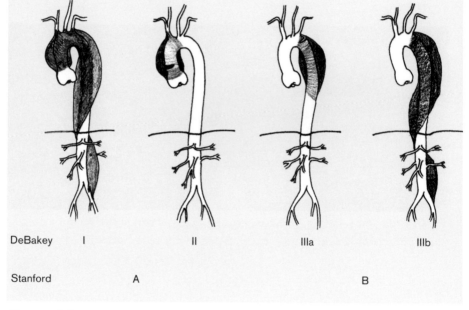

| DeBakey | I | II | IIIa | IIIb |

| Stanford | A | B |

Figure 14. DeBakey and Stanford classifications of thoracic aortic dissection.

22 Describe the pathophysiology of a thoracic aortic dissection

- The entry tear is defined as the point where blood tracks through the intima into the media.
- The dissection is classified by the extent of media stripping from the entry tear to the distal re-entry point.

- The dissection begins with an intimal tear and is propagated by the ingress of blood into the media spiralling through the length of the aorta.
- Multiple re-entry tears are often present in the descending aorta.
- It is important to distinguish the entry tear from the extent of the dissection as surgery for Type A thoracic aortic dissection aims to excise the entry tear but often leaves residual separated layers of the aortic arch and descending aorta. As the entry tear is closed and the layers are joined at the distal ascending aorta, no further blood can enter the false lumen unless additional entry intimal tears exist within the aorta.

23 Where are the entry tears usually located in acute thoracic aortic dissection?

- Ascending aorta (65%) - approximately 2cm above the non-coronary sinus.
- Descending aorta (20%) - proximally on the left anterolateral wall.
- Aortic arch (10%) - opposite the innominate artery on the lesser curve.

24 What are the predisposing factors for aortic dissection?

- A: age, atherosclerosis, aneurysm.
- B: bicuspid aortic valve (fibrillin deficiency), blood pressure (hypertension).
- C: connective tissue disorders (Marfan syndrome, Ehlers-Danlos syndrome).
- D: degenerative (cystic medial degeneration).
- E: trauma, surgery, iatrogenic, pregnancy.

25 What are the clinical features of Type A aortic dissection?

- Pain - tearing retrosternal chest pain radiating into the back or neck.
- Symptoms of organ malperfusion - myocardial ischaemia, stroke or abdominal pain.
- Dyspnoea - secondary to aortic regurgitation, tamponade or haemothorax.
- Hypotension, hypertension or blood pressure differential between the left and right arms.
- Aortic regurgitation murmur.
- Absent peripheral pulses.

26 What are the different investigations available for the diagnosis of acute Type A aortic dissection (Figure 15)?

- Transoesophageal echocardiography (TOE, 98% sensitive) provides clear images and is able to quantify the degree of aortic regurgitation but:

  a)   results are operator-dependent;
  b)   passing the TOE probe may cause anxiety and hypertension;
  c)   there is a blind spot in the distal ascending aorta and proximal aortic arch.

- Computed tomography with contrast enhancement (95% sensitive) is quick, commonly available and can image the pleura, head and neck vessels, and pericardium, but the patient is at risk of contrast nephropathy.

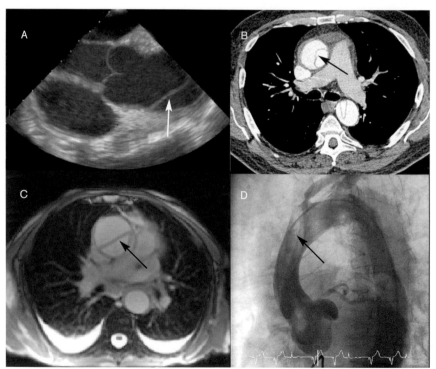

Figure 15. Acute Type A aortic dissection as demonstrated by: A) transoesophageal echocardiography; B) computed tomography; C) magnetic resonance imaging; and D) aortography. The dissection flap (arrows) separates the true and the false lumens.

- Magnetic resonance imaging (99% sensitive) is the gold standard imaging but is not always available.
- Aortography (80% sensitive) was historically the gold standard but now is rarely used and may precipitate aortic rupture.

27 Describe the monitoring required for patients undergoing surgery for Type A aortic dissection

- Arterial lines - pre-arch (right radial artery) and post-arch (femoral or left radial artery).
- Urinary catheter.
- Central venous access.
- Nasopharyngeal temperature probe.
- Cerebral oximetry (near infrared spectroscopy, if available) to detect cerebral malperfusion.

28 How is the right axillary artery cannulated for cardiopulmonary bypass (Figure 16)?

- The patient is placed in a supine position with upper body elevated to 20° and tilted towards the left, so that the skin overlying the infraclavicular fossa is on a horizontal plane.
- A 5cm infraclavicular incision is then made beneath the lateral third of the clavicle.
- The pectoralis major fibres are split with pectoralis minor retracted laterally.
- The axillary artery is mobilised from under the axillary vein avoiding the medial and lateral cords of the brachial plexus.
- A 18Fr straight arterial cannula is then placed into the axillary artery, either directly (using the Seldinger wire technique) or indirectly via an 8mm woven Dacron® graft sutured with 5-0 polypropylene.
- It is important to compare right and left radial artery pressures to ensure adequate cerebral perfusion.
- This technique is not suitable if the patient has an aortic dissection that extends into the brachiocephalic artery.

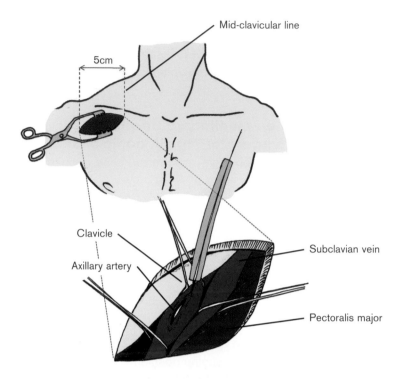

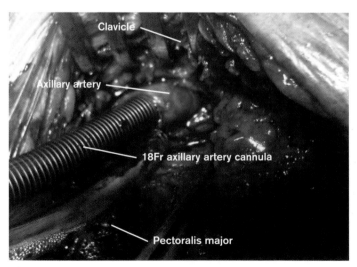

Figure 16. Axillary artery cannulation.

29 What are the principles of surgery for Type A aortic dissection (Figures 17 and 18)?

- Entry tear - resect and replace the site of the aortic entry tear.
- Aortic root - to prevent coronary malperfusion and late aortic root complications, surgery can either:

  a) repair the aortic sinus segments by adhesive reconstruction to obliterate the false lumen; or
  b) replace the aortic root.

- Aortic valve - resuspension or replacement of the aortic valve.
- Aortic arch - hemi-arch or total arch replacement depending on whether the entry tear has extended into the aortic arch.
- Distal anastomotic line - adhesive reconstruction at the distal anastomosis to obliterate the false lumen and restore flow through the true lumen.
- The different surgical options include:

  a) ascending aorta interposition graft;
  b) ascending aorta interposition graft and aortic valve replacement;
  c) ascending aorta interposition graft and resuspension of the aortic valve;
  d) aortic root replacement (Bentall or Cabrol);
  e) valve-sparing aortic root replacement (Yacoub or David);
  f) in addition, hemi-arch or total arch replacement.

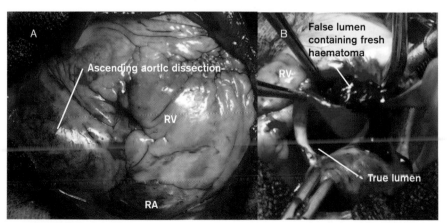

Figure 17. Acute Type A aortic dissection. A) Following opening of the pericardium, a bluish discoloration of the ascending aorta is observed, indicating blood in the aortic wall. B) Following aortotomy, fresh haematoma is observed in the false lumen of the ascending aorta.

- The underlying principle of surgery for these patients is to prevent the life-threatening complications of acute Type A aortic dissection, which include intra-pericardial rupture, tamponade, myocardial ischaemia and aortic regurgitation.
- Mortality without surgery approximates 90%, whereas surgical mortality ranges between 10-20%. Five-year survival of hospital survivors following surgery is 60%.

Acute Type A aortic dissection

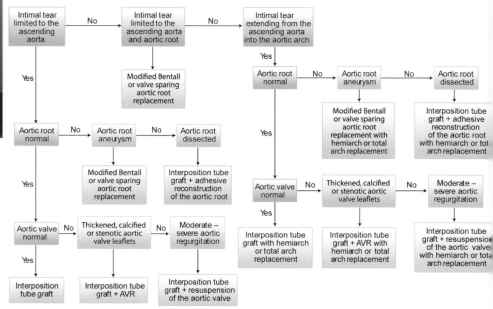

Figure 18. Decision-making algorithm delineating the surgical options for acute Type A aortic dissection.

30 What is the management of a Stanford Type B thoracic aortic dissection (Figure 19)?

- Medical management with blood pressure control - labetalol (α and β-blocker) is used to reduce the force of ventricular contraction, shear stress and absolute blood pressure.

- The rationale for not operating on all Type B aortic dissections is:

   a)   the mortality with medical management is 10% compared with an operative mortality of 27% and an operative paraplegia rate of 24%;

   b)   the 5-year survival is not improved with surgery.

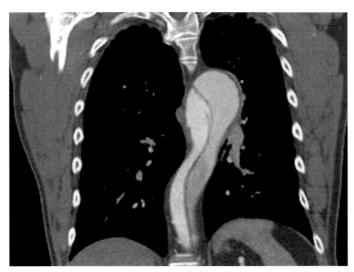

Figure 19. Type B aortic dissection demonstrated on a coronal computed tomography scan.

31   **What are the indications for intervention (surgical or endovascular stent grafting) on an acute Stanford Type B aortic dissection (Figures 20 and 21)?**

- Rupture or impending rupture of the descending thoracic aorta (large mediastinal haematoma, large haemothorax).
- Extension of the dissection with unremitting pain.
- Evidence of limb, visceral or spinal cord hypoperfusion - metabolic acidosis, raised lactate, oliguria or anuria, paraesthesia or paraplegia in the lower limbs.

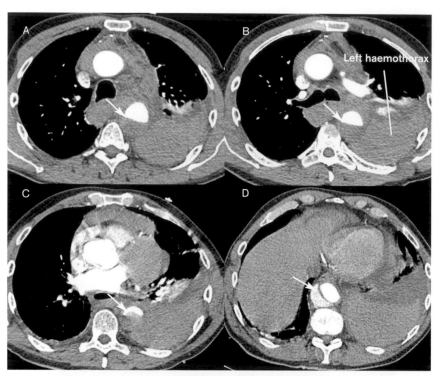

Figure 20. Serial axial computed tomography scans demonstrating a ruptured Type B aortic dissection (arrows) with an associated large left haemothorax.

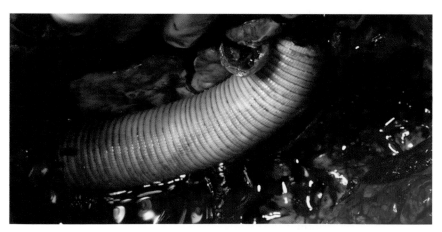

Figure 21. Replacement of the descending aorta using a Dacron® interposition graft, following rupture of a Type B aortic dissection.

344

32 What are the indications for endovascular stent grafting of the thoracic aorta?

- Acute and chronic Stanford Type B aortic dissection.
- Traumatic aortic injury (e.g. transection).
- Descending aortic aneurysms.
- Coarctation of the aorta.
- Aortic arch aneurysms, in conjunction with bespoke branched endografts, *in situ* fenestration or debranching surgery.

33 What are the requirements and complications of endovascular stent graft deployment in the thoracic aorta (Figure 22)?

- Requirements for optimal results following endovascular stent grafting include:

   a) proximal and distal landing zones >1.5cm of normal aorta;
   b) femoral arteries >7mm diameter to allow access for the stent graft;
   c) relatively straight descending thoracic aorta.

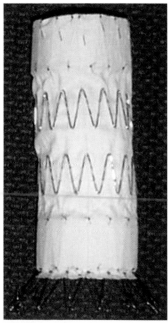 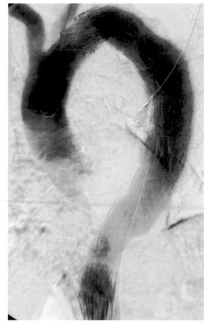

Figure 22. Endovascular stent graft.

- Complications include:

  a) stent complication (endoleak, stent migration) - 10-15%;
  b) local vascular complication - 5-10%;
  c) mortality - 5-10%;
  d) aortic trauma (rupture, dissection, fistula) - 5%;
  e) stroke or paraplegia - 5%.

34 Describe the classification of endoleaks that may occur following endovascular stent grafting

- Endoleak is defined as blood flow between the outside of the stent graft and the diseased vessel wall. It represents a complication of endovascular stent grafting and is classified according to the source of blood:

  a) I: leak at the junction of the aorta and the stent graft due to an inadequate seal;
  b) II: back bleeding vessels within the aneurysmal sac;
  c) III: leak through a defect in the stent graft prosthesis (graft failure);
  d) IV: leak through the pores of the stent graft fabric (graft porosity).

Recommended reading

1. Coady MA, Rizzo JA, Hammond GL, Mandapati D, Darr U, Kopf GS, Elefteriades JA. What is the appropriate size criterion for resection of thoracic aortic aneurysms? *J Thorac Cardiovasc Surg* 1997; 113(3): 476-91.

2. Coselli JS. The use of left heart bypass in the repair of thoracoabdominal aortic aneurysms: current techniques and results. *Semin Thorac Cardiovasc Surg* 2003; 15(4): 326-32.

3. Coselli JS, Lemaire SA, Köksoy C, Schmittling ZC, Curling PE. Cerebrospinal fluid drainage reduces paraplegia after thoracoabdominal aortic aneurysm repair: results of a randomized clinical trial. *J Vasc Surg* 2002; 35(4): 631-9.

4. Elefteriades JA. Natural history of thoracic aortic aneurysms: indications for surgery, and surgical versus nonsurgical risks. *Ann Thorac Surg* 2002; 74(5): S1877-80; discussion S1892-8.

5. Erbel R, Alfonso F, Boileau C, Dirsch O, Eber B, Haverich A, Rakowski H, Struyven J, Radegran K, Sechtem U, Taylor J, Zollikofer C, Klein WW, Mulder B, Providencia LA. Task force on aortic dissection, European Society of Cardiology. Diagnosis and management of aortic dissection. *Eur Heart J* 2001; 22(18): 1642-81.

6.   Khan IA, Nair CK. Clinical, diagnostic, and management perspectives of aortic dissection. *Chest* 2002; 122(1): 311-28.

7.   Sinclair MC, Singer RL, Manley NJ, Montesano RM. Cannulation of the axillary artery for cardiopulmonary bypass: safeguards and pitfalls. *Ann Thorac Surg* 2003; 75: 931-4.

8.   Svensson LG, Kouchoukos NT, Miller DC, Bavaria JE, Coselli JS, Curi MA, Eggebrecht H, Elefteriades JA, Erbel R, Gleason TG, Lytle BW, Mitchell RS, Nienaber CA, Roselli EE, Safi HJ, Shemin RJ, Sicard GA, Sundt TM 3rd, Szeto WY, Wheatley GH 3rd; Society of Thoracic Surgeons Endovascular Surgery Task Force. Expert consensus document on the treatment of descending thoracic aortic disease using endovascular stent-grafts. *Ann Thorac Surg* 2008; 85(1 Suppl): S1-41.

9.   Vilacosta I, San Roman JA. Acute aortic syndrome. *Heart* 2001; 85: 365-8.

10.   White GH, Yu W, May J, Chaufour X, Stephen MS. Endoleak as a complication of endoluminal grafting of abdominal aortic aneurysms: classification, incidence, diagnosis, and management. *J Endovasc Surg* 1997; 4(2): 152-68.

11.   Hiratzka LF, Bakris GL, Beckman JA, Bersin RM, Carr VF, Casey DE Jr, Eagle KA, Hermann LK, Isselbacher EM, Kazerooni EA, Kouchoukos NT, Lytle BW, Milewicz DM, Reich DL, Sen S, Shinn JA, Svensson LG, Williams DM. 2010 AHA/AATS guidelines for the diagnosis and management of patients with thoracic aortic disease. *Circulation* 2010; 121(13): e266-369.

12.   Westaby S, Saito S, Anastasiadis K, Moorjani N, Jin X. Aortic root remodelling in atheromatous aneurysms: the role of selected sinus repair. *Eur J Cardiothorac Surg* 2002; 21(3): 459-64.

Chapter 17

Coronary artery disease

1 **What is the pathophysiology of coronary artery disease (Figure 1)?**

● Coronary artery disease is caused by atherosclerosis, which develops in three stages:

    a) linear fatty streak - focal intimal thickening caused by deposition of lipid-filled macrophages and smooth muscle cells;

    b) fibrolipid plaques - consisting of these lipid-laden cells, an inflammatory core and cholesterol deposits, encased by a fibrous cap, resulting in luminal narrowing;

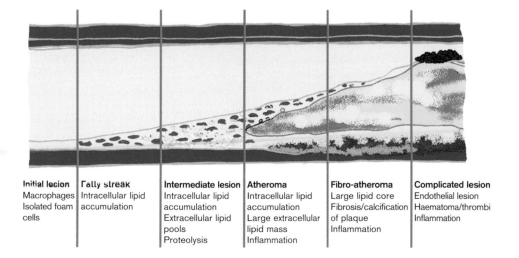

Initial lesion	Fatty streak	Intermediate lesion	Atheroma	Fibro-atheroma	Complicated lesion
Macrophages	Intracellular lipid	Intracellular lipid	Intracellular lipid	Large lipid core	Endothelial lesion
Isolated foam	accumulation	accumulation	accumulation	Fibrosis/calcification	Haematoma/thrombi
cells		Extracellular lipid	Large extracellular	of plaque	Inflammation
		pools	lipid mass	Inflammation	
		Proteolysis	Inflammation		

Figure 1. Development of atherosclerosis.

c) evolution of plaques - plaque rupture and exposure of blood to the contents of a plaque can result in luminal thrombosis or a 'major plaque event'. With smaller amounts of thrombosis, luminal occlusion does not occur but subsequent embolisation of thrombi may trigger arrhythmias or plaque growth by the release of platelet-derived growth factors which stimulate smooth muscle division. Plaque rupture is more likely in soft plaques with low fibrin content than hard plaques, thus soft plaques are potentially more lethal even if they are smaller than hard plaques which have a thick fibrous cap.

- Risk factors for atherosclerosis include smoking, hyperlipidaemia, hypertension, diabetes mellitus, male gender, increasing age and a positive family history of ischaemic heart disease.
- Myocardial ischaemia represents an imbalance between myocardial oxygen supply and demand.
- Myocardial infarction (MI) represents ischaemia-induced cardiomyocyte loss (necrosis) and is caused by coronary artery occlusion secondary to:

a) progressive atherosclerosis;
b) disruption of an unstable plaque with acute thrombosis.

2 What are the principles of treating angina pectoris?

- Conservative - cessation of smoking, healthy diet, blood pressure control, diabetic control.
- Medical - antiplatelet, statin, nitrate, β-blocker, calcium channel blocker, nicorandil (see Chapter 3).
- Percutaneous coronary intervention (PCI) - balloon angioplasty, bare metal stent, drug-eluting stent.
- Surgery - coronary artery bypass grafting (CABG), transmyocardial revascularisation (see below).

3 What is the Canadian Cardiovascular Society (CCS) classification?

- It is a functional classification that relates the patient's symptoms of angina with the ability to perform activities:

a) I: no limitations of physical activity and no symptoms with ordinary activity;
b) II: slight limitation of physical activity with angina precipitated by vigorous activity;

c)   III: marked limitation of physical activity with angina precipitated by routine activity;

d)   IV: inability to perform any activities without angina or symptoms of angina at rest.

4   What is acute coronary syndrome (ACS)?

- Acute coronary syndrome represents a group of clinical conditions that are caused by acute myocardial ischaemia.
- They are grouped together as their management is similar and are only differentiated by blood tests and electrocardiographical changes:

a)   unstable angina (UA) - defined as angina:
  i)   occurring with increasing frequency and severity;
  ii)   occurring at rest or more frequently at night;
  iii)   not relieved quickly with sublingual glyceryl trinitrate (GTN);
b)   non-ST elevation MI (NSTEMI);
c)   ST elevation MI (STEMI).

Table 1. Cardiac enzymes and ECG changes associated with acute coronary syndrome.

	Troponin I (ng/mL)	CK and CK-MB	ECG changes
UA	<0.6	Normal	Transient ST and T-wave changes or normal ECG
NSTEMI	0.6-1.5	<2x normal	Transient ST and T-wave changes or normal ECG
STEMI	>1.5	>2x normal	ST elevation or Q waves

5   How are patients with UA or NSTEMI managed?

- The main principles of managing patients with UA and NSTEMI include:

a)   stabilisation of the atheromatous plaque;
b)   restoration of coronary blood flow;
c)   alleviation of the flow-limiting stenosis.

- Initial medical management of patients with acute coronary syndrome includes:

  a)   analgesia (diamorphine);
  b)   anti-anginal therapy (β-blocker, nitrate, calcium channel blocker);
  c)   dual antiplatelet therapy (aspirin and clopidogrel);
  d)   low-molecular-weight heparin;
  e)   statin.

- Within 6 months following admission with ACS, 30% of patients will be readmitted with recurrent unstable angina, myocardial infarction or death (12%). In view of this, it is important to risk stratify these patients to determine which patient should undergo coronary revascularisation prior to discharge.
- High-risk patients should receive glycoprotein IIb/IIIa inhibitors, undergo urgent coronary angiography and subsequent revascularisation with PCI or CABG. High-risk factors include:

  a)   patient factors:
     i)   age >65;
     ii)   hypertension;
     iii)   diabetes mellitus;
     iv)   previous myocardial infarction;
     v)   left ventricular dysfunction;
     vi)   ongoing pain despite medical therapy;
     vii)   cardiogenic shock;
  b)   ECG changes:
     i)   transient ST elevation or depression during pain;
     ii)   persistent ST depression;
     iii)   deep T-wave inversion;
     iv)   left bundle branch block (LBBB);
     v)   ventricular tachycardia;
  c)   any elevation in cardiac enzymes.

- The remaining patients should undergo investigation with an exercise tolerance test or stress nuclear medicine scanning and if positive proceed to coronary angiography.

6   How is myocardial infarction classified?

- Size:

  a)   microscopic - focal necrosis;

b)   small - <10% of the left ventricle;
c)   medium - 10-30% of the left ventricle;
d)   large - >30% of the left ventricle.

- Location - anterior, septal, inferior, lateral or posterior.
- Time from onset:

a)   acute - 6 hours to 7 days (polymorphonuclear leucocytes);
b)   healing - 7 to 28 days (mononuclear cells and fibroblasts);
c)   healed - >28 days (scar tissue without cellular infiltration).

- ST elevation:

a)   non-ST elevation MI - no transmurality;
b)   ST elevation MI - transmural.

7   **What are the diagnostic features of an acute ST elevation myocardial infarction (STEMI)(Figure 2 and Table 2)?**

- According to the European Society of Cardiology (ESC) and American College of Cardiology (ACC) guidelines, the criteria for acute ST elevation myocardial infarction are a typical rise and fall of cardiac enzymes (troponin or CK-MB) associated with at least one of the following:

a)   ST elevation (>0.1mV except >0.2mV in V1-3 at the J point in two or more contiguous leads) with peaked T wave;
b)   pathological Q waves >0.04sec or >25% of total QRS complex;
c)   ischaemic type chest pain lasting >20 minutes.

Table 2. Elevation of cardiac enzymes associated with acute myocardial infarction.

	Begins to rise (hours)	Peak (hours)	Remains elevated (days)
Tp I	4-6	12-16	5-10
Tp T	4-6	12-16	5-14
CK	4-8	12-24	3
CK-MB	2-6	12-24	2
Myoglobin	2	6-8	24

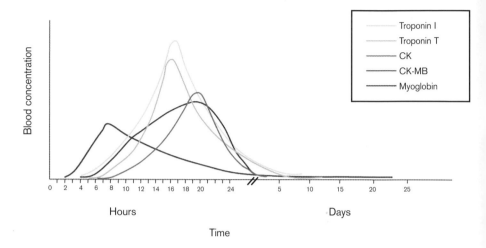

Figure 2. Cardiac enzyme elevation during acute ST elevation myocardial infarction. CK = creatinine kinase; CK-MB = creatinine kinase - muscle brain fraction.

- Elevated cardiac enzymes:

  a) creatinine kinase (normal <140IU/L for women and <170IU/L for men);
  b) creatinine kinase MB (cardiac) isoenzyme (normal <3.0ng/L);
  c) troponin T (normal <0.1ng/mL);
  d) troponin I (normal <0.3ng/mL) - may also be raised with renal impairment.

- LBBB can make ST elevation difficult to interpret.

8 **How are patients with STEMI managed?**

- The main principles of managing patients with STEMI are similar to those with UA and NSTEMI including stabilisation of atheromatous plaque, restoration of coronary blood flow and alleviation of the flow-limiting stenosis.
- Initial medical management of patients with STEMI includes:

  a) oxygen;
  b) analgesia (diamorphine) and anti-emetic (metoclopramide);
  c) antiplatelet therapy (aspirin);
  d) β-blocker;
  e) statin.

- Nitrates, furosemide, atropine and lidocaine may be required for the complications of myocardial infarction including ongoing chest pain, pulmonary oedema, bradycardia or ventricular arrhythmia, respectively.
- Restoration of coronary blood flow is achieved by primary PCI (if available) or thrombolysis (indications include ST elevation or new onset LBBB within 12 hours of the onset of pain or within 24 hours in patients with ongoing pain).
- High-risk rescue PCI or CABG may be required for patients who have ongoing chest pain or ECG changes following thrombolysis.

9 **What are the indications for coronary artery bypass grafting (CABG)?**

AHA guidelines

For asymptomatic patients or patients with mild angina
- Class I:

  a) significant left main stem stenosis (>50%);
  b) left main stem equivalent disease, which represents proximal left anterior descending artery (LAD) and proximal circumflex disease >70%;
  c) three-vessel coronary artery disease (survival benefit is greater in patients with a left ventricular ejection fraction [LVEF] <50%);
  d) one or two-vessel coronary artery disease (including proximal LAD stenosis) and LVEF <50%.

- Class IIa:

  a) one or two-vessel coronary artery disease (including proximal LAD stenosis) and LVEF >50%.

- Class IIb:

  a) one or two-vessel coronary artery disease (without proximal LAD stenosis) but a large area of myocardium at risk, demonstrated on non-invasive testing.

For patients with chronic stable angina
- Class I:

  a) significant left main stem stenosis (>50%);
  b) left main stem equivalent disease;
  c) three-vessel coronary artery disease (survival benefit is greater in patients with LVEF <50%);
  d) one or two-vessel coronary artery disease (including proximal LAD stenosis) and LVEF <50%;
  e) one or two-vessel coronary artery disease (without proximal LAD stenosis) but a large area of myocardium at risk, demonstrated on non-invasive testing.

- Class IIa:

  a) one or two-vessel coronary artery disease (including proximal LAD stenosis) and LVEF >50%;
  b) one or two-vessel coronary artery disease (without proximal LAD stenosis) but a moderate area of myocardium at risk, demonstrated on non-invasive testing.

- Class III (contra-indication):

  a) one or two-vessel coronary artery disease (without proximal LAD stenosis) with no myocardium at risk;
  b) borderline stenosis 50-60% with no myocardium at risk;
  c) insignificant stenosis (<50%).

Unstable angina or non-ST elevation MI

* Class I:

    a)   significant left main stem stenosis (>50%);
    b)   left main stem equivalent disease;
    c)   other coronary disease with ongoing ischaemia unresponsive to maximal non-surgical treatment.

* Class IIa:

    a)   one or two-vessel coronary artery disease (including proximal LAD stenosis) and LVEF >50%.

* Class IIb:

    a)   one or two-vessel coronary artery disease (without proximal LAD stenosis) when PCI is not an option but a large area of myocardium is at risk.

ST elevation MI

* Class I - emergency or urgent CABG is indicated when the patient has suitable coronary anatomy and:

    a)   failed PCI with haemodynamic instability;
    b)   persistent or recurrent ischaemia with a large area of myocardium at risk but not suitable for PCI;
    c)   mechanical complications of myocardial infarction including ventricular septal rupture, mitral regurgitation and left ventricular rupture;
    d)   cardiogenic shock within 36 hours of MI, unless further intervention is futile;
    e)   life-threatening ventricular arrhythmias with left main stem stenosis >50% or three-vessel coronary artery disease.

* Class IIa:

    a)   primary reperfusion within 6-12 hours of MI, in patients not suitable for, or following failed, PCI and thrombolysis.

- Class III (contra-indication):

  a) haemodynamically stable patient with a small area of myocardium at risk.

Poor LV function

- Class I:

  a) significant left main stem stenosis (>50%);
  b) left main stem equivalent disease;
  c) three-vessel coronary artery disease;
  d) one or two-vessel coronary artery disease (including proximal LAD stenosis).

- Class IIa:

  a) significant viable non-contracting revascularisable myocardium (without above anatomy).

- Class III (contra-indication):

  a) no evidence of intermittent ischaemia or viable non-contracting revascularisable myocardium.

Life-threatening ventricular arrhythmias

- Class I:

  a) life-threatening ventricular arrhythmia caused by left main stem stenosis or three-vessel coronary artery disease;
  b) resuscitated sudden death or sustained ventricular tachycardia in patients with one or two-vessel coronary artery disease.

- Class IIa:

  a) life-threatening ventricular arrhythmia caused by one or two-vessel coronary artery disease.

- Class III (contra-indication):

  a) ventricular tachycardia with myocardial scar and no evidence of ischaemia.

CABG after failed PCI

- Class I:

  a) ongoing ischaemia;
  b) threatened occlusion;
  c) haemodynamic compromise.

- Class IIa:

  a) retained foreign body;
  b) haemodynamic compromise with impaired clotting and no previous median sternotomy.

- Class IIb:

  a) haemodynamic compromise with impaired clotting and previous median sternotomy.

- Class III (contra-indication):

  a) no evidence of ischaemia;
  b) no suitable targets for grafting.

Patients with previous CABG

- Class I:

  a) disabling angina pectoris despite maximal non-surgical therapy;
  b) if no grafts are patent, indications are similar to that for primary coronary artery bypass grafting (e.g. left main stem stenosis or three-vessel coronary artery disease).

- Class IIa:

  a) threatened myocardium, demonstrated by non-invasive studies;
  b) atherosclerotic vein grafts with >50% stenosis supplying a large area of myocardium.

10 **What are the recommendations and levels of evidence for revascularisation in patients with lesions suitable for both CABG and PCI and low predicted surgical mortality (Table 3)?**

Table 3. European Society of Cardiology guidelines for revascularisation with PCI and CABG.

Subset of CAD by anatomy	Favours CABG	Favours PCI
1VD or 2VD - non-proximal LAD	IIb C	I C
1VD or 2VD - proximal LAD	I A	IIa B
3VD simple lesions, full revascularisation achievable with PCI, SYNTAX score ≤22	I A	IIa B
3VD simple lesions, incomplete revascularisation achievable with PCI, SYNTAX score >22	I A	III A
Left main (isolated or 1VD, ostium or shaft)	I A	IIa B
Left main (isolated or 1VD, distal bifurcation)	I A	IIb B
Left main + 2VD or 3VD, SYNTAX score ≤32	I A	IIb B
Left main + 2VD or 3VD, SYNTAX score ≥33	I A	III B

CABG = coronary artery bypass grafting; CAD = coronary artery disease; LAD = left anterior descending; PCI = percutaneous coronary intervention; VD = vessel disease

11 **What are the short and long-term survival results for patients undergoing CABG?**

- Short and long-term results for individual patients depend on a number of risk factors but overall quoted figures for isolated CABG are shown below (Table 4).

360

Table 4. Short and long-term results for patients undergoing CABG.	
30-day survival	98-99%
1-year survival	97%
2-year survival	96%
3-year survival	93%
5-year survival	90%
10-year survival	80%
15-year survival	60%
20-year survival	40%
5-year freedom from angina	83%
10-year freedom from angina	63%
10-year freedom from re-operation	90%
20-year freedom from re-operation	75%

12 What is the risk and important predictors of morbidity and mortality following CABG?

- Stroke (3.1%) - aortic atherosclerosis, hypertension, age >70.
- Deep sternal wound infection (2.5%) - obesity, reoperation, bilateral internal mammary artery harvest, diabetes mellitus, operative duration.
- Renal failure (7.7%) - age, left ventricular dysfunction, prior CABG, diabetes mellitus, pre-existing renal impairment (creatinine >140μmol/L).
- Postoperative atrial fibrillation (28%) - age, chronic obstructive pulmonary disease, proximal right coronary artery disease, prolonged aortic cross-clamp time, atrial ischaemia, withdrawal of β-blockers, cross-clamp fibrillation technique (as cardioplegia contains magnesium).
- Postoperative mortality (1-2%) - age, previous cardiac surgery, urgency of operation, left ventricular dysfunction (see EuroSCORE: Table 5).
- Long-term survival - age, diabetes mellitus, number of vessels of coronary artery disease, gender, left ventricular dysfunction.

Table 5. EuroSCORE.

Patient-related factors		Score
Age	(per 5 years or part thereof over 60 years)	1
Gender	Female	1
Chronic pulmonary disease	Long-term use of bronchodilators or steroids for lung disease	1
Extracardiac arteriopathy	Any one or more of the following: claudication, carotid occlusion or >50% stenosis, previous or planned intervention on the abdominal aorta, limb arteries or carotids	2
Neurological dysfunction	Disease severely affecting ambulation or day-to-day functioning	2
Previous cardiac surgery	Requiring opening of the pericardium	3
Serum creatinine	>200µmol/L pre-operatively	2
Active endocarditis	Patient still under antibiotic treatment for endocarditis at the time of surgery	3
Critical pre-operative state	Any one or more of the following: ventricular tachycardia or fibrillation or aborted sudden death, pre-operative cardiac massage, pre-operative ventilation before arrival in the anaesthetic room, pre-operative inotropic support, intra-aortic balloon counterpulsation or pre-operative acute renal failure (anuria or oliguria <10mL/hour)	3

Cardiac-related factors		Score
Unstable angina	Rest angina requiring IV nitrates until arrival in the anaesthetic room	2
LV dysfunction	Moderate LV (EF 30-50%)	1
	Poor LV (EF <30%)	3
Recent myocardial infarct	<90 days	2
Pulmonary hypertension	Systolic PA pressure >60 mmHg	2

Operation-related factors		Score
Emergency	Carried out on referral before the beginning of the next working day	2
Other than isolated CABG	Major cardiac procedure other than or in addition to CABG	2
Surgery on thoracic aorta	For disorder of ascending, arch or descending aorta	3
Post-infarct septal rupture		4

The Additive EuroSCORE (sum total of the score) represents an approximate percentage mortality risk. The Logistic EuroSCORE, which is calculated using a complex algorithm involving the same factors, is thought to be more accurate at predicting the operative mortality risk.

362

13 **How would you manage a patient with a porcelain aorta requiring CABG (Figure 3)?**
- No-touch technique using off-pump or hypothermic fibrillatory arrest (with femoral artery cannulation) with bilateral mammary arteries and a y-graft or sequential anastomosis, as required.
- Hybrid procedure with off-pump LIMA-LAD (left internal mammary artery to left anterior descending artery) anastomosis and PCI to the remaining lesions.
- PCI if the porcelain aorta is discovered pre-operatively.

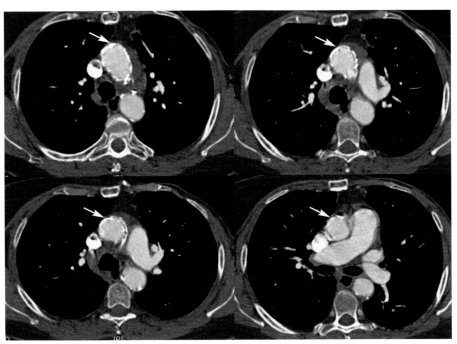

Figure 3. Porcelain aorta. Marked calcification (arrows) of the ascending aorta makes aortic cross-clamping impossible.

14 **Which patients should have a CABG on an in-hospital urgent basis rather than placed on a routine elective waiting list?**
- NSTEMI - high-risk group.
- Critical anatomy - left main stem stenosis, left main equivalent with right coronary artery disease.
- Unstable angina - ongoing symptoms at rest.
- Cardiac instability - pulmonary oedema or ventricular arrhythmias with surgical anatomy.

15 How is a patient with acute post-infarct ventricular septal rupture (VSR) managed?

- According to the AHA guidelines, a patient with a post-infarction ventricular septal rupture should undergo emergency repair, with coronary artery bypass grafting at the same time.
- These patients are haemodynamically optimised without delaying surgery by using an inodilator (such as dobutamine), diuretics and placing an intra-aortic balloon pump (IABP). This reduces the systemic vascular resistance and the left to right shunt, thereby maintaining cardiac output and organ perfusion.
- In patients who present with cardiogenic shock and multi-organ failure, it may be prudent to optimise them with medical therapy as emergency surgery carries a very high mortality in this cohort.

16 What is the long-term survival of patients with post-infarct VSR?

- In patients medically treated with post-infarct VSR, the survival is shown in Table 6.

Table 6. Long-term survival of patients with medically treated post-infarct VSR.

1 day	75%
1 week	50%
2 weeks	35%
1 month	20%
1 year	5%

- In comparison, the operative mortality for these patients is 30-40%, with a 5-year survival of 75% in hospital survivors and an NYHA symptom status I-II in 80%.

17 What are the operative risk factors for patients undergoing surgery for post-infarct VSR?

- Cardiogenic shock.
- Left main stem stenosis.
- Right heart failure.

- Renal impairment.
- Inferior myocardial infarction.
- Increased age.

18 What is the operative technique for a post-infarct VSR (Figure 4)?

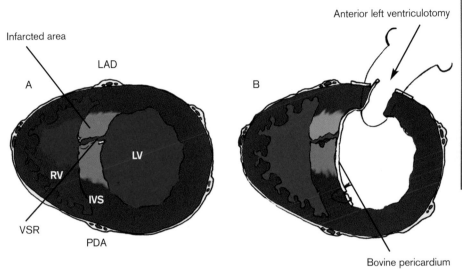

Figure 4. Surgical repair of a post-infarct ventricular septal rupture. A) Antero-septal myocardial infarction with associated ventricular septal rupture. B) Following an anterior ventriculotomy, the rupture is excluded from the left ventricular cavity using a bovine pericardial patch, which is brought out through the ventriculotomy. C) Two-layered closure of the ventriculotomy, supported by Teflon® strips. PDA = posterior descending artery; LAD = left anterior descending artery; LV = left ventricle; RV = right ventricle; IVS = interventricular septum; VSR = ventricular septal rupture.

- A left ventriculotomy is made through the infarcted anterior or inferior left ventricular wall 2-3cm parallel to the left anterior descending artery or posterior descending artery, respectively.
- A glutaraldehyde-fixed bovine pericardial patch is then sutured to healthy endocardium deep in the left ventricle, to exclude the infarct and VSR from the high-pressure area of the left ventricle.
- The ventriculotomy is closed in two layers, buttressed by Teflon® strips and biological glue.
- Using this technique left ventricular geometry and volume can be restored.

19 How is a patient with a post-infarct left ventricular false aneurysm managed?

- Acute rupture is invariably fatal.
- In patients who present subacutely, the infarct exclusion technique (as described with post-infarct VSR repair) can be used.
- Alternatively, the left ventricle can be closed in two layers buttressed by Teflon® strips and biological glue.

20 How is a patient with post-infarct papillary muscle rupture managed?

- Surgery is the treatment of choice. Although operative mortality is high (20-50%), it compares favourably with medical treatment (75% mortality at 24 hours and 95% at 48 hours).
- Pre-operatively, these patients are haemodynamically optimised without delaying surgery by using an inodilator (such as dobutamine), and diuretics, and placing an IABP. This reduces the systemic vascular resistance, thereby helping to maintain cardiac output and organ perfusion until surgical correction.
- Operative techniques include:

  a) re-implantation of the papillary muscle in patients with partial rupture;
  b) mitral valve replacement in patients with complete papillary muscle rupture.

21 **In addition to the LIMA, what are the conduit options for patients with long saphenous varicose veins undergoing CABG?**

- Right internal mammary artery.
- Left and right radial arteries.
- Sequential grafts.
- Short saphenous vein.
- Hybrid procedure with LIMA-LAD followed by PCI.

22 **What is the long-term patency of coronary artery bypass conduits (Figure 5 and Table 7)?**

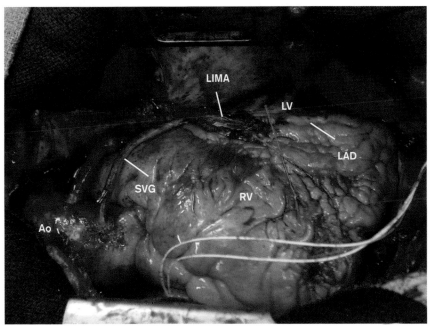

Figure 5. Operative image following completion of coronary artery bypass grafting surgery with the LIMA anastomosed to the LAD and SVG anastomosed to the diagonal, obtuse marginal and posterior descending artery. LIMA = left internal mammary artery; LAD = left anterior descending artery; SVG = saphenous vein graft; Ao = aorta; RV = right ventricle; LV = left ventricle.

Table 7. Long-term patency of coronary artery bypass conduits.		
LIMA	95%	10-year patency
Free LIMA	90%	10-year patency
RIMA	90%	10-year patency
Free RIMA	80%	10-year patency
Radial artery	80%	9-year patency
Gastroepiploic artery	63%	10-year patency
Inferior epigastric artery	80%	1-year patency
Long saphenous vein	80%	9-year patency
Short saphenous vein	60%	3-year patency
Cephalic vein	45%	5-year patency
Cryopreserved homograft vein	15%	1-year patency

23 What is the evidence for using the radial artery as a conduit for CABG?

- Several non-randomised retrospective studies have shown improved patency using radial artery as compared to long saphenous vein as the second graft in addition to the left internal mammary artery.
- This difference in long-term patency, however, has not been confirmed in the prospective, randomised controlled trials that have compared the two conduits, including the RAPCO study (Radial Artery Patency and Clinical Outcome), which showed the 5-year patency of saphenous vein grafts to be 94% compared to radial artery grafts at 87%. Subsequent data from the same trial showed the longer-term patency to be approximately 80% in both groups at 9 years.
- Radial artery grafts have been shown to have better patency on left-sided coronary targets with >70% stenosis.

24 What are the principles of using the left internal mammary artery to left anterior descending artery graft (LIMA-LAD)?

- The use of the LIMA-LAD, in addition to saphenous vein grafts, confers a 10% survival benefit at 10 years, compared to those who have saphenous vein grafts alone.
- The use of the left internal mammary artery as a conduit to bypass the left anterior descending artery has also been shown to improve peri-operative mortality, and freedom from angina, myocardial infarction and re-intervention.

25 When should the internal mammary artery be harvested as a skeletonised conduit (Figure 6)?

- Use of bilateral skeletonised mammary arteries can reduce the incidence of mediastinitis and sternal dehiscence as compared to bilateral pedicled mammary arteries, especially in diabetic patients.
- In the only prospective, randomised trial comparing the two techniques of internal mammary harvest, skeletonisation was shown to reduce postoperative pain and improve sternal perfusion. There was, however, no difference in conduit length or arterial flow.
- Harvesting the mammary artery using a skeletonised technique, however, takes more time and may lead to increased endothelial damage and vasoreactivity.
- Furthermore, some studies have demonstrated reduced long-term patency of skeletonised mammary arteries.

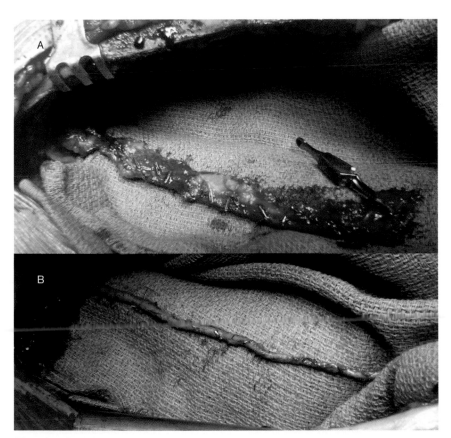

Figure 6. Left internal mammary artery. A) Pedicled. B) Skeletonised.

26 What is the evidence for using bilateral internal mammary arteries as a conduit for CABG?

- Large retrospective studies and a meta-analysis have demonstrated a survival advantage, improved long-term patency and greater freedom from re-intervention using the right internal mammary artery as the second conduit for CABG as opposed to saphenous vein.
- Bilateral internal mammary artery harvest, however, is associated with an increased incidence of sternal dehiscence as compared to patients that only had a single internal mammary artery harvested.
- Long-term survival and patency results of bilateral internal mammary artery use are awaited from the prospective, randomised Arterial Revascularisation Trial (ART).

27 What are the principles of off-pump coronary artery bypass grafting (OPCAB)(Figure 7)?

- The heart is appropriately positioned using deep pericardial sutures, an apical suction device (such as the Starfish®) and a coronary artery stabilising device (such as the Octopus®).
- The right pleural cavity may be opened to allow large hearts to be displaced into the right pleural space thus preventing mechanical

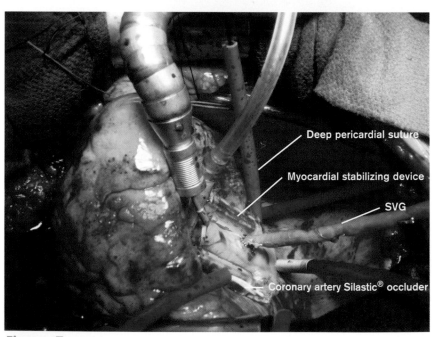

Figure 7. Off-pump coronary artery bypass grafting. SVG = saphenous vein graft.

compression of the right heart during grafting of the circumflex territory.

- Haemodynamic stability is maintained using a deep Trendelenburg position, fluid boluses and vasopressors.
- Following clearing of the epicardial fat, a snare is placed proximally to encircle the coronary artery.
- The coronary artery is then occluded, opened and the diameter of the vessel measured.
- An appropriately sized shunt (just smaller than the diameter of the vessel) is placed and the snare released.
- Coronary artery bypass grafting can then be performed with the aid of a Blower/Mister to enhance visualisation.

28 What is the evidence for OPCAB surgery?

- Although retrospective, non-randomised studies have shown improved morbidity and mortality using OPCAB as compared to CABG using standard cardiopulmonary bypass, these changes have not been consistently shown in the prospective randomised trials.
- The majority of these studies, however, have shown a reduced intensive care unit and hospital length of stay, need for blood transfusion and release of cardiac enzymes.
- Meta-analyses, however, have shown a reduced long-term patency and number of vessels revascularised with OPCAB as compared to CABG using standard cardiopulmonary bypass. Furthermore, certain coronary arteries (small, intramuscular, calcified vessels) may not be accessible during OPCAB and there is a high mortality when these patients need to be converted to cardiopulmonary bypass.

29 What are the principles of transmyocardial revascularisation (TMR)(Figure 8)?

- TMR uses yttrium aluminium garnet (YAG) or carbon dioxide (CO_2) laser energy to create transmural myocardial channels, thereby directing oxygenated blood from the left ventricle into ischaemic myocardium mimicking the myocardial perfusion of the reptilian heart. The myocardial injury caused by the laser is also thought to improve myocardial blood supply by inducing angiogenesis.
- TMR can be used for patients with symptomatic coronary artery disease, on maximal medical treatment, who are not amenable to CABG or PCI.
- Studies have shown that TMR leads to an improvement in angina symptoms, exercise tolerance and myocardial perfusion but no increase in survival at 1 year.

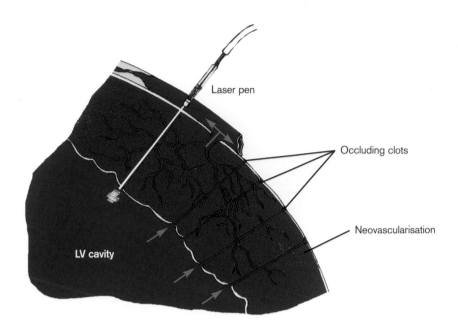

Figure 8. Transmyocardial revascularization. LV = left ventricular.

● Attempts at percutaneous TMR failed to show any improvement in symptoms or exercise tolerance.

30 How are patients with carotid artery stenosis undergoing CABG managed?

● Carotid screening is recommended in patients:

   a)   with a carotid bruit;
   b)   with a previous neurological event;
   c)   aged over 65 years;
   d)   with left main stem stenosis;
   e)   with a smoking history;
   f)   with peripheral vascular disease.

● The post-CABG risk of stroke is 2% in patients with a carotid stenosis <50%, 10% with a 50-80% stenosis, 15% with a stenosis >80% and 20% with an untreated high-grade bilateral carotid stenosis.

- According to the AHA guidelines (Class IIa), carotid endarterectomy is recommended prior to or concomitant with CABG for patients with asymptomatic unilateral stenosis >80% or symptomatic carotid stenosis.
- Carotid artery stenting can be used as an alternative to endarterectomy for patients with carotid artery stenosis.

31 What are the principles of drug-eluting stents (DES)?

- DES incorporate a drug (such as sirolimus or paclitaxel) that is released slowly over months, which impairs the cellular proliferation and fibromuscular hyperplasia healing response to stent deployment and balloon barotrauma.
- Complications of stent deployment include:

  a) immediate complications, such as occlusion (stent thrombosis), embolism, dissection, side-branch occlusion and wire fracture;

  b) emergency CABG (0.3%), mortality (0.5%), MI (0.8%), local vascular problems (2%);

  c) in-stent stenosis, secondary to neointimal hyperplasia, which is reduced in DES as compared to bare metal stents;

  d) late stent thrombosis, which is more common with DES as the polymer has inhibited endothelialisation of the stent, hence when dual antiplatelet therapy is stopped, there is an increased risk of thrombosis.

32 What did the VA coronary artery bypass grafting trial show?

- VA = Veterans Administration.
- The VA trial was a prospective, randomised controlled study between 1972-1974 in 686 men with coronary artery disease, including those with impaired left ventricular function (EF <35%), left main stem stenosis and aged >65 years old.
- The patients were randomised to either:

  a) group I (n=354) - optimal medical treatment;

  b) group II (n=332) - coronary artery bypass grafting and optimal medical treatment.

- For those undergoing CABG, the study demonstrated:

  a) an overall survival advantage at 7 years follow-up (CABG 77% vs. medical treatment 70%) but not at 11 years (CABG 58% vs. medical treatment 57%);

  b) a survival advantage for patients with impaired left ventricular function and three-vessel disease at 7 years follow-up (CABG 76% vs. medical treatment 52%) and at 11 years (CABG 50% vs. medical treatment 38%);

  c) a survival advantage for patients with left main stem stenosis (CABG 80% vs. medical treatment 64%) at 7 years.

33 What did the ECSS trial show?

- ECSS = European Coronary Surgery Study.
- The ECSS trial was a prospective, randomised controlled study between 1973-1976 in 768 men with coronary artery disease, including those with good left ventricular function (EF <50% excluded) and two or more-vessel disease (single-vessel disease excluded).

- The patients were randomised to either:

  a) group I (n=373) - optimal medical treatment;

  b) group II (n=395) - coronary artery bypass grafting and optimal medical treatment.

- For those undergoing CABG, the study demonstrated:

  a) an overall survival advantage at 5 years (CABG 92% vs. medical treatment 83%) and 12 years follow-up (CABG 71% vs. medical treatment 67%) but with the two groups becoming more convergent with time;

  b) a decreased recurrence of angina (CABG 51% vs. medical treatment 80%);

  c) a survival advantage for patients with proximal LAD stenosis (CABG 88% vs. medical treatment 79%) at 8 years;

  d) a survival advantage for patients with three-vessel coronary artery disease (CABG 92% vs. medical treatment 77%) at 8 years.

- The convergence was attributed to saphenous vein graft stenosis, progression of the original native lesions, new coronary artery lesions and cross-over of patients from the medical group to the surgical group.

34 **What did the CASS trial show?**
- CASS = Coronary Artery Surgery Study.
- The CASS trial was a prospective, randomised controlled study between 1975-1979 in 780 patients (16% females) with coronary artery disease, excluding those with impaired left ventricular function (EF <35%) or aged >65 years old.
- The patients were randomised to either:

  a) group I (n=390) - optimal medical treatment;
  b) group II (n=390) - coronary artery bypass grafting and optimal medical treatment.

- At 10-year follow-up, for those undergoing CABG, the study demonstrated:

  a) no significant overall survival difference;
  b) a survival advantage for patients with impaired left ventricular function (CABG 80% vs. medical treatment 59%) and especially with three-vessel coronary disease.

35 **What did the Yusuf meta-analysis show?**
- This meta-analysis collected data from 7 prospective, randomised studies between 1972-1984 that compared coronary artery bypass grafting surgery with optimal medical management for patients with coronary artery disease.
- The study demonstrated a significant overall survival advantage and freedom from angina for patients in the CABG group at 5, 7 and 10 years but with the two groups becoming more convergent over time:

  a) 5-year survival - CABG 90% vs. optimal medical treatment 84%;
  b) 7-year survival - CABG 84% vs. optimal medical treatment 78%;
  c) 10-year survival - CABG 74% vs. optimal medical treatment 69%.

- In addition, subgroup analysis demonstrated a significant survival advantage for patients undergoing CABG, with left main stem stenosis, proximal LAD stenosis or three-vessel coronary artery disease.
- There was no significant difference between surgery and medical treatment for patients with one or two-vessel disease (without proximal LAD stenosis).

36 What did the BARI trial show?

- BARI = Bypass Angioplasty Revascularisation Investigation.
- The BARI trial was a prospective, randomised controlled study between 1988-1991 in 1829 patients with coronary artery disease (41% with three-vessel disease).
- The patients were randomised to either:

   a)   group I (n=915) - percutaneous transluminal coronary (balloon) angioplasty (PTCA);

   b)   group II (n=914) - coronary artery bypass grafting.

- At mean 5-year follow-up, for those undergoing CABG, the study demonstrated:

   a)   no overall survival advantage;

   b)   a decreased need for repeat revascularisation (CABG 8% vs. PTCA 54%);

   c)   a survival advantage for diabetic patients (CABG 81% vs. PTCA 65%).

37 What did the RITA trial show?

- RITA = Randomised Intervention Treatment of Angina trial.
- The RITA trial was a prospective, randomised controlled study between 1988-1991 in 1011 patients with coronary artery disease (12% with three-vessel disease), excluding patients with left main stem stenosis.
- The patients were randomised to either:

   a)   group I (n=510) - percutaneous transluminal coronary (balloon) angioplasty (PTCA);

   b)   group II (n=501) - coronary artery bypass grafting.

- At mean 5-year follow-up, for those undergoing CABG, the study demonstrated:

   a)   no overall survival advantage;

   b)   a decreased need for repeat revascularisation (CABG 12% vs. PTCA 53%);

   c)   a decreased recurrence of angina (CABG 34% vs. PTCA 49%).

38 What did the ARTS trial show?

- ARTS = Arterial Revascularization Therapies Study.
- The ARTS trial was a prospective, randomised controlled study between 1997-1998 in 1205 patients with coronary artery disease (30% with three-vessel disease), excluding patients with left main stem stenosis.
- The patients were randomised to either:

  a) group I (n=600) - percutaneous coronary intervention with bare metal stents;
  b) group II (n=605) - coronary artery bypass grafting.

- At mean 5-year follow-up, for those undergoing CABG, the study demonstrated:

  a) no overall survival advantage;
  b) a decreased need for repeat revascularisation (CABG 9% vs. PTCA 30%);
  c) a decreased recurrence of angina (CABG 16% vs. PTCA 21%);
  d) this difference was more marked in patients with diabetes mellitus.

39 What did the SoS trial show?

- SoS = Stent or Surgery.
- The SoS trial was a prospective, randomised controlled study between 1997-1998 in 988 patients with coronary artery disease (42% with three-vessel disease and 1% with left main stem stenosis).
- The patients were randomised to either:

  a) group I (n=488) - percutaneous coronary intervention with bare metal stents;
  b) group II (n=500) - coronary artery bypass grafting.

- At mean 2-year follow-up, for those undergoing CABG, the study demonstrated:

  a) decreased mortality (CABG 2% vs. PCI 5%);
  b) a decreased need for repeat revascularisation (CABG 6% vs. PCI 21%);
  c) a decreased recurrence of angina (CABG 21% vs. PCI 34%).

40 What did the SYNTAX trial show?
- SYNTAX = Synergy between PCI with TAXUS and cardiac surgery.
- The SYNTAX trial was a prospective, randomised controlled study between 2005-2007 in 1800 patients with three-vessel coronary artery disease or left main stem stenosis.
- The patients were randomised to either:

  a) group I (n=897) - percutaneous coronary intervention with drug (paclitaxel)-eluting stents;
  b) group II (n=903) - coronary artery bypass grafting.

- At mean 1-year follow-up, for those undergoing CABG, the study demonstrated:

  a) decreased major adverse cardiac or cerebrovascular events (CABG 12.4% vs. PCI 17.8%);
  b) a decreased need for repeat revascularisation (CABG 6% vs. PCI 13%);
  c) an increased rate of stroke (CABG 2.2% vs. PCI 0.6%);
  d) no difference for death or myocardial infarction.

- At mean 3-year follow-up, the difference in the stroke rate was no longer significant (CABG 3.4% vs. PCI 2.0%). The CABG group, however, still had significantly decreased major adverse cardiac or cerebrovascular events (CABG 20.2% vs. PCI 28.0%), MI (CABG 3.6% vs. PCI 7.1%) and repeat revascularisation (CABG 10.7% vs. PCI 19.7%) rates.
- The study concluded that CABG remains the standard of care for patients with three-vessel or left main coronary artery disease.

41 What did the ROOBY trial show?
- ROOBY = Randomized On/Off Bypass Study.
- The ROOBY trial was a prospective randomised study in 2203 patients undergoing urgent or elective coronary artery bypass grafting (CABG).
- The patients were randomised to:

  a) group I (n=1104) - off-pump CABG; or
  b) group II (n=1099) - on-pump CABG.

- The study demonstrated:

  a)   12.4% of patients in the off-pump group required intra-operative conversion to on-pump CABG;

  b)   no difference in short-term (30-day) outcomes, including death, reoperation, stroke, renal failure or additional mechanical support;

  c)   higher composite outcome of death, myocardial infarction and repeat revascularisation after 1 year in the off-pump group (off-pump 9.9% vs. on-pump 7.4%);

  d)   lower graft patency at 1 year in the off-pump group (off-pump 82.6% vs. on-pump 87.8%).

- The study concluded that patients undergoing off-pump CABG had worse composite outcomes and graft patencies at 1 year.

Recommended reading

1.   Loop FD, Lytle BW, Cosgrove DM, Stewart RW, Goormastic M, Williams GW, Golding LA, Gill CC, Taylor PC, Sheldon WC, Proudfit W. Influence of the internal-mammary-artery graft on 10-year survival and other cardiac events. *N Engl J Med* 1986; 314: 1-6.

2.   The Veterans Administration Coronary Artery Bypass Surgery Cooperative Study Group. Eleven-year survival in the Veterans Administration randomized trial of coronary bypass surgery for stable angina. *N Engl J Med* 1984; 311: 1333-9.

3.   Varnauskas E. Twelve-year follow-up of survival in the randomized European Coronary Surgery Study. *N Engl J Med* 1988; 319: 332-7.

4.   Alderman EL, Bourassa MG, Cohen LS, Davis KB, Kaiser GG, Killip T, Mock MB, Pettinger M, Robertson TL. Ten-year follow-up of survival and myocardial infarction in the randomized Coronary Artery Surgery Study. *Circulation* 1990; 82: 1629-46.

5.   Yusuf S, Zucker D, Peduzzi P, Fisher LD, Takaro T, Kennedy JW, Davis K, Killip T, Passamani E, Norris R, Morris C, Mathur V, Varnauskas E, Chalmers TC. Effect of coronary artery bypass graft surgery on survival: overview of 10-year results from randomised trials by the Coronary Artery Bypass Graft Surgery Trialists Collaboration. *Lancet* 1994; 344: 563-70.

6.   The Bypass Angioplasty Revascularization Investigation (BARI) Investigators. Comparison of coronary bypass surgery with angioplasty in patients with multivessel disease. *N Engl J Med* 1996; 335: 217-25.

7.   Coronary angioplasty versus coronary artery bypass surgery: the Randomized Intervention Treatment of Angina (RITA) trial. *Lancet* 1993; 341: 573-80.

8.   Serruys PW, Ong AT, van Herwerden LA, Sousa JE, Jatene A, Bonnier JJ, Schönberger JP, Buller N, Bonser R, Disco C, Backx B, Hugenholtz PG, Firth BG, Unger F. Five-year outcomes after coronary stenting versus bypass surgery for the

treatment of multivessel disease: the final analysis of the Arterial Revascularization Therapies Study (ARTS) randomized trial. *J Am Coll Cardiol* 2005; 46(4): 575-81.

9. SoS Investigators. Coronary artery bypass surgery versus percutaneous coronary intervention with stent implantation in patients with multivessel coronary artery disease (the Stent or Surgery trial): a randomised controlled trial. *Lancet* 2002; 360(9338): 965-70.

10. Cleveland JC, Shroyer AL, Chen AY, Peterson E, Grover FL. Offpump coronary artery bypass grafting decreases risk-adjusted mortality and morbidity. *Ann Thorac Surg* 2001; 72: 1282-8.

11. Angelini GD, Taylor FC, Reeves BC, Ascione R. Early and midterm outcome after off-pump and on-pump surgery in Beating Heart Against Cardioplegic Arrest Studies (BHACAS 1 and 2): a pooled analysis of two randomised controlled trials. *Lancet* 2002; 359: 1194-9.

12. van Dijk D, Nierich AP, Jansen EW, Nathoe HM, Suyker WJ, Diephuis JC, van Boven WJ, Borst C, Buskens E, Grobbee DE, Robles De Medina EO, de Jaegere PP; Octopus Study Group. Early outcome after off-pump versus on-pump coronary bypass surgery: results from a randomized study. *Circulation* 2001; 104: 1761-6.

13. Puskas JD, Williams WH, Duke PG, Staples JR, Glas KE, Marshall JJ, Leimbach M, Huber P, Garas S, Sammons BH, McCall SA, Petersen RJ, Bailey DE, Chu H, Mahoney EM, Weintraub WS, Guyton RA. Off-pump coronary artery bypass grafting provides complete revascularization with reduced myocardial injury, transfusion requirements, and length of stay: a prospective randomized comparison of two hundred unselected patients undergoing off-pump versus conventional coronary artery bypass grafting. *J Thorac Cardiovasc Surg* 2003; 125: 797-808.

14. Boodhwani M, Lam BK, Nathan HJ, Mesana TG, Ruel M, Zeng W, Sellke FW, Rubens FD. Skeletonized internal thoracic artery harvest reduces pain and dysesthesia and improves sternal perfusion after coronary artery bypass surgery: a randomized, double-blind, within-patient comparison. *Circulation* 2006; 114(8): 766-73.

15. Hayward PA, Gordon IR, Hare DL, Matalanis G, Horrigan ML, Rosalion A, Buxton BF. Comparable patencies of the radial artery and right internal thoracic artery or saphenous vein beyond 5 years: results from the Radial Artery Patency and Clinical Outcomes trial. *J Thorac Cardiovasc Surg* 2010; 139(1): 60-5.

16. Buxton BF, Raman JS, Ruengsakulrach P, Gordon I, Rosalion A, Bellomo R, Horrigan M, Hare DL. Radial artery patency and clinical outcomes: five-year interim results of a randomized trial. *J Thorac Cardiovasc Surg* 2003; 125(6): 1363-71.

17. Patel MR, Dehmer GJ, Hirshfeld JW, Smith PK, Spertus JA. ACCF/SCAI/STS/AATS/AHA/ASNC 2009 Appropriateness Criteria for Coronary Revascularization. *Circulation* 2009; 119(9): 1330-52.

18. Eagle KA, Guyton RA, Davidoff R, Edwards FH, Ewy GA, Gardner TJ, Hart JC, Herrmann HC, Hillis LD, Hutter AM Jr, Lytle BW, Marlow RA, Nugent WC, Orszulak TA; American College of Cardiology; American Heart Association. ACC/AHA 2004 guideline update for coronary artery bypass graft surgery. *Circulation* 2004; 110(14): e340-437.

19. Taggart DP, D'Amico R, Altman DG. Effect of arterial revascularisation on survival: a systematic review of studies comparing bilateral and single internal mammary arteries. *Lancet* 2001; 358(9285): 870-5.

20. Taggart DP, Lees B, Gray A, Altman DG, Flather M, Channon K; ART Investigators. Protocol for the Arterial Revascularisation Trial (ART). A randomised trial to compare survival following bilateral versus single internal mammary grafting in coronary revascularisation [ISRCTN46552265]. *Trials* 2006; 7: 7.

21. Lytle BW, Blackstone EH, Loop FD, Houghtaling PL, Arnold JH, Akhrass R, McCarthy PM, Cosgrove DM. Two internal thoracic artery grafts are better than one. *J Thorac Cardiovasc Surg* 1999; 117(5): 855-72.

22. Parolari A, Alamanni F, Polvani G, Agrifoglio M, Chen YB, Kassem S, Veglia F, Tremoli E, Biglioli P. Meta-analysis of randomized trials comparing off-pump with on-pump coronary artery bypass graft patency. *Ann Thorac Surg* 2005; 80(6): 2121-5.

23. Lim E, Drain A, Davies W, Edmonds L, Rosengard BR. A systematic review of randomized trials comparing revascularization rate and graft patency of off-pump and conventional coronary surgery. *J Thorac Cardiovasc Surg* 2006; 132(6): 1409-13.

24. Serruys PW, Morice MC, Kappetein AP, Colombo A, Holmes DR, Mack MJ, Ståhle E, Feldman TE, van den Brand M, Bass EJ, Van Dyck N, Leadley K, Dawkins KD, Mohr FW; SYNTAX Investigators. Percutaneous coronary intervention versus coronary artery bypass grafting for severe coronary artery disease. *N Engl J Med* 2009; 360(10): 961-72.

25. Alpert JS, Thygesen K, Antman E, Bassand JP. Myocardial infarction redefined: a consensus document of the Joint European Society of Cardiology/American College of Cardiology Committee for the redefinition of myocardial infarction. *J Am Coll Cardiol* 2000; 36: 959-69.

26. Anderson JL, Adams CD, Antman EM, Bridges CR, Califf RM, Casey DE Jr, Chavey WE 2nd, Fesmire FM, Hochman JS, Levin TN, Lincoff AM, Peterson ED, Theroux P, Wenger NK, Wright RS, Smith SC Jr, Jacobs AK, Halperin JL, Hunt SA, Krumholz HM, Kushner FG, Lytle BW, Nishimura R, Ornato JP, Page RL, Riegel B. ACC/AHA 2007 guidelines for the management of patients with unstable angina/non-ST-elevation myocardial infarction: *J Am Coll Cardiol* 2007; 50: e1-e157.

27. Stone GW, Teirstein PS, Rubenstein R, Schmidt D, Whitlow PL, Kosinski EJ, Mishkel G, Power JA. A prospective, multicenter, randomized trial of percutaneous transmyocardial laser revascularization in patients with nonrecanalizable chronic total occlusions. *J Am Coll Cardiol* 2002; 39(10): 1581-7.

28. Spertus JA, Jones PG, Coen M, Garg M, Bliven B, O'Keefe J, March RJ, Horvath K. Transmyocardial CO_2 laser revascularization improves symptoms, function, and quality of life: 12-month results from a randomized controlled trial. *Am J Med* 2001; 111(5): 341-8.

29. Madsen JC, Daggett WM Jr. Repair of postinfarction ventricular septal defects. *Semin Thorac Cardiovasc Surg* 1998; 10(2): 117-27.

30. David TE, Armstrong S. Surgical repair of postinfarction ventricular septal defect by infarct exclusion. *Semin Thorac Cardiovasc Surg* 1998; 10(2): 105-10.

31. Nashef SA, Roques F, Michel P, Gauducheau E, Lemeshow S, Salamon R. European system for cardiac operative risk evaluation (EuroSCORE). *Eur J Cardiothorac Surg* 1999; 16(1): 9-13.

32. Shroyer AL, Grover FL, Hattler B, Collins JF, McDonald GO, Kozora E, Lucke JC, Baltz JH, Novitzky D; Veterans Affairs Randomized On/Off Bypass (ROOBY) Study Group. On-pump versus off-pump coronary-artery bypass surgery. *N Engl J Med* 2009; 361(19): 1827-37.

33.   Wijns W, Kolh P. Guidelines on myocardial revascularization: The Task Force on Myocardial Revascularization of the European Society of Cardiology (ESC) and the European Association for Cardio-Thoracic Surgery (EACTS). *Eur Heart J* 2010; 31(20): 2501-55.

Chapter 18

Heart failure

1 What is heart failure?

- Heart failure is a complex clinical syndrome resulting from any structural or functional cardiac disorder, that impairs the ability of the ventricle to fill with or eject blood, and results in a cardiac output which is inadequate to meet the metabolic demands of the body.

2 What are the symptoms of left heart failure?

- Dyspnoea, orthopnoea and paroxysmal nocturnal dyspnoea.
- Fatigue and reduced exercise tolerance.
- Weight loss and muscle wasting, which may progress to cachexia.
- Cold peripheries.
- Systemic embolism.

3 What are the symptoms of right heart failure?

- Peripheral oedema.
- Ascites.
- Hepatic congestion and pain.
- Distended varicose veins.
- Epistaxis.

4 What are the signs of heart failure?

- Peripheral cyanosis with cold peripheries.
- Low pulse volume, resting tachycardia or pulsus alternans (in severe cases).
- Hypotension with low pulse pressure.
- Raised systemic venous pressure, resulting in a prominent jugular venous pulse, and prominent veins over the chest, abdomen and legs.
- Displaced apex beat.
- Right ventricular heave.
- 3rd heart sound (gallop rhythm).

- Pleural effusions.
- Smooth hepatomegaly.
- Ascites.
- Peripheral oedema.

5 What is the New York Heart Association (NYHA) classification?

- It is a functional classification that relates the patient's symptoms (dyspnoea or fatigue) and the ability to perform activities:

a) I: no limitations of physical activity and no symptoms with ordinary activity;

b) II: slight limitation of physical activity but comfortable at rest or mild exertion;

c) III: marked limitation of physical activity and comfortable only at rest;

d) IV: symptoms of heart failure at rest.

384

6 How is heart failure classified?

- According to the American Heart Association (AHA) classification of heart failure:

a) stage A: asymptomatic patient at risk of developing heart failure (e.g. hypertension or coronary artery disease);

b) stage B: asymptomatic patient with ventricular changes of heart failure (e.g. left ventricular hypertrophy or systolic dysfunction);

c) stage C: patients with a current or past history of symptomatic heart failure associated with structural changes;

d) stage D: patients with refractory heart failure.

7 What is the pathophysiology of chronic heart failure?

- The inadequate cardiac output associated with heart failure triggers neuro-endocrine activation, including:

a) activation of the sympathetic nervous system;

b) activation of the renin-angiotensin system;

c) the release of endogenous noradrenaline, antidiuretic hormone (vasopressin) and endothelin.

This results in fluid retention and an inappropriately high afterload.

- In response to fluid overload associated with heart failure, atrial and brain natriuretic peptides (ANP and BNP) are released. Their actions include:

  a)   natriuresis and diuresis;
  b)   arterial and venous dilation;
  c)   inhibition of ADH and aldosterone release.

  Their effects, however, are overwhelmed by the neuro-endocrine activation.

8   **What are the main causes of heart failure?**

- Increased pre-load (volume overload), secondary to mitral or aortic regurgitation, atrial or ventricular septal defects.
- Reduced contractility, secondary to coronary artery disease, dilated cardiomyopathy, restrictive cardiomyopathy or myocarditis.
- Increased afterload (pressure overload), secondary to aortic stenosis, hypertension or aortic coarctation.
- Impaired cardiac rhythm, secondary to atrial or ventricular tachy-arrhythmias.
- Impaired ventricular filling, secondary to pericardial tamponade, constrictive pericarditis or mitral stenosis.
- High-output heart failure, secondary to anaemia, sepsis, arterio-venous fistula, hyperthyroidism or pregnancy.

9   **What are the principles of treatment in heart failure and the studies that investigated their therapeutic efficacy?**

- Treat the underlying cause:

  a)   coronary artery bypass grafting (CASS);
  b)   mitral valve surgery;
  c)   aortic valve replacement.

- Reduce pre-load:

  a)   diuretics;
  b)   aldosterone antagonism (RALES).

- Left ventricular volume reduction (SAVER, RESTORE and STICH).
- Improve contractility - mechanical or biological:

  a)   cardiac resynchronization therapy (MUSTIC);
  b)   implantable cardioverter defibrillator (MADIT);

c)   ventricular assist devices (REMATCH);
d)   dynamic cardiomyoplasty (C-SMART);
e)   cardiac transplantation (COCPIT);
f)   cellular cardiomyoplasty (MAGIC).

- Reduce afterload:

a)   angiotensin-converting   enzyme   inhibitors   (SOLVD,
        CONSENSUS);
b)   angiotensin receptor blockers (CHARM, Val-HeFT);
c)   β-blockers (COPERNICUS);
d)   intra-aortic balloon pump;
e)   ventricular septal myectomy (Morrow operation) for
        hypertrophic cardiomyopathy.

(Please refer to the abbreviation list on pages x-xvi for the full trial names.)

10 What is viable myocardium?

- Viable myocardium is defined as cardiac muscle amenable to revascularisation. This includes:

a)   hibernating myocardium;
b)   stunned myocardium;
c)   ischaemic myocardium.

11 What is hibernating myocardium?

- Hibernating myocardium is defined as the state of myocardial hypocontractility during chronic hypoperfusion, which recovers functionally upon revascularisation.

12 What is myocardial stunning?

- Myocardial stunning is defined as cardiac dysfunction following a period of ischaemia-reperfusion. It may last up to 2 weeks.

13 How is hibernating myocardium identified?

- Dobutamine stress echocardiography - a biphasic response (demonstrating increased contractility with low-dose dobutamine but not with high-dose dobutamine) is indicative of hibernating myocardium.

- Magnetic resonance imaging (MRI) - signs indicative of hibernating myocardium include:

  a)   absence of myocardial thinning (<6mm) on perfusion MRI;
  b)   delayed hyperenhancement on gadolinium-enhanced MRI;
  c)   a biphasic response on dobutamine stress MRI.

- Positron emission tomography (PET) scanning - normal uptake with ^{18}FDG (marker of metabolism) but decreased uptake of ^{13}N ammonia or ^{15}O water (markers of perfusion).
- ^{201}Thallium nuclear medicine scan - increased uptake on late redistribution.

14 **What are the indications for coronary artery bypass grafting in patients with heart failure?**

- Indications include:

  a)   coronary artery disease with reasonable target vessels to graft;
  b)   myocardial ischaemia (evidenced by chest pain);
  c)   myocardial viability (evidenced by hibernating myocardium - see above); >20% of left ventricle demonstrating viability.

- The evidence for treating these patients was provided by the CASS Registry, with the 5-year survival for patients with ischaemic cardiomyopathy (coronary artery disease and ejection fraction <25%) being 41% for patients treated medically and 62% for those undergoing surgery.
- Further evidence may be provided by the STICH trial hypothesis I.
- The survival advantage from coronary artery bypass surgery in these patients increases as the ejection fraction decreases.
- The relative contra-indications to coronary artery bypass surgery in these patients include:

  a)   poor target vessels;
  b)   pulmonary hypertension (>60mm Hg);
  c)   significantly impaired right ventricular function.

15 **What are the main principles of biventricular pacing (cardiac resynchronization therapy, Figure 1)?**

- Ventricular dyssynchrony often results from left bundle branch block (LBBB) as earlier contraction of the right ventricle and paradoxical

A LBBB   B   Biventricular pacing

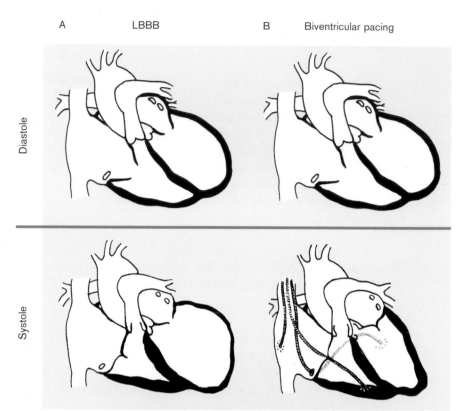

Diastole

Systole

Figure 1. Biventricular pacing. A) Left bundle branch block (LBBB) causes delayed left ventricular contraction with paradoxical septal motion in systole. B) Biventricular pacing induces synchronous contraction of the left and right ventricles and improved contribution of the septum to left ventricular contraction.

ventricular septal motion leads to impaired left ventricular filling and impaired left ventricular systolic function.

- Biventricular pacing induces simultaneous left and right ventricular contraction, thereby increasing the efficacy of ventricular contractility without increasing myocardial oxygen consumption.
- Biventricular pacing is indicated in patients with:

a)   heart failure for at least 6 weeks on maximal medical therapy;
b)   NYHA functional status III or IV;
c)   left ventricular ejection fraction <35%;
d)   QRS interval >150ms.

16 What are the indications for an implantable cardio-defibrillator in heart failure?

- Primary prevention, in patients who have sustained a previous myocardial infarction with an ejection fraction of <35%, with:

  a)   non-sustained ventricular tachycardia; or
  b)   inducible ventricular tachycardia on electro-physiological studies.

- Secondary prevention, in patients with haemodynamically significant ventricular tachyarrhythmias and an ejection fraction of <35%.
- It is important to treat any underlying causes including drug toxicity, electrolyte disturbance, and reversible ischaemia, before implanting a cardio-defibrillator device.

17 What is partial left ventriculectomy (Batista procedure, Figure 2)?

- The Batista procedure involves resection of the posterolateral left ventricular wall between the anterior and posterior papillary muscles from the apex to the mitral valve annulus. The papillary muscles may also be resected or re-implanted to ensure an adequate portion of the left ventricle is removed. Subsequent mitral valve annuloplasty or replacement may be required to ensure competency of the valve.
- The principal aim of the procedure is to reduce left ventricular volume and wall stress (Laplace's law), thereby improving overall ventricular contractility.
- Although initial results from Batista suggested improved survival and symptoms, subsequent studies in ischaemic cardiomyopathic patients failed to show a sustained benefit of this procedure. This may have been caused by resection of viable sections of the lateral left ventricular wall.

A

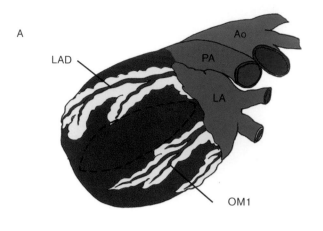

B

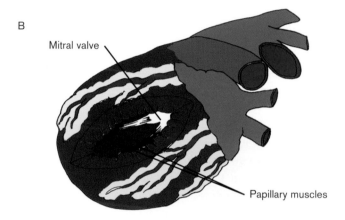

C

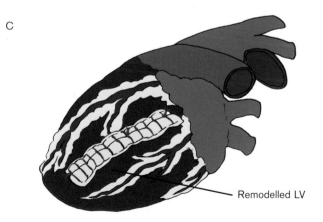

Figure 2. Batista procedure. A) Lateral view of the left ventricle. B) Resection of the lateral left ventricular wall between the LAD and OM1, whilst preserving the papillary muscles of the mitral valve. C) Remodelled left ventricle with a two-layered ventriculotomy closure. OM1 = 1st obtuse marginal artery; LAD = left anterior descending artery; Ao = aorta; PA = pulmonary artery; LA = left atrium; LV= left ventricle.

18 What is dynamic cardiomyoplasty (Figure 3)?

- Dynamic cardiomyoplasty involves mobilisation of the latissimus dorsi muscle on its neurovascular pedicle. Following transposition into the chest through a small left thoracotomy, the muscle is wrapped around the left and right ventricles.

- Concomitant implantation of a pacemaker coupled to a neurotransmitter electrically stimulates the muscle to contract in synchrony with ventricular systole.

- Over time, pacing of the skeletal muscle induces transformation from fast twitch to slow twitch muscle, which is less fatigable.

- The mechanisms of action of dynamic cardiomyoplasty include:

  a) augmenting muscular pump function resulting in increased stroke volume;

  b) girdling of the ventricles as an external constraint device, resulting in reduced ventricular dilation and wall stress (Laplace's law);

391

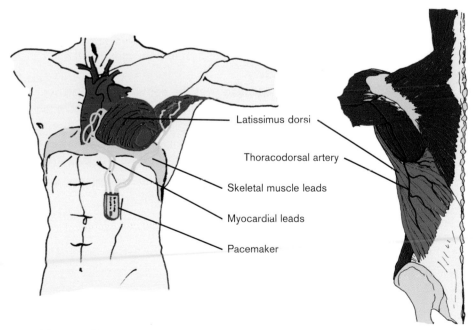

Latissimus dorsi

Thoracodorsal artery

Skeletal muscle leads

Myocardial leads

Pacemaker

Figure 3. Dynamic cardiomyoplasty. The left latissimus dorsi muscle is transposed into the left hemi-thorax and wrapped around the left and right ventricles.

c) arresting the remodelling process of heart failure, resulting in reduced deterioration in ventricular systolic and diastolic function.

● The Cardiomyoplasty-Skeletal Muscle Assist Randomised Trial (C-SMART) was a prospective, randomised controlled trial that compared dynamic cardiomyoplasty with medical therapy alone. It was, however, terminated due to poor recruitment of approximately 100 patients and showed no survival benefit after 12 months with dynamic cardiomyoplasty.

19 What are the principles of the surgical ventricular restoration procedure (Figures 4 and 5)?

● The surgical ventricular restoration procedure excludes areas of non-functioning left ventricle, resulting in reduced left ventricular volume and wall stress (Laplace's law), and return of an elliptical shape to the left ventricle.

● During the procedure, coronary artery disease and mitral valve disease are also addressed.

● The operative procedure is usually performed for akinesia or dyskinesia of the anterior left ventricular wall and involves:

a) a left ventriculotomy through scar tissue, 2cm lateral to the left anterior descending artery;
b) subtotal endocardial resection over the septum and posterior wall, and cryotherapy at the limits of the resection for patients with recurrent ventricular arrhythmias;
c) a circumferential endoventricular (Fontan) circular suture is passed 1-2cm outside the limit of healthy muscle and then tied around a balloon mannequin to reduce the size of the left ventricle to a diastolic volume of 50-60mL/m^2;
d) the residual apical defect is closed with a Dacron® patch to produce an elliptical-shaped left ventricle;
e) the ventriculotomy is then closed with two-layered 2/0 Prolene® buttressed by Teflon® strips.

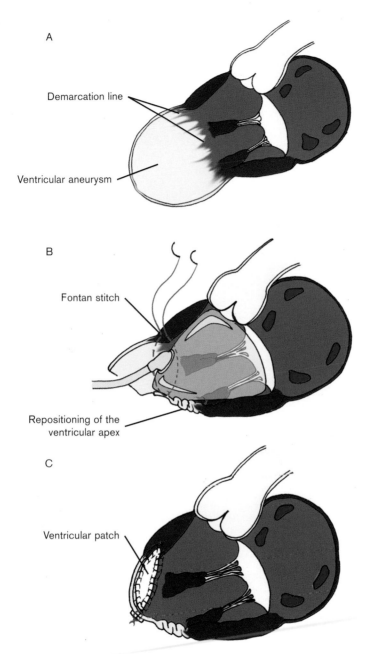

A

Demarcation line

Ventricular aneurysm

B

Fontan stitch

Repositioning of the
ventricular apex

C

Ventricular patch

Figure 4. Surgical ventricular restoration. A) Aneurysmal dilation of the antero-apical left ventricular wall with a line of demarcation between viable muscle and scar tissue. B) Following ventriculotomy, a balloon mannequin is placed and inflated within the left ventricle. The left ventricular apex is then repositioned using a Fontan stitch and plication of the scar tissue. C) An elliptical shape of the left ventricle is produced by using a Dacron® patch attached from the ventricular septum to the ventriculotomy.

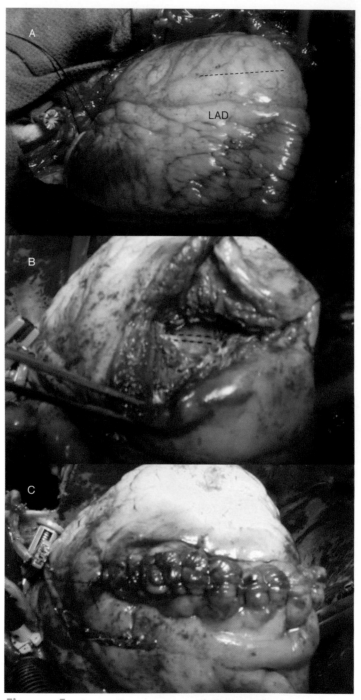

Figure 5. Operative images of the surgical ventricular restoration procedure. A) A linear incision is made 2cm lateral to the left anterior descending artery. B) Following remodelling of the left ventricle, a Dacron® patch is placed from the ventricular septum to the ventriculotomy. C) Two-layered ventriculotomy closure.

20 Describe the mechanisms of action of passive ventricular constraint devices (Figure 6)

- Passive constraint devices (such as CorCap®) are designed to promote reverse ventricular remodelling by reducing further ventricular dilation and hence ventricular wall stress (Laplace's law).
- The Acorn Clinical Trial was a multi-centre, prospective, randomised trial with 300 patients using a passive ventricular constraint device, which showed improvement in quality of life, composite endpoint (death, progression of heart failure), left ventricular dilation, left ventricular end-systolic volume and left ventricular sphericity index.

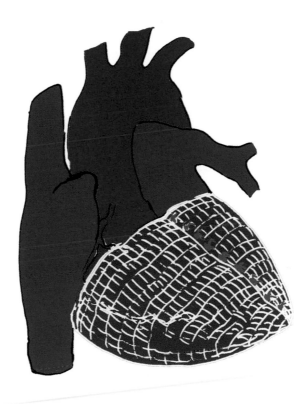

Figure 6. Passive ventricular constraint device.

21 What is the long-term survival of patients following cardiac transplantation?

- 1 month - 93%.
- 1 year - 85%.
- 3 year - 78%.
- 5 year - 72%.
- 7 year - 66%.
- 10 year - 55%.
- Whilst on a waiting list, patients have a 25% mortality but 50-60% of patients receive a heart within 2 years.

22 What are the components of the heart failure survival score (HFSS)?

- Ischaemic cardiomyopathy.
- Heart rate.
- Left ventricular ejection fraction.
- Mean arterial blood pressure.
- Interventricular conduction delay.
- Peak myocardial oxygen consumption (VO_2 max).
- Serum sodium.
- Using a complex algorithm, the heart failure survival score is calculated and patients are categorized according to risk (Table 1).
- Patients with a medium or high-risk HFSS would benefit from transplantation as the 1-year survival for transplantation is approximately 85%.

Table 1. One-year survival according to the heart failure survival score.

Risk	HFSS	1-year survival
Low risk	>8.1	93%
Medium risk	7.2-8.1	73%
High risk	<7.2	43%

23 What are the indications for cardiac transplantation?

- According to the International Society for Heart and Lung Transplantation (ISHLT):

  a) definite indications:

      i) high-risk heart failure survival score;

      ii)   peak myocardial oxygen consumption <10mL/kg/min after reaching the anaerobic threshold;

      iii)   NYHA class IV heart failure, refractory to maximal medical treatment;

      iv)   recurrent hospitalisation for heart failure;

      v)   refractory ischaemia, a left ventricular ejection fraction of <20% and coronary artery disease not amenable to revascularisation;

      vi)   recurrent symptomatic ventricular arrhythmias refractory to medical treatment, implantable cardio-defibrillator or surgery;

b)   probable indications:

      i)   medium-risk heart failure survival score;

      ii)   NYHA class III heart failure, refractory to medical treatment;

      iii)   recent hospitalisations for heart failure;

      iv)   peak myocardial oxygen consumption <14mL/kg/min and severe functional limitations;

      v)   recurrent unstable ischaemia, a left ventricular ejection fraction of <25% and coronary artery disease not amenable to revascularisation;

c)   inadequate indications:

      i)   low-risk heart failure survival score;

      ii)   peak myocardial oxygen consumption >15mL/kg/min without other indications;

      iii)   a left ventricular ejection fraction of <20% alone;

      iv)   history of NYHA class III/IV symptoms alone;

      v)   history of ventricular arrhythmias alone.

24 What are the contra-indications for cardiac transplantation?

- Age >65 years.
- Active infection.
- Diabetes with end-organ damage or brittle diabetes.
- Significant symptomatic carotid or peripheral vascular disease.
- Active or recent malignancy. Ideally the patient should have a 5-year disease-free interval.
- Excessive obesity.
- Chronic renal failure with a creatinine level of >250mmol/L or creatinine clearance of <50mL/min.
- Hepatic impairment, with a bilirubin level of >25mmol/L or an ALT/AST ratio >2, not due to congestion.
- Significant chronic lung disease.

- Irreversible pulmonary hypertension, with a:

  a) systolic pulmonary artery pressure >60mmHg;
  b) pulmonary vascular resistance >5 woods units;
  c) transpulmonary gradient <18mmHg.

- Evidence of drug abuse within 6 months.
- High risk of non-compliance or lack of family and social support.
- Active psychiatric illness.
- Recent peptic ulcer disease.
- Significant coagulopathy.

25 Describe the donor criteria for cardiac transplantation (Figure 7)

- Brain stem death.
- Consent (donor card or family approval).

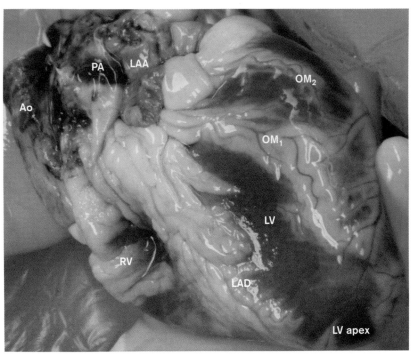

Figure 7. Explanted heart prior to cardiac transplantation. Ao = aorta; PA = pulmonary artery; LAA = left atrial appendage; LV = left ventricle; RV = right ventricle; LAD = left anterior descending artery; OM$_{1/2}$ = 1st / 2nd obtuse marginal artery.

- Absence of:

  a) coronary artery disease or previous myocardial infarction;
  b) other cardiac disease including refractory ventricular arrhythmias;
  c) malignancies (except central nervous system tumours);
  d) refractory infection.

26 Describe the criteria used for matching donor to recipient in cardiac transplantation

- Geographical location, to limit the organ ischaemia time.
- Candidate status:

  a) Ia: patients requiring mechanical circulatory support for acute haemodynamic decompensation, mechanical ventilation, high-dose intravenous inotropes or with evidence of a significant device-related complication;
  b) Ib: patients with a ventricular-assist device implanted or on a continuous infusion of intravenous inotropes;
  c) II: all other patients.

- ABO blood group compatibility.
- Human leucocyte antigen (HLA) compatibility.
- Matching patient's size (height and weight).
- Time on waiting list.
- Cytomegalovirus (CMV) positive donors given to CMV positive recipients.
- Organ matching is usually arranged through a central transplant co-ordination list, such as the United Network for Organ Sharing (UNOS).

27 Describe the operative sequence for cardiac transplantation (Figure 8)

- The recipient procedure begins about 90 minutes before the donor heart is due to arrive, to minimize the organ ischaemia time.
- Following a median sternotomy, cardiopulmonary bypass is instituted via the ascending aorta and snared venous cannulae, which are positioned directly into both venae cavae.
- The donor heart is inspected for a foramen ovale, palpable coronary artery disease or dilated cardiac chambers. If the donor heart is

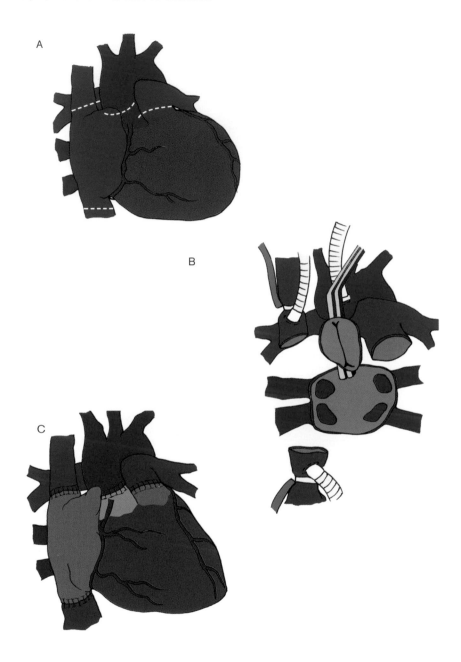

Figure 8. Cardiac transplantation. A) Dilated native heart excised with incisions (dotted lines) in the inferior vena cava, superior vena cava, aorta, pulmonary artery and left atrium (not seen). B) Pericardial cavity with native great vessels following explantation of the native heart. C) Implantation of donor heart with anastomosis of the left atrium (not seen), inferior vena cava, superior vena cava, pulmonary artery and aorta.

suitable for transplantation, the recipient heart can then be explanted using the following steps:

a) the right atrium is excised at the junction with the inferior and superior venae cavae;

b) the aorta and pulmonary artery are divided just above the sino-tubular junction;

c) the left atrium is excised to leave an island of pulmonary veins.

- The donor heart is then implanted in the following order (modified bicaval technique):

a) left atrium;
b) inferior vena cava;
c) superior vena cava;
d) pulmonary artery;
e) aorta.

28 What are the complications of cardiac transplantation and immunosuppression?

- Early graft failure.
- Rejection (see below).
- Infection.
- Allograft vasculopathy - 50% over 5 years.
- Malignancy - especially lymphomas and malignant tumours of the skin (e.g. Kaposi's sarcoma).

29 What is the classification of organ rejection?

- Hyperacute rejection, which is a complement-mediated response by pre-existing antibodies that are circulating in the recipient. They bind to donor ABO blood group antigens.
- Acute rejection, where the T-lymphocytes respond to differences between the human leucocyte antigens (HLA) of the donor and recipient.
- Chronic rejection, which manifests itself as allograft vasculopathy with diffuse initmal hyperplasia in the coronary arteries of a transplanted heart.

30 What are the agents used for immunosuppression following cardiac transplantation?

- Short induction phase (first 3 days following transplantation):

  a)   anti-thymocyte globulin (ATG);
  b)   azathioprine;
  c)   corticosteroids.

- Permanent maintenance phase:

  a)   cyclosporine A or tacrolimus, which are calcineurin inhibitors that inhibit the transcription of interleukin-2 (IL-2) and T-lymphocyte signal transduction;
  b)   azathioprine or mycophenolate mofetil (MMF), which are purine synthesis inhibitors;
  c)   corticosteroids, which inhibit the production of cytokines (such as IL-1, TNF-α and interferons).

- Newer agents include:

  a)   OKT3, which is a monoclonal antibody that binds to the CD3 receptor on T-lymphocytes;
  b)   daclizumab and basiliximab, which are monoclonal antibodies that bind to the IL-2 receptors of T-lymphocytes;
  c)   sirolimus (rapamycin), which stops IL-2-induced activation of T-lymphocytes.

31 How are left ventricular assist devices (LVAD) classified (Figure 9)?

- Mechanism of action:

  a)   pulsatile - electric or pneumatic, such as the Thoratec HeartMate I® or Novacor®;
  b)   non-pulsatile (continuous flow) - centrifugal or axial flow, such as the Thoratec Heart Mate II®, Jarvik 2000 or Micromed DeBakey VAD®.

- Location:

  a)   totally implantable - thoracic or abdominal;
  b)   paracorporeal;
  c)   percutaneous.

HeartMate I®   HeartMate II®

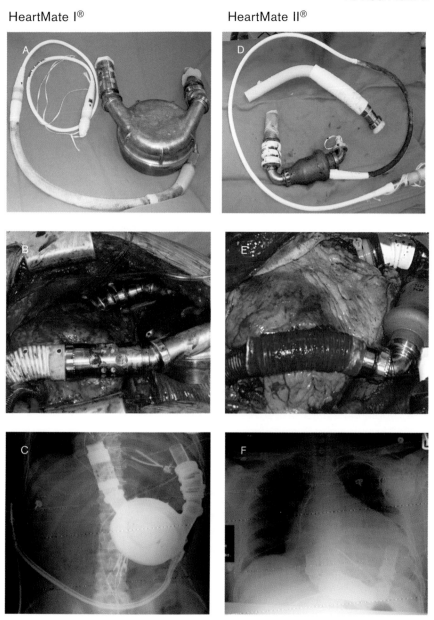

Figure 9. Left ventricular assist devices. A) Pre-operative, B) intra-operative, and C) radiographical images of a pulsatile left ventricular assist device (Thoratec HeartMate I®). D) Pre-operative, E) Intra-operative and F) radiographical images of an axial flow left ventricular assist device (Thoratec HeartMate II®).

- Power source and driveline:

  a)   transabdominal;
  b)   transcranial;
  c)   transcutaneous.

32 What are the main uses of a left ventricular assist device?

- Bridge to transplantation, which has been shown to increase the survival of patients following cardiac transplantation.
- Bridge to recovery, following an acute myocardial injury, post-cardiac surgery or viral myocarditis.
- Destination therapy, for patients with end-stage heart failure ineligible for cardiac transplantation.

33 What are the complications of left ventricular assist devices?

- Mortality (5-10% at 30 days).
- Bleeding.
- Infection (driveline, pocket).
- Right ventricular failure.
- Thrombo-embolic events.
- Haemolysis.
- Device malfunction (rare).

34 What did the REMATCH trial show?

- REMATCH = Randomised Evaluation of Mechanical Assistance for the Treatment of Congestive Heart Failure.
- The REMATCH trial was a prospective, randomised controlled study in 129 patients with:

  a)   end-stage heart failure (NYHA class IV);
  b)   a left ventricular ejection fraction <25%;
  c) VO_2 max <12mL/min/kg.

- The patients were randomised to either:

  a)   group I (n=68) - left ventricular assist device (Thoratec HeartMate I®); or
  b)   group II (n=61) - optimal medical therapy.

- The study demonstrated a survival advantage for patients in the LVAD group:

  a) 1-year survival - LVAD 52% vs. optimal medical treatment 25%;

  b) 2-year survival - LVAD 23% vs. optimal medical treatment 8%.

- There were, however, more adverse serious events in the LVAD group, such as infection, bleeding, haemolysis, thrombo-embolism, neurological dysfunction and device failure.
- The study concluded that LVAD therapy is an acceptable alternative in selected patients who are not candidates for cardiac transplantation.

35 What did the MADIT trial show?

- MADIT = Multicenter Automatic Defibrillator Implantation Trial.
- The MADIT trial was a prospective, randomised controlled study in 196 patients with:

  a) previous myocardial infarction;

  b) a left ventricular ejection fraction of <35%;

  c) a documented episode of asymptomatic unsustained ventricular tachycardia or an inducible, non-suppressible ventricular arrhythmia on electrophysiologic study.

- The patients were randomised to either an implanted defibrillator (ICD, n=95) or conventional medical therapy with anti-arrhythmic drugs (n=101).
- The study demonstrated an overall 27% reduction in mortality in patients in the ICD group (15 deaths) compared to standard medical therapy (39 deaths).
- The study concluded that an ICD leads to improved survival in patients with a previous myocardial infarction, low ejection fraction and at high risk for ventricular tachyarrhythmia.

36 What did the MUSTIC trial show?

- MUSTIC = Multisite Stimulation in Cardiomyopathies.
- The MUSTIC trial was a prospective, randomised controlled study in 48 patients with:

  a) severe heart failure (NYHA III or IV);

  b) a left ventricular ejection fraction of <35%;

  c) normal sinus rhythm with a QRS interval >150msec.

- Patients received transvenous atrio-biventricular pacemakers and the study compared the response to 3-month periods with or without pacing in the same patients.
- The study concluded that biventricular pacing leads to an improved quality of life and exercise tolerance (improved by 23%), and reduced hospitalisations.

37 What did the STICH trial (hypothesis 2) show?

- STICH = Surgical Treatment for Ischaemic Heart Failure.
- The STICH trial was a prospective, randomised study in 2800 patients with:

   a)   coronary artery disease amenable to revascularisation;
   b)   a left ventricular ejection fraction of <35%;
   c)   dominant akinesia or dyskinesia of the anterior left ventricular wall amenable to surgical ventricular restoration.

- Patients were sub-divided into different strata and then randomised to:

   a)   medical therapy alone;
   b)   coronary artery bypass grafting (CABG) and medical therapy;
   c)   surgical ventricular restoration (SVR), coronary artery bypass grafting and medical therapy.

- Hypothesis 1 - CABG with intensive medical therapy improves long-term survival compared to survival with medical therapy alone.
- Hypothesis 2 - SVR when added to CABG decreases the rate of death or hospitalisation for a cardiac event as compared with CABG alone.
- The results of the hypothesis 2 study at a median of 48-month follow-up showed no significant difference in:

   a)   primary outcome (death from any cause or hospitalisation for cardiac causes);
   b)   acute myocardial infarction;
   c)   stroke;
   d)   symptoms (angina class, NYHA dyspnoea class, 6-minute walk test).

38 What did the RESTORE group show?

- RESTORE = Reconstructive Endoventricular Surgery returning Torsion Original Radius Elliptical shape to the left ventricle.

- The RESTORE group assessed the effects of surgical ventricular restoration with a prospective registry study in 1198 patients with:

  a)   previous anterior myocardial infarction;
  b)   significant ventricular dilation (left ventricular end-systolic volume index >60mL/m²);
  c)   a regional asynergic (non-contractile) LV circumference of >35%.

- The study demonstrated:

  a)   overall 30-day mortality was 5.3% (8.7% with mitral repair, 4.0% without repair);
  b)   overall 5-year survival was 69%;
  c)   5-year freedom from hospital admissions for heart failure was 78%;
  d)   improvement in NYHA functional status with 85% of patients in class I-II postoperatively;
  e)   left ventricular ejection fraction improved from 29% to 39%;
  f)   left ventricular end-systolic volume index decreased from 80 to 57mL/m².

- The study concluded that surgical ventricular restoration improves ventricular function and symptom status in patients with ischaemic cardiomyopathy.

39 What did the Heartmate II® trial show?

- The Heartmate II® trial was a prospective randomised study in 200 patients with advanced heart failure who were ineligible for transplantation.
- The patients were randomised, in a 2:1 ratio, to:

  a)   group I (n=134) - implantation of a continuous flow left ventricular assist device (Thoratec Heartmate II®); or
  b)   group II (n=66) - implantation of a pulsatile flow left ventricular assist device (Thoratec Heartmate XVE®).

- The study demonstrated:

  a)   survival advantage at 2 years for patients in the continuous flow LVAD (Heartmate II®) group (Heartmate II® 58% vs. Heartmate I® 24%);
  b)   reduced adverse events for patients in the continuous flow LVAD (Heartmate II®) group,

- The study concluded that treatment with a continuous flow LVAD in patients with advanced heart failure significantly improved the probability of survival free from mortality, stroke and device failure as compared to a pulsatile flow device.

Recommended reading

1. Dor V, Sabatier M, Di Donato M, Montiglio F, Toso A, Maioli M. Efficacy of endoventricular patch plasty in large postinfarction akinetic scar and severe left ventricular dysfunction: comparison with a series of large dyskinetic scars. *J Thorac Cardiovasc Surg* 1998; 116: 50-9.

2. Athanasuleas CL, Stanley AW Jr, Buckberg GD, Dor V, DiDonato M, Blackstone EH. Surgical Anterior Ventricular Endocardial Restoration (SAVER) in the dilated remodelled ventricle after anterior myocardial infarction: RESTORE group [Reconstructive Endoventricular Surgery, returning Torsion Original Radius Elliptical shape to the LV]. *J Am Coll Cardiol* 2001; 37: 1199-209.

3. Athanasuleas CL, Buckberg GD, Dor V, RESTORE group. Surgical ventricular restoration in the treatment of congestive heart failure due to post-infarction ventricular dilation. *J Am Coll Cardiol* 2004; 44: 1439-45.

4. Menicanti L, Castelvecchio S, Ranucci M, Frigiola A, Santambrogio C, de Vincentiis C, Brankovic J, Di Donato M. Surgical therapy for ischemic heart failure: single centre experience with surgical anterior ventricular restoration. *J Thorac Cardiovasc Surg* 2007; 134: 433-41.

5. Bolling SF, Pagani FD, Deeb GM, Bach DS. Intermediate-term outcome of mitral reconstruction in cardiomyopathy. *J Thorac Cardiovasc Surg* 1998; 115: 381-8.

6. Batista RJ, Verde J, Nery P, Bocchino L, Takeshita N, Bhayana JN, Bergsland J, Graham S, Houck JP, Salerno TA. Partial left ventriculectomy to treat end-stage heart disease. *Ann Thorac Surg* 1997; 64: 634-8.

7. Batista R. Partial left ventriculectomy: the Batista procedure. *Eur J Cardiothorac Surg* 1999; 15: 12-9.

8. Jones RH, Velazquez EJ, Michler RE, Sopko G, Oh JK, O'Connor CM, Hill JA, Menicanti L, Sadowski Z, Desvigne-Nickens P, Rouleau JL, Lee KL; STICH Hypothesis 2 Investigators. Coronary bypass surgery with or without surgical ventricular reconstruction. *N Engl J Med* 2009; 360(17): 1705-17.

9. Rose EA, Gelijns AC, Moskowitz AJ, Heitjan DF, Stevenson LW, Dembitsky W, Long JW, Ascheim DD, Tierney AR, Levitan RG, Watson JT, Meier P, Ronan NS, Shapiro PA, Lazar RM, Miller LW, Gupta L, Frazier OH, Desvigne-Nickens P, Oz MC, Poirier VL; Randomized Evaluation of Mechanical Assistance for the Treatment of Congestive Heart Failure (REMATCH) Study Group. Long-term mechanical left ventricular assistance for end-stage heart failure. *N Engl J Med* 2001; 345(20): 1435-43.

10. Cazeau S, Leclercq C, Lavergne T, Walker S, Varma C, Linde C, Garrigue S, Kappenberger L, Haywood GA, Santini M, Bailleul C, Daubert JC; Multisite Stimulation in Cardiomyopathies (MUSTIC) Study Investigators. Effects of multisite

biventricular pacing in patients with heart failure and intraventricular conduction delay. *N Engl J Med* 2001; 344(12): 873-80.

11. McCarthy PM, Starling RC, Wong J, Scalia GM, Buda T, Vargo RL, Goormastic M, Thomas JD, Smedira NG, Young JB. Early results with partial left ventriculectomy. *J Thorac Cardiovasc Surg* 1997; 114(5): 755-63.

12. Bolling SF, Pagani FD, Deeb GM, Bach DS. Intermediate-term outcome of mitral reconstruction in cardiomyopathy. *J Thorac Cardiovasc Surg* 1998; 115(2): 381-6.

13. Moss AJ, Zareba W, Hall WJ, Klein H, Wilber DJ, Cannom DS, Daubert JP, Higgins SL, Brown MW, Andrews ML; Multicenter Automatic Defibrillator Implantation Trial II Investigators. Prophylactic implantation of a defibrillator in patients with myocardial infarction and reduced ejection fraction. *N Engl J Med* 2002; 346: 877-83.

14. Granger CB, McMurray JJ, Yusuf S, Held P, Michelson EL, Olofsson B, Ostergren J, Pfeffer MA, Swedberg K; CHARM Investigators and Committees. Effects of candesartan in patients with chronic heart failure and reduced left-ventricular systolic function intolerant to angiotensin-converting-enzyme inhibitors: the CHARM-Alternative trial. *Lancet* 2003; 362: 772-6.

15. Pitt B, Zannad F, Remme WJ, Cody R, Castaigne A, Perez A, Palensky J, Wittes J. The effect of spironolactone on morbidity and mortality in patients with severe heart failure. Randomized Aldactone Evaluation Study Investigators. *N Engl J Med* 1999; 341(10): 709-17.

16. Digitalis Investigation Group. The effect of digoxin on mortality and morbidity in patients with heart failure. *N Engl J Med* 1997; 336: 525-33.

17. Hunt SA, Abraham WT, Chin MH, Feldman AM, Francis GS, Ganiats TG, Jessup M, Konstam MA, Mancini DM, Michl K, Oates JA, Rahko PS, Silver MA, Stevenson LW, Yancy CW. 2009 focused update incorporated into the ACC/AHA 2005 Guidelines for the Diagnosis and Management of Heart Failure in Adults. *Circulation* 2009; 119(14): e391-479.

18. Killip T, Passamani E, Davis K. Coronary Artery Bypass Surgery Study (CASS): a randomized trial of coronary bypass surgery. Eight years follow-up and survival in patients with reduced ejection fraction. *Circulation* 1985, 72: V102-9.

19. Deng MC, De Meester JM, Smits JM, Heinecke J, Scheld HH. Effect of receiving a heart transplant: analysis of a national cohort entered on to a waiting list, stratified by heart failure severity. Comparative Outcome and Clinical Profiles in Transplantation (COCPIT) Study Group. *BMJ* 2000; 321(7260): 540-5.

20. Packer M, Fowler MB, Roecker EB, Coats AJ, Katus HA, Krum H, Mohacsi P, Rouleau JL, Tendera M, Staiger C, Holcslaw TL, Amann-Zalan I, DeMets DL; Carvedilol Prospective Randomized Cumulative Survival (COPERNICUS) Study Group. *Circulation* 2002; 106(17): 2194-9.

21. SOLVD Investigators. Effect of enalapril on survival in patients with reduced left ventricular ejection fractions and congestive heart failure. *N Engl J Med* 1991; 325: 293-302.

22. Chachques JC, Marino JP, Lajos P, Zegdi R, D'Attellis N, Fornes P, Fabiani JN, Carpentier A. Dynamic cardiomyoplasty: clinical follow-up at 12 years. *Eur J Cardiothorac Surg* 1997; 12(4): 560-7.

23. Slaughter MS, Rogers JG, Milano CA, Russell SD, Conte JV, Feldman D, Sun B, Tatooles AJ, Delgado RM 3rd, Long JW, Wozniak TC, Ghumman W, Farrar DJ, Frazier OH; HeartMate II Investigators. Advanced heart failure treated with continuous-flow left ventricular assist device. *N Engl J Med* 2009; 361(23): 2241-51.

Chapter 19

Arrhythmia surgery

1 **How is atrial fibrillation classified?**
- Atrial fibrillation (AF) is defined as uncoordinated atrial activity at a rate of 300-500 bpm.
- It is classified as:

    a)   isolated AF (single episode);
    b)   recurrent AF (≥2 episodes):
        i)   paroxysmal AF, which lasts less than 7 days and reverts spontaneously;
        ii)   persistent AF, which does not terminate spontaneously and requires drugs or DC cardioversion to restore sinus rhythm;
        iii)   permanent AF, which does not revert into sinus rhythm using drugs or DC cardioversion.

2 **What is the incidence of atrial fibrillation?**
- AF occurs in 1% of the population.
- It increases with age with an incidence of 0.2-0.3% at 25-35, 3-4% at 55-65 and 6-9% at 65-90.
- It is the commonest arrhythmia, occurring in 33% of all patients with an arrhythmia.

3 **What are the common causes of atrial fibrillation?**
- Idiopathic (primary).
- Mitral valve disease and subsequent left atrial dilation.
- Ischaemic heart disease.
- Hypertension.
- Post-cardiac surgery.
- Alcohol.
- Thyrotoxicosis.

4 **Which patients in atrial fibrillation should be anticoagulated?**

● According to the American Heart Association (AHA) guidelines, class I indications for anticoagulation in patients with atrial flutter or atrial fibrillation (paroxysmal, persistent, or permanent) are shown in Table 1.

Table 1. AHA guidelines for anticoagulation in patients with atrial flutter or atrial fibrillation.	
Prosthetic mechanical valves	Warfarin (INR 2.5-3.5)
1 high-risk factor for thrombo-embolism	Warfarin (INR 2.0-3.0)
More than 1 moderate-risk factor for thrombo-embolism	Warfarin (INR 2.0-3.0)
1 moderate-risk factor for thrombo-embolism	Aspirin 81-325mg or Warfarin (INR 2.0-3.0)
Low-risk factor for thrombo-embolism	Aspirin 81-325mg
INR = international normalised ratio	

412

● High-risk factors include prior thrombo-embolism (stroke, transient ischaemic attack or systemic embolism) and rheumatic mitral stenosis.
● Moderate-risk factors include age >75 years, hypertension, heart failure, impaired left ventricular systolic function (ejection fraction <35%) and diabetes mellitus.
● Low-risk factors include female gender, age 65-75 years, coronary artery disease, thyrotoxicosis.
● For patients with lone AF aged <60 years, anticoagulation is not recommended.

5 **What are the risk factors for atrial fibrillation following cardiac surgery?**

● Age.
● Withdrawal of β-blockers.
● Electrolyte imbalance (potassium, magnesium).
● Hypoxia.
● Ischaemia.
● Pericardial effusion.
● Infection, e.g. pneumonia.

6 What is the pathophysiology of atrial fibrillation (Figure 1)?

- Atrial fibrillation is induced by focal areas of automaticity (mainly around the pulmonary veins) and is maintained by multiple macro re-entry circuits within both atria.

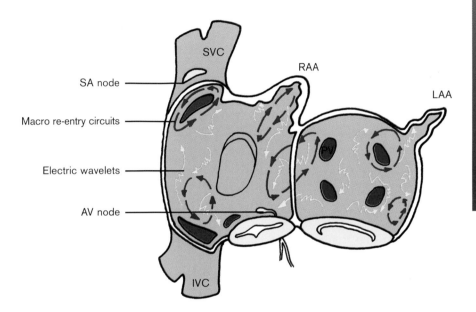

413

Figure 1. Pathophysiology of atrial fibrillation. Macro re-entrant circuits (red) maintain the uncoordinated activity of the electric wavelets (yellow). RAA = right atrial appendage; LAA = left atrial appendage; SA node = sino-atrial node; AV node = atrioventricular node; PV = pulmonary vein; SVC = superior vena cava; IVC = inferior vena cava.

- The requirements of AF are:

  a) triggers - atrial ectopic foci, changes in atrial wall tension;
  b) substrate - atrial abnormality (inflammation/fibrosis);
  c) modulating factors - autonomic nervous system.

- Treatment of paroxysmal AF requires stopping the induction pathways (focal areas of automaticity) by pulmonary vein isolation.
- Treatment of persistent AF, however, requires eliminating the maintaining pathways (macro re-entry circuits) using the Cox-maze procedure.

7 What are the sequelae of atrial fibrillation?

- Irregular heartbeat resulting in palpitations and patient anxiety.
- Compromised haemodynamics causing a 30% loss of cardiac output and in the long-term this may result in cardiomyopathy.
- Stasis of blood flow producing thrombo-embolism causing a stroke or pulmonary embolism.

8 What are the treatment options for patients with atrial fibrillation?

- Pharmacological for chemical cardioversion and rate control, e.g. amiodarone, digoxin, β-blocker, calcium channel blocker.
- DC cardioversion.
- Catheter ablation using transvenous radiofrequency ablation has a 60% success rate. It is, however, associated with complications including pulmonary vein stenosis, systemic embolisation, pericardial effusion, tamponade and phrenic nerve paralysis.
- Surgical ablation, which has a 75-80% success rate (see below).

414

9 What are the surgical options for the treatment of atrial fibrillation?

- Cut and sew - surgical incisions using the lesion set described by Cox in the maze III operation.
- Radiofrequency ablation, which employs an alternating current at 350kHz-1MHz to heat tissue to 70-80°C for 1 minute, creates a 3-6mm lesion using unipolar or bipolar devices. Transmurality is indicated by electrical conductance and impedance monitoring.
- Microwave, which uses high-frequency electromagnetic radiation to induce oscillation of water molecules.
- Cryoablation, which uses nitrous oxide as a cooling agent for 2 minutes at -60°C to produce a transmural lesion that can be visualised as an 'iceball' (Figure 2).
- Ultrasound, which uses high-frequency sound waves (2-20MHz) emitted by piezoelectric crystals to cause thermal heating and disruption of cell membranes.
- Laser, which uses a monochromatic, phase coherent beam to cause heating and cellular destruction.

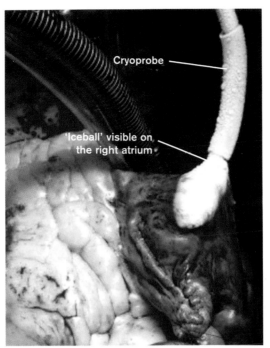

Figure 2. Ice ball visible on the surface of the right atrium during cryoablation.

10 What are the principles of the maze operation?

- A 'maze' is created with a set of blind alleys with one entrance and one exit for atrial electrical activation, thereby directing the electrical impulse along one specified route from the sino-atrial node to the atrioventricular node by interrupting conduction routes and re-entrant pathways (Figure 3).

- Using the maze procedure as opposed to the Guiraudon 'corridor' procedure, atrial transport can be better maintained.

- Left atrial appendage excision is often performed in association with the maze procedure to reduce the area of blood stasis and subsequent thrombus formation.

- The maze procedure is less likely to be successful in patients with large left atria (>5cm) or with longstanding AF (>5 years).

A

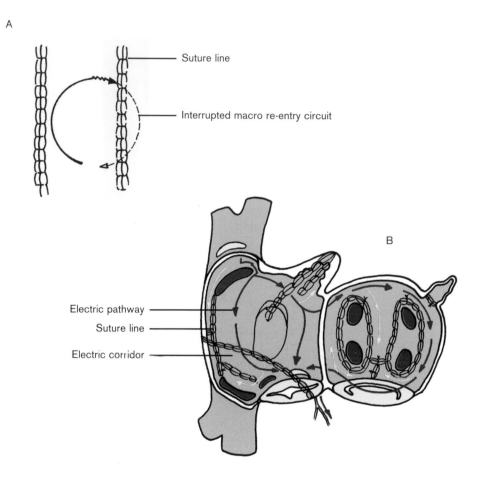

Suture line

Interrupted macro re-entry circuit

B

Electric pathway
Suture line
Electric corridor

Figure 3. Mechanism of atrial ablation. A) Two parallel lines of fibrous tissue (scar tissue) interrupt the myocardial continuity and avoid the propagation of the electrical wave. The lines are close enough to stop the macro re-entrant circuit. The scar lesion can be obtained by healing of a surgical incision or by alternative sources of energy that create transmural myocardial injury. B) A pre-determined set of lesions creates a 'maze', which allows the linear propagation of the electrical impulse through a series of 'channels' (red and yellow arrows).

11 ## What are the lesion sets for the maze procedure, when performed with mitral valve surgery (Figure 4)?

- The full maze procedure consists of lesion sets involving the left and right atrium. In certain patients, however, only a left heart maze is carried out using a cryoablation or radiofrequency ablation clamp or probe device with lesions:

  a) around the right superior and inferior pulmonary veins;

  b) around the left superior and inferior pulmonary veins. To gain access to the left pulmonary veins, the heart needs to be retracted cephalad and to the right. Often the ligament of Marshall (black arrow), between the left superior pulmonary vein (LSPV) and the left pulmonary artery (LPA), also needs to be divided;

  c) from the left superior pulmonary vein to the left atrial appendage, which is then excluded from the atrial cavity with a direct suture;

  d) from the right inferior pulmonary vein to the left inferior pulmonary vein;

  e) from the connecting lesion between the left and right inferior pulmonary veins to the middle of the posterior mitral valve annulus;

  f) from the left atriotomy to the middle of the posterior mitral valve annulus.

- For completion of the full maze procedure, the right atrial lesion set is performed. Initially, incisions in the right atrium (1, 2 and 3) are made to allow insertion of the cryoablation or radiofrequency ablation clamp device to create lesions from the:

  g) right atrial free wall to the superior vena cava;

  h) right atrial free wall to the inferior vena cava;

  i) right atrial free wall to the anteroposterior commissure of the tricuspid valve;

  j) right atrial appendage to the anteroseptal commissure of the tricuspid valve;

  k) right atrial appendage to the right atrial free wall, ensuring a 2-3cm gap is left to allow for electrical conduction.

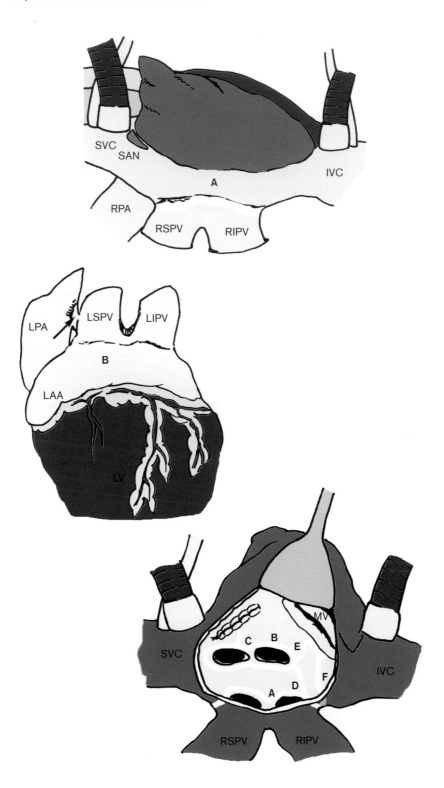

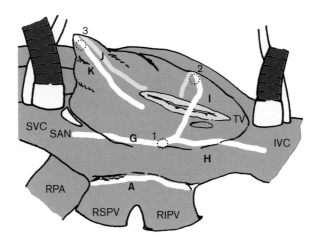

Figure 4. Left (A-F) and right (G-K) atrial maze lesion sets. LAA = left atrial appendage; LV = left ventricle; LPA = left pulmonary artery; LSPV = left superior pulmonary vein; LIPV = left inferior pulmonary vein; SVC = superior vena cava; IVC = inferior vena cava; RSPV = right superior pulmonary vein; RIPV = right inferior pulmonary vein; MV = mitral valve; TV = tricuspid valve; RPA = right pulmonary artery; SAN = sino-atrial node.

12 How is atrial flutter managed (Figure 5)?

- Atrial flutter is caused by a single macro re-entry circuit.
- Patients usually present with a variable block (e.g. 2:1, 3:1 or 4:1), which represents an atrial rate of 300 bpm and a ventricular response of 150, 100 or 75 bpm, respectively.
- Treatment options include amiodarone, calcium channel blockers, DC cardioversion, catheter ablation or surgical ablation of the flutter isthmus.
- The atrial flutter isthmus runs from the inferior vena caval opening along the Eustachian valve and the coronary sinus, to the tricuspid valve.

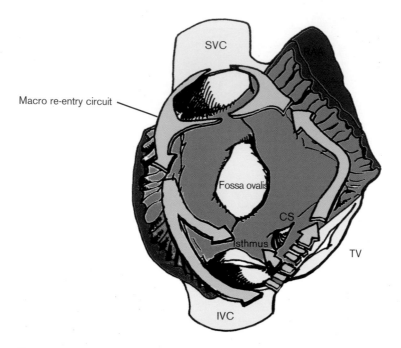

Figure 5. Macro re-entrant circuit of atrial flutter. The electric impulse crosses the isthmus between the orifices of the inferior vena cava (IVC) and the coronary sinus (CS). An ablation lesion is placed at this point, effectively blocking the electric loop. RAA = right atrial appendage; TV = tricuspid valve; SVC = superior vena cava.

13 What is the Vaughan-Williams classification of anti-arrhythmic drugs (Table 2)?

Table 2. Vaughan-Williams classification of anti-arrhythmic drugs.		
I	Fast sodium channel blockade	1a - quinidine, procainamide, disopyramide
		1b - lidocaine, phenytoin
		1c - flecainide, propafenone
II	β-sympathetic blockade	β-blockers, bretylium, guanethidine
III	Potassium channel blockade	amiodarone, sotalol, bretylium
IV	Slow calcium channel blockade	verapamil, diltiazem, adenosine

Recommended reading

1. Fuster V, Rydén LE, Cannom DS, Crijns HJ, Curtis AB, Ellenbogen KA, Halperin JL, Le Heuzey JY, Kay GN, Lowe JE, Olsson SB, Prystowsky EN, Tamargo JL, Wann S, Smith SC Jr, Jacobs AK, Adams CD, Anderson JL, Antman EM, Halperin JL, Hunt SA, Nishimura R, Ornato JP, Page RL, Riegel B, Priori SG, Blanc JJ, Budaj A, Camm AJ, Dean V, Deckers JW, Despres C, Dickstein K, Lekakis J, McGregor K, Metra M, Morais J, Osterspey A, Tamargo JL, Zamorano JL. ACC/AHA/ESC 2006 Guidelines for the management of patients with atrial fibrillation. *Circulation* 2006; 114(7): e257-354.

2. Cox JL, Schuessler RB, Boineau JP. The development of the Maze procedure for the treatment of atrial fibrillation. *Semin Thorac Cardiovasc Surg* 2000; 12: 2-14.

3. Haissaguerre M, Jais P, Shah DC, *et al*. Spontaneous initiation of atrial fibrillation by ectopic beats originating in the pulmonary veins. *N Engl J Med* 1998; 339: 659-66.

4. Cox JL, Boineau JP, Schuessler RB, Jaquiss RD, Lappas DG. Modification of the Maze procedure for atrial flutter and atrial fibrillation. I. Rationale and surgical results. *J Thorac Cardiovasc Surg* 1995; 110: 473-84.

5. Bakir I, Casselman FP, Brugada P, Geelen P, Wellens F, Degrieck I, Van Praet F, Vermeulen Y, De Geest R, Vanermen H. Current strategies in the surgical treatment of atrial fibrillation: review of the literature and Onze Lieve Vrouw Clinic's strategy. *Ann Thorac Surg* 2007; 83(1): 331-40.

6. Viola N, Williams MR, Oz MC, Ad N. The technology in use for the surgical ablation of atrial fibrillation. *Semin Thorac Cardiovasc Surg* 2002; 14(3): 198-205.

7. Cox JL. The longstanding, persistent confusion surrounding surgery for atrial fibrillation. *J Thorac Cardiovasc Surg* 2010; 139(6): 1374-86.

Chapter 20

Pericardial disease, cardiac tumours and cardiac trauma

1 **What are the clinical features of pericardial tamponade?**
- Haemodynamic compromise with acute dyspnoea and tachypnoea.
- Low pulse volume with pulsus paradoxus (see below).
- Low or undetectable blood pressure.
- Raised jugular venous pulse (JVP) with prominent x descent but no y descent.
- Kussmaul's sign (inspiratory rise of JVP) is not common.
- Muffled heart sounds.
- Oliguria or anuria.

2 **What is pulsus paradoxus?**
- Pulsus paradoxus is defined as an abnormally excessive fall in systolic blood pressure on inspiration >10mmHg (Figure 1).

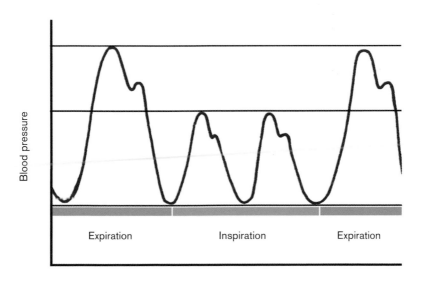

Figure 1. Pulsus paradoxus.

- Normally on inspiration there is a slight fall in systolic blood pressure (<5mmHg).
- In cardiac tamponade, the increased venous return that occurs on inspiration causes filling of the right heart, thereby displacing the interventricular septum to the left (rigid box with tamponade), resulting in less filling possible in the left heart producing a reduced cardiac output and systemic blood pressure.
- Other causes of pulsus paradoxus include constrictive pericarditis and status asthmaticus.

3 What are the typical findings on investigations with pericardial tamponade (Figure 2)?

- ECG - low voltage QRS complexes, electric alternans (due to the heart moving within a fluid-filled sac).

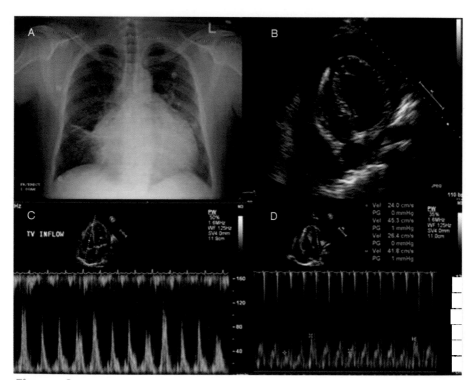

Figure 2. A) Chest radiograph and B) echocardiogram (apical 4 chamber) demonstrating a large pericardial collection. M-mode echocardiography demonstrating marked respiratory C) tricuspid valve and D) mitral valve inflow variation.

- CXR - symmetrical globular enlargement of the heart.
- Echocardiography:

  a) large pericardial collection;
  b) heart swinging freely within the pericardial sac;
  c) early diastolic collapse of the right ventricle;
  d) late diastolic collapse of the right atrium;
  e) marked respiratory tricuspid valve (>40%) and mitral valve (>25%) inflow variation.

4 **What is the treatment for pericardial tamponade?**
- Depending on the stability of the patient and the underlying cause:

  a) paraxiphoid pericardiocentesis;
  b) subxiphoid drainage of the pericardial collection;
  c) anterolateral thoracotomy drainage of the pericardial collection with a pericardial window;
  d) re-opening of median sternotomy.

5 **What are the causes of constrictive pericarditis?**
- Idiopathic, which is the major cause in the developed world.
- Infection - tuberculosis, viral (Coxsackie), fungal (*Histoplasma*).
- Mediastinal radiotherapy, which is dose-dependent (e.g. for lymphoma).
- Post-cardiac surgery (incidence 0.2-0.3%).
- Rare causes include tumour (mesothelioma), drugs (procainamide, hydralazine), sarcoidosis, amyloidosis, carcinoid syndrome, uraemia, trauma and myocardial infarction.

6 **What are the clinical features of constrictive pericarditis?**
- Symptoms of left and right heart failure, including dyspnoea, fatigue, weakness, anorexia, peripheral oedema and ascites.
- Raised jugular venous pressure.
- Ascites.
- Peripheral oedema.
- Hepatosplenomegaly.
- Displaced apex beat.
- Muffled heart sounds.
- Narrowed pulse pressure.
- Kussmaul's sign.
- Pulsus paradoxus may be present.

7 **What are the diagnostic findings of constrictive pericarditis (Figure 3)?**

- CXR - pericardial calcification and bilateral pleural effusions.
- Echocardiogram - impaired diastolic ventricular filling, thickened echobright pericardium, and dilated right atrium, inferior vena cava and hepatic veins.
- Doppler echocardiography - increased E:A ratio (rapid early filling and diastasis) and decreased inspiratory flow reduction in the hepatic veins.
- Coronary angiography - radiation-induced coronary artery disease.
- CT/MRI - thickened pericardium >4mm (compared to normal thickness 1-2mm).

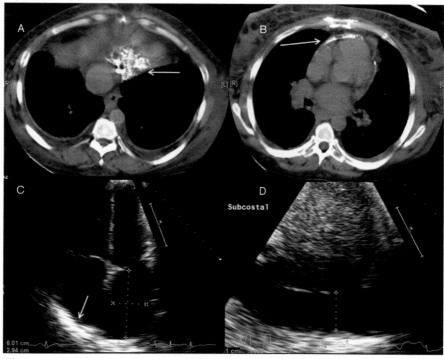

Figure 3. A, B) Computed tomography and C) echocardiography demonstrating calcified pericardium associated with constrictive pericarditis (arrows). D) Echocardiography demonstrating a dilated inferior vena cava on subcostal transthoracic views.

- Cardiac catheterisation - allows differentiation of constrictive pericarditis from restrictive cardiomyopathy:

  a) equalisation (within 5mmHg) of raised left and right ventricular end-diastolic pressures at any phase of respiration;
  b) equalisation of raised (>10mmHg) left and right atrial pressures with prominent x and y descents;
  c) square root sign - dip and plateau pattern of ventricular pressure with most of the diastolic filling occurring in early diastole, due to raised venous pressure, which then halts abruptly in mid-diastole;
  d) left ventricular systolic function is usually normal but may be impaired in severe cases;
  e) pulmonary artery systolic pressure <50mmHg;
  f) right ventricular end-diastolic to systolic pressure ratio >1:3;
  g) these findings can be masked by hypovolaemia but can be revealed with rapid fluid transfusion.

427

8 How is constrictive pericarditis (CP) differentiated from restrictive cardiomyopathy (RCM)?

- Certain features occur in both RCM and CP:

  a) increased EA ratio on the mitral valve inflow pattern;
  b) dip and plateau ventricular waveform;
  c) prominent x and y descents on the atrial waveform.

- Patients with RCM are more likely to have:

  a) pulmonary hypertension (pulmonary artery systolic pressure >50mmHg);
  b) reduced left ventricular function (EF <40%);
  c) endomyocardial biopsy evidence of an infiltrative process.

- Patients with CP are more likely to have:

  a) equalization of left and right ventricular end-diastolic pressure (<5mmHg);
  b) Kussmaul's sign;
  c) right ventricular end-diastolic to systolic pressure ratio >1:3;
  d) CT or echocardiographic evidence of a thickened pericardium.

9 **What are the principles of pericardiectomy (Figure 4)?**

- The aim is to achieve complete removal of all thickened pericardium and epicardium from the left and right ventricle and diaphragm, whilst preserving both phrenic nerves.
- Cardiopulmonary bypass and cardioplegic arrest are usually required for clearance of the posterior pericardium.
- Although incomplete resection of the pericardium overlying the atria risks residual constrictive haemodynamics, removal of densely adherent atrial tissue is not always necessary as the pathophysiology mainly affects ventricular filling.
- Operative mortality is 10-15% with a 5-year survival of 70% following pericardiectomy.

10 **What are the causes of restrictive cardiomyopathy (SAILS)?**

- Scleroderma.
- Amyloidosis.
- Iron storage diseases.
- Loeffler's eosinophilic endocarditis / endomyocardial fibrosis.
- Sarcoidosis.

11 **How are cardiac neoplasms classified?**

- Primary tumours, of which 75% are benign and 25% malignant.
- Secondary tumours from metastatic spread (lymphoma, breast, lung, melanoma, sarcoma) and direct spread (oesophagus, lung, breast, thymus) to the heart are 30 times more common than primary cardiac tumours.
- Subdiaphragmatic tumours originating from the kidneys, uterus, liver and adrenals, may also 'invade' the atrium via the inferior vena cava (Figure 5).

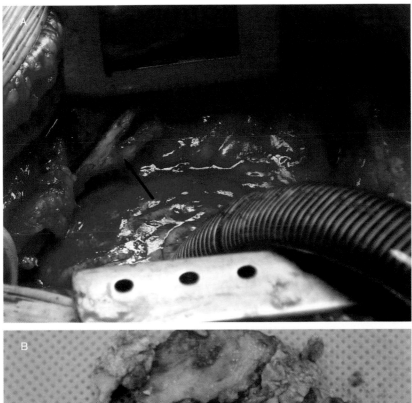

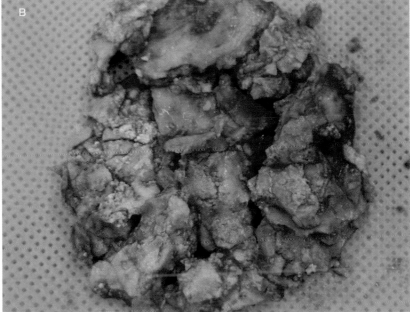

Figure 4. Pericardiectomy for constrictive pericarditis. A) Operative image following a median sternotomy demonstrating a markedly thickened fibrous and parietal pericardium (arrow). B) Resected fragments of thickened and calcified pericardium following pericardiectomy.

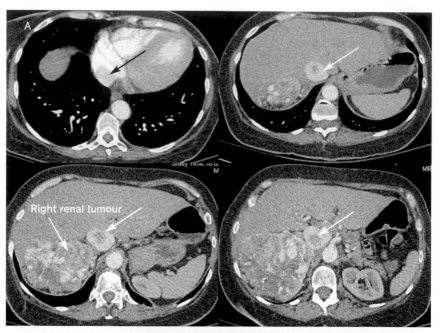

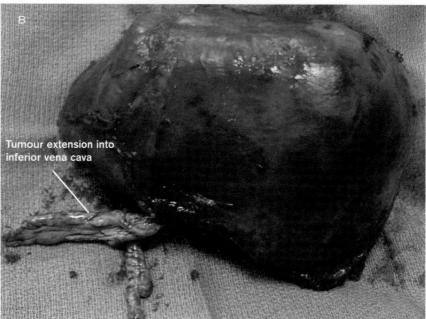

Figure 5. Renal cell carcinoma of the right kidney extending into the inferior vena cava and right atrium. A) Serial axial computed tomography images demonstrating a large right renal tumour and a 'filling defect' (arrows) in the inferior vena cava and right atrium. B) Excised right kidney with tumour extension into the inferior vena cava.

12 What are the most frequent primary benign cardiac tumours?

- Myxoma (see below).
- Lipoma, which present as well encapsulated tumours throughout the heart (especially the right atrium), commonly in obese, elderly, female patients. Surgery is usually indicated for symptomatic patients caused by obstruction to cardiac flow.
- Fibroelastoma (Figure 6), which usually occur on cardiac valves (especially mitral and aortic) or in ventricles as masses with frond-like projections. They can be asymptomatic, obstruct flow or embolise, and therefore are treated by resection.
- Rhabdomyoma, which are the commonest benign primary cardiac tumour in children, and present as multicentric, pedunculated tumours in either ventricle, with obstructive symptoms, valvular regurgitation or arrhythmias.
- Other primary benign cardiac tumours include fibroma, haemangioma, teratoma, neurofibroma and lymphangioma.

431

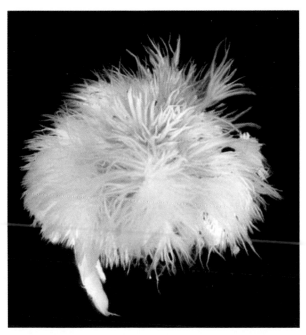

Figure 6. Fibroelastoma.

13 What are the most frequent primary malignant cardiac tumours?

- Angiosarcoma, which are frequently located in the atria and present with caval or valvular obstruction. Patients usually have distant metastases at the time of presentation and this is associated with a poor prognosis (median survival is approximately 6 months).
- Rhabdomyosarcoma, which are multicentric tumours that occur in all locations throughout the heart. They are usually treated by resection followed by adjuvant chemotherapy and radiotherapy. Median survival is approximately 12 months.
- Other primary malignant cardiac tumours include fibrous histiocytoma, fibrosarcoma, leiomyosarcoma and liposarcoma.
- Most sarcomas are incurable but cardiac transplantation can be considered for those without metastatic spread.

14 What is the epidemiology of cardiac myxomas?

- Cardiac myxomas occur with an incidence of 1:500,000 with 5% familial.
- They are commonest in patients aged 40-60 with a female predominance (70%).
- They account for 40% of benign cardiac tumours in adults and 15% in children.
- The majority of cardiac myxomas are located in the left atrium (75%) usually originating from the interatrial septum, with 20% in the right atrium and 5% in the ventricles or attached to valves.

15 What is Carney's syndrome?

- Carney's syndrome is an autosomal dominant familial form of atrial myxoma.
- It occurs with a male predominance at an earlier age than the non-familial form, often in childhood.
- They commonly occur in both atria and are multicentric (65%) with frequent recurrence (40%).
- They are associated with adrenocortical nodular masses, Sertoli cell testicular tumours and spotty mucocutaneous pigmentation.

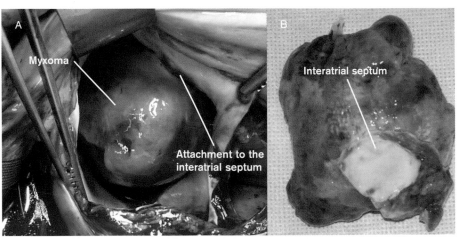

Figure 7. Myxoma A) within the cavity of the left atrium attached to the interatrial septum and B) following resection with attached interatrial septum.

16 What is the pathology of cardiac myxomas (Figure 7)?

- Cardiac myxomas are neoplasms of endocardial origin, derived from either pluripotent mesenchymal cells or endocardial nerve cells.
- They often appear as ovoid, pedunculated masses, which are friable, mucoid, gray-white in colour and smooth or granular in appearance.
- Histological analysis of cardiac tumours reveals an acid mucopolysaccharide matrix with polygonal cells, capillary-like structures and haemorrhagic areas.

17 What are the clinical features of cardiac myxomas (Figure 8)?

- Patients with cardiac myxomas present with symptoms related to:

  a) obstruction to blood flow;
  b) interference with valvular function;
  c) systemic embolisation;
  d) constitutional symptoms - fever, weight loss, malaise, myalgia, anaemia.

- Diastolic murmur (mimics mitral or tricuspid stenosis).
- Early diastolic tumour 'plop'.
- Pan-systolic murmur of mitral or tricuspid regurgitation (wrecking ball effect).

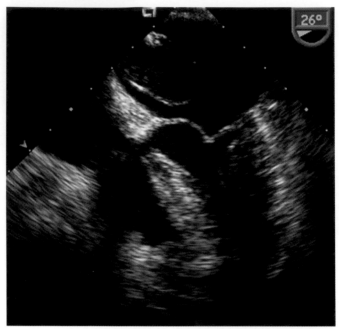

Figure 8. Echocardiographic image demonstrating a left atrial myxoma attached to the interatrial septum.

18 What are the principles of surgery for patients with left atrial myxomas?

- Following a median sternotomy, cardiopulmonary bypass is instituted using bicaval cannulation and snares, with minimal cardiac manipulation to avoid tumour embolisation.
- The myxoma is approached via a standard left atriotomy, a trans-septal atrial incision or a Dubost bi-atrial incision.
- Ideally the tumour is resected en bloc with clear resection margins and if the interatrial septum is involved, it may be closed with a pericardial patch.
- Irrigate the atrial cavity with saline to wash away any residual neoplastic cells (avoid using cell-saver or bypass suction).
- Assess valvular function for any 'wrecking ball' effect causing regurgitation.
- A recurrence rate of <5% occurs due to:

  a) inadequate resection;
  b) tumour seeding at the primary operation; or
  c) multicentric tumours.

19 What is the pathophysiology of traumatic aortic rupture (aortic transection)?

- Traumatic aortic rupture usually occurs following a deceleration injury, which causes strain at the points of anatomical fixation of the thoracic aorta.
- As the descending aorta is held in place by the intercostal arteries and the ligamentum arteriosum, aortic transection usually occurs at the aortic isthmus (between the left subclavian artery and the ligamentum arteriosum) in 80-90% of cases with the remaining at the origin of the aortic arch branches.
- The majority (80-90%) of patients with traumatic aortic rupture die at the scene of injury, with 50% of survivors dying within the next 48 hours.
- The adventitia and surrounding fascia of the thoracic aorta can maintain luminal continuity following traumatic aortic rupture.
- In certain situations, it is necessary to diagnose and treat other life-threatening injuries first and if this is the case the systolic blood pressure needs to be kept <110mmHg.

20 What are the clinical features of traumatic aortic rupture?

- The diagnosis of traumatic aortic rupture should be considered in all patients that have sustained severe blunt thoracic trauma, especially in those with upper rib (1st-3rd), sternal and scapula fractures.
- Retrosternal or interscapular pain caused by stretching or dissection of the aortic adventitia.
- Haemodynamic compromise producing tachycardia, hypotension and oliguria.
- Peri-aortic haematoma causing compression of surrounding structures resulting in dysphagia, stridor, dyspnoea or hoarseness.

21 What are the typical radiological findings with traumatic aortic injury (Figure 9)?

- Chest radiograph:

  a)   widened (>8cm) superior mediastinum (note most trau chest radiographs are anterior-posterior in projection, wh artificially enlarges the mediastinal silhouette);

  b)   fractures of the superior thoracic cage (1st-3rd ribs, sternu scapula);

  c)   obliteration of the aortic knob;

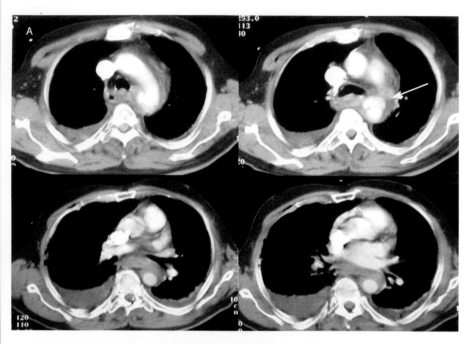

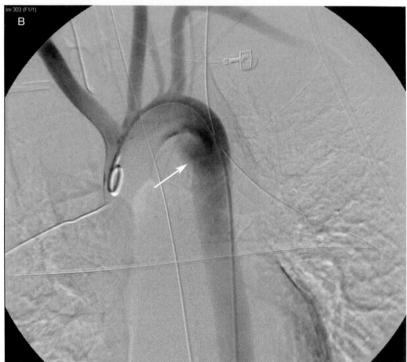

Figure 9. A) Computed tomography and B) angiography images demonstrating transection (arrow) of the proximal descending aorta (just distal to the origin of the the left subclavian artery), with extravasation of contrast and an irregular luminal contour.

d)   left apical pleural cap;

e)   left pleural effusion or haemothorax;

f)   deviation of the oesophagus (nasogastric tube) to the right;

g)   deviation of the trachea (endotracheal tube) to the right;

h)   displacement of the left hilum downwards;

i)   widening of the paratracheal and paraspinal stripe.

- CT scan:

a)   disruption of the aortic lumen;

b)   extravasation of radio-opaque contrast;

c)   peri-aortic haematoma.

22 What are the surgical options for treating traumatic aortic rupture?

- The patient is positioned for a left thoracotomy with the pelvis slightly rotated to gain access to the left femoral vessels, if required.

- The aortic isthmus is then carefully dissected and following clamping of the aortic arch (between the left subclavian artery and left common carotid artery), the left subclavian artery and the distal descending thoracic aorta, an interposition graft is anastomosed to the thoracic aorta, using a number of different adjunct techniques:

a)   clamp and sew technique, which avoids the need for cardiopulmonary bypass and systemic heparinisation, but is associated with an increased risk of paraplegia if the clamp time exceeds 30 minutes;

b)   Gott shunt, using heparin-bonded tubing to bypass the area of aorta undergoing surgery, from the ascending aorta or left ventricular apex to the descending aorta or femoral artery (Figure 10);

c)   left heart bypass, using heparin-bonded tubing between the left atrial appendage and the left femoral artery with a centrifugal pump (no oxygenator or heat exchanger) at ~2L/min and no need for systemic heparinisation;

d)   total cardiopulmonary bypass from the femoral vein to the femoral artery, which allows better control of collateral flow with improved surgical visualisation but requires administration of systemic heparin.

- Endovascular stenting should also be considered for patients with traumatic aortic rupture.

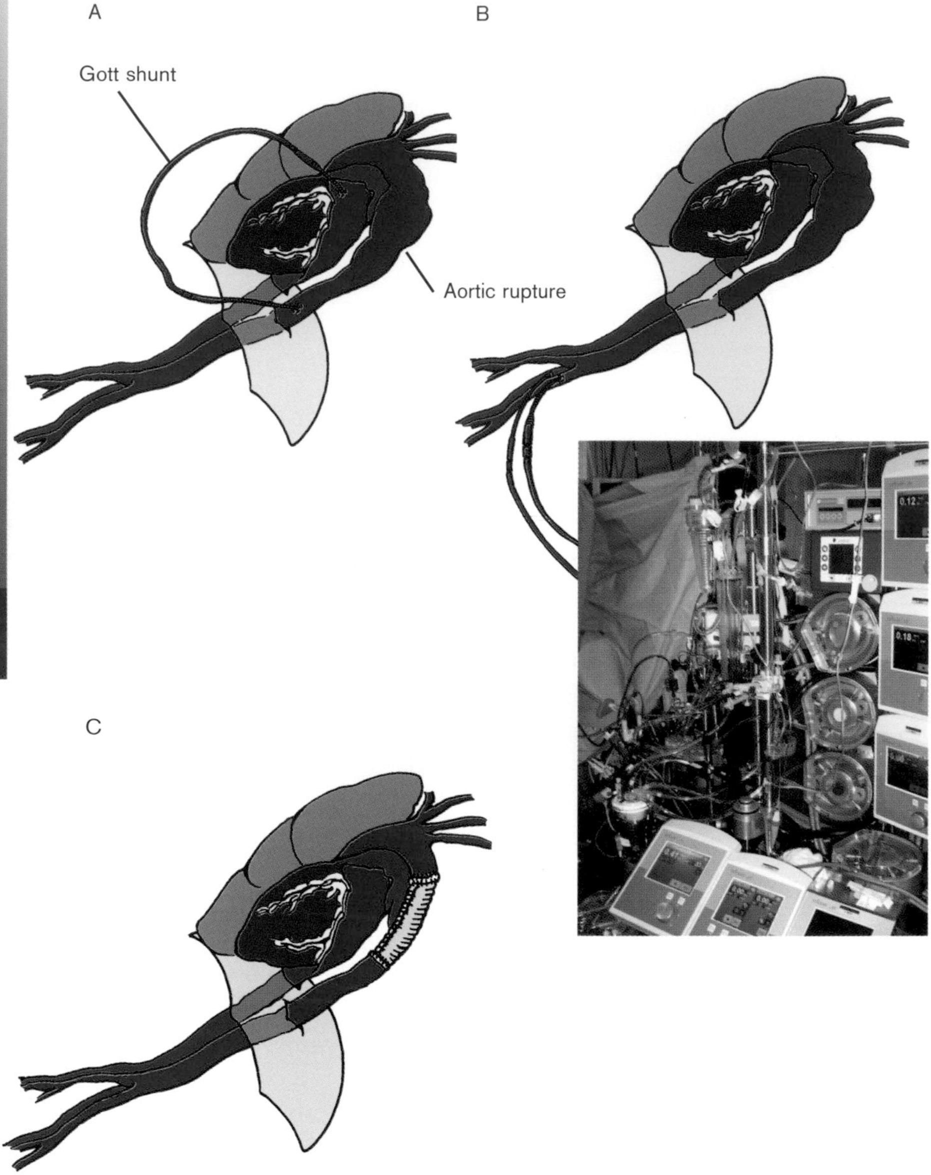

A

B

Gott shunt

Aortic rupture

C

Figure 10. A) Gott shunt bypassing blood from the left atrium to the descending aorta using heparin-bonded tubing. B) Total cardiopulmonary bypass from the femoral vein to the femoral artery. C) Completed descending thoracic aortic interposition graft.

23 What are the indications for an emergency resuscitative thoracotomy?

- According to the Advanced Trauma Life Support (ATLS®) guidelines, following penetrating trauma (not blunt trauma) within 10 minutes of pulseless electrical activity (PEA).
- It is performed by a left anterolateral thoracotomy through the 4th intercostal space.
- Through this access, the therapeutic options include:

  a) evacuation of the pericardium;
  b) open cardiac massage;
  c) clamping of the descending aorta (to stop distal bleeding and increase coronary and cerebral perfusion).

24 What are the principles of treating blunt cardiac trauma?

- Patients with blunt cardiac trauma are managed as per the ATLS® guidelines with particular attention to cardiac dysrhythmias, tamponade and myocardial contusion.
- These patients should be monitored in a high dependency area with serial ECGs, echocardiograms, cardiac enzymes, chest radiographs and CT scans.
- Blunt cardiac trauma may result in left pleuropericardial tears, right atrial disruption at the caval junctions, atrial or ventricular septal defects or aortic regurgitation.

25 What are the principles of treating penetrating cardiac trauma (Figure 11)?

- Prompt diagnosis of cardiac tamponade is essential by clinical signs (haemodynamic compromise, Beck's triad, Kussmaul's sign, pulsus paradoxus) and echocardiography.
- Patients need prompt decompression by paraxiphoid pericardiocentesis and then operative closure of the penetrating cardiac wound.
- Access to the heart is obtained by a left anterolateral thoracotomy in emergency situations, otherwise a median sternotomy gives better access to the pericardium and great vessels if time permits.
- Once the mediastinum is accessed, the pericardium is opened, any clots or liquid evacuated, open cardiac massage performed and any bleeding point occluded.
- Atrial and ventricular lacerations are treated with direct suture and may be buttressed by Teflon® strips.

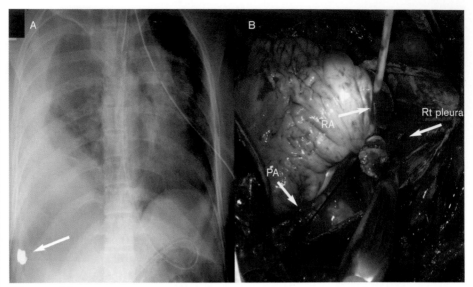

Figure 11. Penetrating cardiac trauma caused by a gun-shot wound to the thorax. A) Chest radiograph demonstrating a right haemothorax and the bullet (arrow) lying in the right costophrenic angle. B) Operative image following a median sternotomy illustrating the path of the bullet with a repaired main pulmonary artery, a tear in the right atrium occluded by a Foley catheter and a hole in the right pleura.

- Coronary artery lacerations may need ligation and bypass grafting.
- If a posterior cardiac injury is observed, it is important to avoid air embolism when lifting the heart.

Recommended reading

1. Kabbani SS, LeWinter MM. Pericardial diseases. *Curr Treat Options Cardiovasc Med* 2002; 4(6): 487-95.

2. Inglessis II, Dec GW. Constrictive pericarditis. *Curr Treat Options Cardiovasc Med* 1999; 1(1): 63-71.

3. Xenos ES, Abedi NN, Davenport DL, Minion DJ, Hamdallah O, Sorial EE, Endean ED. Meta-analysis of endovascular vs open repair for traumatic descending thoracic aortic rupture. *J Vasc Surg* 2008; 48(5): 1343-51.

4. Svensson LG, Kouchoukos NT, Miller DC, Bavaria JE, Coselli JS, Curi MA, Eggebrecht H, Elefteriades JA, Erbel R, Gleason TG, Lytle BW, Mitchell RS, Nienaber CA, Roselli EE, Safi HJ, Shemin RJ, Sicard GA, Sundt TM 3rd, Szeto WY, Wheatley GH 3rd; Society of Thoracic Surgeons Endovascular Surgery Task Force. Expert consensus document on the treatment of descending thoracic aortic disease using endovascular stent-grafts. *Ann Thorac Surg* 2008; 85(1 Suppl): S1-41.

Chapter 21

Cardiac anaesthesia and intensive care management

1   **Describe the monitoring used during cardiac anaesthesia**
- Electrocardiogram - limb leads and V5.
- Arterial oxygen saturations.
- End-tidal carbon dioxide levels.
- Arterial blood pressure (invasive and non-invasive).
- Central venous pressure.
- Central (core) and peripheral temperature.
- Urine output.
- Cardiac output, using invasive (Swan-Ganz catheter) and non-invasive techniques (LiDCO).
- Pulmonary artery pressure.
- Transoesophageal echocardiogram.

2   **What are the principles of cardiac anaesthesia?**
- Prior to arrival in the anaesthetic room, most elective patients have fasted for 6-8 hours and have been given a premedication. An example includes using a benzodiazepine (such as temazepam) and an opiate (such as morphine), to reduce anxiety-induced tachycardia and hypertension, and to help facilitate analgesia.
- There are three components to anaesthesia, which include:

    a)   hypnosis to produce a reversible state of non-awareness and amnesia, using:
        i)   intravenous sedatives, such as propofol;
        ii)   inhaled anaesthetic agents, such as isoflurane;
    b)   analgesia to reduce the responses to pain encountered during surgery. Typically, an opiate such as fentanyl or remifentanyl is used, in preference over morphine, as it has less cardiac side effects and is short-acting;
    c)   muscle relaxation using:
        i)   non-depolarising agents (such as vecuronium or rocuronium), which are competitive inhibitors of the acetylcholine receptor at the neuromuscular junction. They have an onset time of 2-3 minutes, last between 20

to 60 minutes and can be reversed by an anti-cholinesterase (such as neostigmine); or

ii) a depolarising agent (such as suxamethonium), which non-competitively binds with the acetylcholine receptor resulting in depolarisation of the neuromuscular junction. It has a rapid onset of action producing paralysis that lasts for 5-10 minutes and cannot be reversed.

- The conduct of anaesthesia includes three phases:

a) induction:
  i) hypnosis - propofol;
  ii) analgesia - fentanyl or remifentanyl;
  iii) muscle relaxation - suxamethonium;
b) maintenance:
  i) hypnosis - propofol and isoflurane;
  ii) analgesia - fentanyl or remifentanyl;
  iii) muscle relaxation - vecuronium or rocuronium;
c) reversal.

- During the different stages of cardiac anaesthesia it is important to minimise myocardial oxygen consumption by controlling the heart rate and blood pressure, and optimising preload and afterload. This allows the myocardial work to be kept to a minimum in patients with cardiac disease.

3 Describe the American Society of Anesthesiologists (ASA) pre-operative scoring system

- Grade I: healthy patient.
- Grade II: mild systemic disease but no functional limitation.
- Grade III: moderate systemic disease with definite functional limitation.
- Grade IV: severe systemic disease with a constant threat to life.
- Grade V: moribund patient, not expected to survive 24 hours with or without surgery.

4 Describe the different grades of intubation

- The different grades of intubation are determined by the degree to which the vocal cords and upper airway can be visualised at the time of intubation and guides future anaesthetists to the degree of difficulty of intubation:

a) Grade I: vocal cords visible;
b) Grade II: vocal cords partially visible;

c)   Grade III: vocal cords not visible; only the epiglottis can be seen;

d)   Grade IV: vocal cords and epiglottis not visible.

- In the pre-anaesthesia assessment, the difficulty of intubation is assessed using the Mallampati system, by asking the patient to open their mouth wide open:

  a)   I: faucial pillars, soft palate and uvula visible;

  b)   II: faucial pillars and soft palate visible;

  c)   III: only the soft palate visible;

  d)   IV: none of the above soft tissues are visible.

5 What are important considerations when transferring a patient from the operating room to the intensive care unit?

- Before transfer, it is important to ensure that the patient is monitored (arterial pressure, central venous pressure, oxygen saturation, cardiac rate and rhythm), haemodynamically stable and not bleeding.
- All intravenous infusions should be checked and refilled if appropriate.
- During transfer, it is important to have:

  a)   monitoring directly visible by the anaesthetist;

  b)   respiratory equipment including an oxygen tank, connection tubing and a 3L self-inflating reservoir bag connected to the endotracheal tube;

  c)   intravenous infusions and boluses available of sedatives, inotropes and antihypertensives;

  d)   a portable cardiac defibrillator.

- On admission to ITU, all monitoring is recalibrated, the drains are connected to 20cm H_2O wall suction and a full set of investigations are ordered (including full blood count, urea and electrolytes, coagulation screen, arterial blood gas, electrocardiogram and chest radiograph).
- There should be a clear hand-over of the patient to the intensive care unit team, including pre-operative findings, the intra-operative procedure and a postoperative plan.

6 Describe the standard monitoring in the intensive care unit following cardiac surgery

- Electrocardiogram - limb leads and V5.
- Arterial oxygen saturation.
- End-tidal carbon dioxide levels.

- Arterial blood pressure (invasive and non-invasive).
- Central venous pressure.
- Central (core) and peripheral temperature.
- Urine output and fluid input.
- Mediastinal drainage.
- Pulmonary artery pressure and cardiac output measurements.

7   What are the common causes of mediastinal bleeding in the immediate postoperative period?

- Surgical:

  a) anastomotic suture lines and cannulation sites;
  b) side branches of arterial or venous conduits;
  c) sternal sites, including the periosteum, sternal wire holes and bone marrow;
  d) raw surfaces, including the internal mammary artery bed, pericardium and thymus.

- Coagulopathy:

  a) residual heparin, secondary to inadequate protamine reversal or heparin rebound;
  b) thrombocytopaenia, secondary to a low platelet count pre-operatively and haemodilution on cardiopulmonary bypass (which can drop platelet counts by 20-50%, especially with long bypass times);
  c) platelet dysfunction, secondary to pre-operative medications (aspirin, ticlopidine, clopidogrel) and damage caused by cardiopulmonary bypass (especially with deep hypothermia);
  d) coagulation factor depletion, secondary to pre-operative factors (residual warfarin effect, hepatic dysfunction and von Willebrand disease) and haemodilution with cardiopulmonary bypass and cell salvage;
  e) fibrinolysis, secondary to pre-operative thrombolytic agents and plasminogen activation on cardiopulmonary bypass.

8   What are the principles of managing mediastinal bleeding post-cardiac surgery?

- Assessment to help distinguish surgical causes from coagulopathy:

  a) blood tests - haemoglobin, activated clotting time (ACT), international normalized ratio (INR), activated partial thromboplastin time ratio (APTTR), platelet count, fibrinogen levels and thrombo-elastogram (TEG);

444

b) radiology - chest radiograph and echocardiogram (TOE preferably) to check for pleural and pericardial collections;

c) drainage - rate of bleeding (sudden or gradual, 'dump' when rolled) and patency of tubes;

d) haemodynamic status, especially to identify tamponade.

- Treatment:

a) correct hypothermia;

b) calcium chloride 1g (10mL of 10%) intravenously if ionised calcium is low (<1.2mmol/L);

c) treat hypertension;

d) consider increasing the positive end expiratory pressure (PEEP) to 12cm H_2O, which increases the intrathoracic pressure to 'tamponade' the bleeding;

e) protamine should be given in patients with mediastinal bleeding and an APTTR >1.3 or ACT >110% of baseline. Doses of 25-100mg should be given slowly depending on the degree of residual heparin effect;

f) platelets should be given in patients with mediastinal bleeding and a platelet count <100 x 10^9 per litre or if platelet dysfunction is indicated on the thrombo-elastogram. One unit of platelets (50mL) should increase the platelet count by 7-10 x 10^9 per litre. The standard transfusion dose recommended is 1 unit per 10kg. One pool of platelets contains 6-10 units of platelets. They are stored at room temperature, can be used for 5 days and should be ABO compatible but do not need to be cross-matched;

g) fresh frozen plasma (FFP) should be given in patients with mediastinal bleeding and an INR >1.3. FFP contains all coagulation factors but no platelets. The standard dose is 2-4U (5-10mL/kg), as each unit contains 250mL. It is stored at -18°C, thawed over 20 minutes and should be used within 2 hours. FFP should be ABO compatible but does not need to be cross-matched. It is also used to treat heparin resistance with anti-thrombin III (ATIII) deficiency. Beriplex® can also be used as a concentrated form of coagulation factors with 500-1000 units representing 2-4U of FFP;

h) cryoprecipitate should be given in patients with mediastinal bleeding and a fibrinogen level <150mg/dL. It contains fibrinogen, Factor VII, Factor VIII and Factor XIII. One pool (200mL) contains five units and should increase the fibrinogen levels by 50mg/dL. The standard dose is 0.1U/kg (1-2 pools for a 70kg patient). Cryoprecipitate should be ABO compatible but does not need to be cross-matched;

i) blood should be given if the haemoglobin is <8g/dL. One unit of packed red blood cells (300-350mL) should increase the haemoglobin by 1g/dL. Large volumes of stored blood may cause hypocalcaemia, hyperkalaemia and a dilutional coagulopathy. Blood should be ABO compatible and cross-matched;

j) cell saver blood, which has been washed of all platelets and coagulation factors;

k) desmopressin can be used to increase the release of von Willebrand Factor from endothelial stores to aid platelet function. Some studies have shown its effectiveness in patients taking antiplatelet agents up to the time of surgery;

l) urgent mediastinal re-exploration is required for tamponade, haemodynamically significant hypovolaemia or persistent mediastinal bleeding (>500mL/hr for 1 hour, >400mL/hr for 2 hours or >300mL/hr for 3 hours).

9 **What are the common causes of low cardiac output syndrome and sustained hypotension in the immediate postoperative period?**

● Reduced preload, caused by:

a) hypovolaemia, secondary to haemorrhage, polyuria or inadequate fluid replacement;

b) restricted cardiac filling, secondary to tamponade or tension pneumothorax;

c) tachyarrhythmias, which reduce ventricular diastolic filling time and loss of atrial transport (in patients with atrial fibrillation);

d) vasodilation (see below).

● Impaired myocardial contractility, secondary to:

a) negative inotropes, such as calcium channel blockers and β-blockers;

b) hypoxia, hypercarbia, acidosis, hyperkalaemia and hypothermia;

c) myocardial stunning, caused by cardiopulmonary bypass and pre-operative myocardial damage;

d) coronary ischaemia (coronary or conduit spasm or thrombosis);

e) mechanical causes, such as incomplete valve repair, systolic anterior motion of the mitral valve and valve thrombosis.

- Reduced afterload, caused by:

  a) rewarming;
  b) vasoplegia, secondary to cardiopulmonary bypass-induced systemic inflammatory response syndrome (SIRS);
  c) protamine;
  d) blood products;
  e) glyceryl trinitrate and sodium nitroprusside;
  f) sepsis;
  g) anaphylaxis.

- Excessive afterload, caused by hypothermia, acidosis, pressors and pain can also cause low cardiac output by increasing the workload of the heart.
- The most serious causes of low cardiac output in the immediate postoperative period include massive bleeding, tamponade and myocardial ischaemia. The treatment of all three causes may require returning to the operating theatre immediately.
- It is also important to consider pre-operative (recent myocardial infarction, pulmonary hypertension) and intra-operative causes (poor myocardial protection, residual valvular regurgitation and incomplete de-airing) that may be contributing to postoperative low cardiac output syndrome.

10 What are the principles in managing low cardiac output syndrome?

- The ideal goal in managing low cardiac output syndrome is to identify and treat the underlying aetiology and achieve a cardiac index >2.5L/min/m².
- If cardiac output monitoring is not available, the following can be used as markers of adequate organ perfusion:

  a) mean arterial blood pressure >70mmHg;
  b) urine output >1mL/kg/hr;
  c) skin temperature >36.5°C;
  d) base excess >-2mmol/L.

- Optimise preload:

  a) fluid resuscitation to achieve right and left atrial filling pressures of 10-14mmHg. Some patients require high filling pressures, such as those with left ventricular hypertrophy, diastolic dysfunction, pulmonary hypertension and tricuspid regurgitation;

b) urgently treat tension pneumothorax and cardiac tamponade with needle thoracocentesis and re-sternotomy, respectively;

c) anti-arrhythmics and electrical cardioversion to restore sinus rhythm and aid rate control in the presence of tachyarrhythmias.

- Optimise myocardial contractility:

    a) treat acidosis, hypoxia, hypercarbia and hyperkalaemia;

    b) support the myocardium with positive inotropic agents such as epinephrine, dopamine and milrinone;

    c) coronary vasodilators such as glyceryl trinitrate, may be required for coronary artery or arterial conduit spasm;

    d) reoperation for occluded coronary artery bypass grafts or severe valvular regurgitation may be necessary.

- Optimise afterload with vasodilators (glyceryl trinitrate, sodium nitroprusside) or vasoconstrictors (noradrenaline, vasopressin) depending on the underlying aetiology.

- Increase the heart rate if the patient has bradycardia or heart block, using the epicardial pacing leads placed at surgery.

- Intra-aortic balloon pumps should also be considered as an efficient method of improving myocardial oxygen supply without increasing myocardial oxygen consumption.

- In certain situations, left ventricular assist devices are required to support the heart until the myocardium recovers.

11 What are the causes of right ventricular failure following cardiac surgery?

- Right ventricular dysfunction, caused by:

    a) poor myocardial protection during cardiopulmonary bypass;

    b) right ventricular stunning following ischaemia reperfusion injury;

    c) ischaemia, secondary to right coronary artery disease or a graft problem;

    d) pre-operative right ventricular dysfunction.

- Pulmonary hypertension, secondary to:

    a) left heart disease, such as severe mitral regurgitation or left ventricular failure;

    b) pulmonary disease;

    c) pulmonary embolism;

    d) adult respiratory distress syndrome (ARDS).

12 **What are the principles of management of patients with right ventricular failure post-cardiac surgery?**

● Optimise right ventricular preload:

    a) volume;
    b) atrioventricular sequential pacing;
    c) restore sinus rhythm, if possible.

● Optimise right ventricular contractility:

    a) epinephrine;
    b) phosphodiesterase inhibitor, such as milrinone.

● Optimise right ventricular afterload:

    a) correct hypoxia, hypercarbia and acidosis, which cause pulmonary vasoconstriction;
    b) phosphodiesterase inhibitor, such as sildenafil or milrinone;
    c) inhaled nitric oxide (20-40 parts per million);
    d) nesiritide (recombinant brain natriuretic peptide);
    e) right ventricular assist device.

13 **What are the indications for an intra-aortic balloon pump in the peri-operative period with regards to cardiac surgery?**

● Elective in patients with significantly impaired pre-operative cardiac function.
● Peri-operative ischaemia.
● Unloading of the left ventricle following a mechanical complication of myocardial infarction, such as a ventricular septal rupture or acute myocardial regurgitation.
● Low cardiac output syndrome, unresponsive to inotropic support.
● Acute myocardial deterioration, as a bridge to revascularization, left ventricular assist device or transplantation.
● Contra-indications to intra-aortic balloon pump insertion include the presence of:

    a) aortic regurgitation;
    b) aortic dissection;
    c) severe peripheral atherosclerosis.

14 **Describe the North American Society of Pacing and Electrophysiology / British Pacing and Electrophysiology Group (NASPE/BPEG) five-position pacemaker classification system**
- I: chamber paced - O (none), A (atrium), V (ventricle), D (dual A+V), S (single A or V).
- II: chamber sensed - O (none), A (atrium), V (ventricle), D (dual A+V), S (single A or V).
- III: response to sensing - O (none), T (triggered), I (inhibited), D (dual).
- IV: programmability - O (none), R (rate modulation).
- V: multisite pacing - O (none), A (atrium), V (ventricle), D (dual A+V).

15 **What are the typical temporary epicardial pacemaker settings following cardiac surgery?**
- Rate 90 bpm.
- Atrial output 5mA.
- Atrial sensitivity 1.0mV.
- Ventricular output 5mA.
- Ventricular sensitivity 2.0mV.
- Atrioventricular delay (AVD) 150msec.
- Mode DDD (see above).

16 **What are the different ventilation modes available?**
- Volume-preset modes:

    a) assist control ventilation (AC), where the ventilator delivers a breath triggered by the patient's respiratory effort or at preset intervals if no breath occurs;

    b) intermittent mandatory ventilation (IMV), where the patient receives positive pressure ventilation at a preset tidal volume and respiratory rate;

    c) synchronised intermittent mandatory ventilation (SIMV), where the patient breathes spontaneously but at preset intervals the next spontaneous breath is augmented by the ventilator to a preset tidal volume.

- Pressure-preset modes:

    a) pressure controlled ventilation (PCV), where the peak airway pressure and inspiratory time are set at a fixed respiratory rate;

b) pressure support ventilation (PS), where the patient's inspiratory effort is augmented by a selected level of inspiratory pressure. Hence, the patient sets the respiratory rate, flow rate and inspiratory time.

17 What are the typical ventilator settings in a patient following cardiac surgery?

- Synchronized intermittent mandatory ventilation (SIMV) or assist control (AC).
- Inspired oxygen concentration (FiO_2) is initially set at 100% following transfer and is then progressively weaned to 40% whilst maintaining the PaO_2 >10kPa.
- Tidal volume (TV) 6-10mL/kg. Higher tidal volumes should be used with caution as they can cause over-stretching of an anastomosed internal mammary artery.
- Respiratory rate (RR) 12-18 breaths/minute.
- Minute volume (= respiratory rate x tidal volume) 100-120mL/kg/min. If the patient develops hypercapnia, it can be treated by increasing the minute volume (by raising either the respiratory rate or the tidal volume).
- Positive end expiratory pressure (PEEP) 5cmH$_2$O. This helps to reduce atelectasis. Higher levels can be used to help 'tamponade' mediastinal bleeding (up to 12cm H$_2$O) but should be used with caution as these levels can impair venous return and ventricular function.
- I:E ratio 1:2. In patients with chronic obstructive pulmonary disease, a ratio of 1:3 may help to reduce the risk of air trapping.
- Peak inflation pressures <35cmH$_2$O. Higher peak airway pressures suggest airway resistance, secondary to a mucous plug, a kinked endotracheal tube, bronchospasm or coughing.

18 What are the exclusion criteria for fast-tracking patients to early extubation following cardiac surgery?

- Poor left ventricular function, recent myocardial infarction or pulmonary oedema.
- Redo sternotomy (previous cardiac surgery).
- Severe respiratory dysfunction (FEV_1 <75% of predicted).
- Severe pulmonary hypertension (systolic pulmonary artery pressure >60mmHg).
- Severe renal or hepatic insufficiency.
- Previous cerebrovascular accident.

- Problematic intubation.
- Prolonged operation or deep hypothermic circulatory arrest.
- High-dose inotropic requirement intra-operatively.
- On-going mediastinal bleeding.
- If patients are deemed appropriate for fast tracking for early extubation, shorter-acting anaesthetic agents are used, and early analgesia and rapid weaning of inotropes are employed.
- If the patient is haemodynamically stable, with good ventilation parameters and mediastinal bleeding is under control, the aim is to extubate within 4-6 hours.

19 What are the disadvantages of prolonged ventilation?

- Cardiovascular side effects of sedatives and narcotics, necessitating increased pressor and volume requirements.
- Impaired right ventricular function from positive pressure ventilation.
- Ventilator-associated morbidity (such as pneumonia).
- Cost.

20 What are the disadvantages of early extubation?

- Increased work of breathing, resulting in increased myocardial oxygen demand.
- Increased pain and higher metabolism, resulting in increased cardiac work.

21 What are the criteria for extubation following cardiac surgery?

- Cardiac:

  a) cardiac index >2.2L/min/m^2;
  b) mean arterial blood pressure >70mmHg;
  c) no haemodynamically significant arrhythmias.

- Respiratory:

  a) partial pressure of oxygen in arterial blood (PaO$_2$) >10kPa and arterial oxygen saturation (SaO$_2$) >92% with an FiO$_2$ <50%;
  b) PEEP <5cm H$_2$O;
  c) respiratory rate <20 per minute;
  d) pressure support <10cm H$_2$O.

- Mediastinal drainage <50mL/hr with haemoglobin >8g/dL.
- Urine output >1mL/kg/hr.
- Neurological:

  a)   awake with stimulation and no residual neuromuscular blockade;
  b)   able to lift head off the bed;
  c)   able to cough and clear secretions to maintain own airway.

- Core temperature >36°C.
- Once the sedation has been stopped, the patient's ventilator settings are maintained with an FiO_2 at 50% and PEEP of 5mmHg, and the IMV rate is reduced by two breaths every 30 minutes checking arterial blood gases and then removing the endotracheal tube if the patient maintains cardiorespiratory stability. Alternatively, a trial of continuous positive airway pressure (CPAP) with the endotracheal tube *in situ* is performed to assess whether the patient is able to self-ventilate.
- Poor prognostic factors for weaning include:

  a)   tidal volume <5mL/kg;
  b)   minute volume <10L/min;
  c)   maximum inspiratory pressure <-20cm H_2O;
  d)   shallow breathing index (respiratory rate/tidal volume) >100.

22 What are the common causes of hypoxia and respiratory impairment in the immediate postoperative period?

- Poor gas exchange:

  a)   atelectasis, caused by:
     i)   general anaesthesia;
     ii) compression of the lung during left internal mammary artery harvesting;
     iii) reduced surfactant production during cardiopulmonary bypass;
     iv) inadequate lung expansion following extubation due to pain;
     v)   retained secretions or sputum plug, associated with pre-operative smoking or pneumonia;

b) pulmonary oedema, caused by:
  i) left ventricular dysfunction;
  ii) systemic inflammatory response caused by cardiopulmonary bypass;
  iii) massive transfusion of blood products;
c) pleural effusion, secondary to:
  i) heart failure;
  ii) undrained postoperative blood;
d) bronchospasm secondary to:
  i) pre-operative asthma or chronic obstructive pulmonary disease (COPD);
  ii) medications, such as β-blockers;
  iii) anaphylaxis;
e) pneumothorax;
f) diaphragmatic dysfunction, secondary to phrenic nerve injury caused by:
  i) iced cold slush;
  ii) direct trauma to the phrenic nerve during pericardiectomy or pericardial window formation;
  iii) injury during harvesting of the internal mammary artery.

• Inadequate oxygen delivery:

a) low inspired oxygen concentration (FiO_2);
b) inadequate ventilator settings, such as low PEEP or ventilator malfunction;
c) misplaced endotracheal tube;
d) low cardiac output syndrome;
e) anaemia;
f) increased oxygen demand with shivering or sepsis.

23 What are the principles of management of patients with respiratory impairment post-cardiac surgery?

• Assessment to identify underlying cause:

a) respiratory examination - inspect, palpate, percuss and auscultate;
b) arterial blood gases - pH, PaO_2, $PaCO_2$, base deficit;
c) chest radiograph - lung pathology, endotracheal tube placement;
d) ventilator settings - FiO_2, PEEP, RR, TV, pressure support, peak airway pressures.

- Treatment for specific aetiology:

  a) atelectasis:
     i) chest physiotherapy;
     ii) CPAP or increase PEEP;
     iii) antibiotics;
     iv) bronchoscopic clearance of secretions and plugs;
  b) pulmonary oedema:
     i) diuresis for cardiogenic aetiology;
     ii) for non-cardiogenic aetiology, use an adult respiratory distress syndrome (ARDS) protocol with low tidal volumes to reduce the risk of barotrauma. Prone ventilation and nitric oxide may also be needed;
  c) pleural effusion - thoracocentesis or chest drain;
  d) bronchospasm - nebulisers (β-agonists and ipratropium bromide);
  e) pneumothorax - chest drain;
  f) phrenic nerve injury - supportive care with chest physiotherapy or diaphragmatic plication in severe cases;

  g) inadequate oxygen delivery or ventilation:
     i) increase FiO_2 or PEEP for a low PaO_2;
     ii) increase RR or TV for a low $PaCO_2$;
     iii) manual ventilation for ventilator malfunction;
     iv) reposition endotracheal tube (ideally 2cm above the carina);
     v) low cardiac output syndrome - optimise preload, contractility and afterload;
     vi) anaemia - give blood if haemoglobin is <8g/dL.

24 What are the criteria that suggest a diagnosis of adult respiratory distress syndrome (ARDS)?

- Acute onset of severe hypoxia refractory to oxygen therapy, with a PaO_2: FiO_2 ratio of <200mmHg.
- Bilateral infiltrates on the chest radiograph.
- Absence of cardiogenic pulmonary oedema (pulmonary capillary wedge pressure <18mmHg).
- Reduced pulmonary compliance.
- Predisposing aetiology such as cardiopulmonary bypass, sepsis, aspiration, trauma and fat embolism.

25 What are the effects of cardiopulmonary bypass on postoperative fluid balance?

● Excess fluid in the interstitial space secondary to:

a) increased capillary permeability caused by systemic inflammatory response;

b) vasodilation, caused by rewarming;

c) reduced intravascular oncotic pressure, caused by haemodilution of plasma proteins and increased capillary leak.

● Increased total body fluid secondary to:

a) cardiopulmonary bypass prime volume (1.5-2.0L);

b) activation of the renin-angiotensin system, resulting in water retention;

c) anti-diuretic hormone production, stimulated by intravascular hypovolaemia (excess fluid in the interstitial space), resulting in water retention;

d) stress response producing cortisol, resulting in sodium and water retention.

26 What are the risk factors for renal impairment in the immediate postoperative period?

● Pre-operative risk factors:

a) pre-operative creatinine >150μmol/L;

b) increasing age;

c) left ventricular dysfunction;

d) emergency operations;

e) low cardiac output states (post-MI or mechanical complications of MI);

f) hypertension;

g) diabetes mellitus;

h) renal artery disease;

i) sepsis;

j) pre-operative nephrotoxins, such as contrast dye, gentamicin, non-steroidal anti-inflammatory drugs and angiotensin-converting enzyme inhibitors.

- Intra-operative risk factors:

  a) prolonged cardiopulmonary bypass time;
  b) periods of systemic hypoperfusion or circulatory arrest;
  c) aprotinin therapy.

- Postoperative risk factors:

  a) acute tubular necrosis caused by hypovolaemia or low cardiac output syndrome;
  b) excessive vasoconstriction;
  c) sepsis;
  d) nephrotoxins (as above).

- Normal values of renal function vary depending on the laboratory:

  a) serum creatinine 60-120μmol/L;
  b) serum urea 3.5-6.5mmol/L;
  c) creatinine clearance 90-140mL/min;
  d) glomerular filtration rate 90-140mL/min.

- Creatinine clearance can be measured with 24-hour urine collection or estimated using the Cockcroft-Gault formula:

  a) actual creatinine clearance $= \dfrac{U_{Cr} \times U_{vol}}{P_{Cr} \times 24 \times 60}$

  b) estimated creatinine clearance for men
  $= \dfrac{(140\text{-age}) \times \text{wt in kg}}{72 \times P_{Cr}}$

  c) estimated creatinine clearance for women
  $= \dfrac{0.85 \times (140\text{-age}) \times \text{wt in kg}}{72 \times P_{Cr}}$

  where U_{Cr} = urinary creatinine concentration, U_{vol} = urine volume over 24 hours, P_{Cr} = plasma creatinine (in mg/dL).

27 What are the principles of managing established renal failure in the immediate postoperative period?

- Identify and treat the underlying cause, if feasible (consider a renal ultrasound).
- Optimise the patient's haemodynamic status, especially to restore the pre-operative mean arterial pressure.

- Monitor daily weights and fluid balance.
- Monitor electrolytes, acid-base status and glucose levels.
- Eliminate nephrotoxic drugs.
- Adjust drugs that are excreted by the kidney, such as digoxin and antibiotics.
- Consider removing the urinary catheter if the patient is anuric.
- Renal replacement therapy to treat hyperkalaemia, acidosis, volume overload or uraemia.

28 What are the principles of renal replacement therapy?

- There are two common techniques used in patients after cardiac surgery:

a) haemodialysis. Blood and crystalloid fluid flow on either side of a semi-permeable membrane, thereby allowing solutes to be removed by diffusion, with molecules moving from a higher to a lower concentration. Larger molecules are not efficiently removed as smaller molecules move faster. Fluid in the dialysis compartment moves in a counter-current direction, thereby maintaining a concentration gradient;

b) haemofiltration. Water is pushed across a filter by a pressure gradient and carries dissolved solutes with it (solute drag). Larger molecules (up to 20,000MW) are removed at a similar rate.

- Both require double-lumen central venous access.
- Although arteriovenous renal replacement therapy is also possible, it is rarely performed in patients with a low cardiac output state as it is dependent on arterial pressure.
- As circulating inflammatory mediators are also removed from the plasma, the patient may not exhibit a pyrexial reaction in the presence of sepsis.
- Although renal replacement therapy can be performed without anticoagulation, heparin is usually used to reduce the risk of the filter or membrane clotting.
- In patients with hypotension, renal replacement therapy may not be possible because of large fluid shifts.

29 What are the causes of hypothermia during cardiac surgery?

- Peripheral vasodilation, caused by anaesthetic agents.
- Reduced metabolic heat production.

- Increased heat loss.
- Thermoregulatory threshold lowered by 3-4°C during general anaesthesia.
- Neuromuscular blocking drugs prevent shivering.
- Cooling effect of cold anaesthetic gases.
- Cooling effect of cold intravenous fluid infusion.
- Active cooling on cardiopulmonary bypass using a heat exchanger.

30 What are the effects of hypothermia in the immediate postoperative period following cardiac surgery?

- Vasoconstriction, causing increased cardiac afterload and therefore myocardial oxygen consumption.
- Increased risk of arrhythmias.
- Coagulopathy.
- Left shift of the oxygen dissociation curve, thereby impairing tissue oxygen delivery.
- Increased postoperative stress response, producing hyperglycaemia.

459

Recommended reading

1. Westaby S, Pillai R, Parry A, O'Regan D, Giannopoulos N, Grebenik K, Sinclair M, Fisher A. Does modern cardiac surgery require conventional intensive care? *Eur J Cardiothorac Surg* 1993; 7: 313-8.

2. Fry AC, Farrington K. Management of acute renal failure. *Postgrad Med J* 2006; 82(964): 106-16.

3. Field ML, Rengarajan A, Khan O, Spyt T, Richens D. Preoperative intra-aortic balloon pumps in patients undergoing coronary artery bypass grafting. *Cochrane Database Syst Rev* 2007; 24(1): CD004472.

Chapter 22

Postoperative management

1   **What are the causes of postoperative hypertension?**
- Anxiety and pain.
- Inotropes (dopamine, noradrenaline, adrenaline, vasopressin).
- Vasoconstriction and shivering from hypothermia.
- Hyperdynamic syndrome following aortic valve replacement or coronary artery bypass grafting (following afterload reduction or revascularisation, respectively).
- Abnormal baroreceptor function following aortic dissection.
- Autonomic neuropathy associated with diabetes.

2   **What are the commonest arrhythmias in the postoperative period?**
- Sinus tachycardia.
- Atrial fibrillation.
- Heart block (especially following valve surgery).
- Ventricular and atrial ectopics.
- Ventricular tachycardia.
- Sinus bradycardia.

3   **What are the causes of sinus tachycardia following cardiac surgery?**
- Withdrawal of β-blockade.
- Fever and sepsis.
- Anxiety and pain.
- Hypovolaemia.
- Inotropes (dopamine, noradrenaline, adrenaline, isoprenaline).
- Anaemia.

4   **What are the causes of acidosis following cardiac surgery?**
●   Metabolic acidosis:

    a)   reduced tissue perfusion producing lactic acidosis, secondary to:
        i)   hypovolaemia;
        ii)   low cardiac output;
        iii)   myocardial dysfunction;
        iv)   excessive vasoconstriction (noradrenaline, vasopressin, methylene blue, hypothermia);
        v)   sepsis;
    b)   increased metabolic activity (adrenaline, sepsis);
    c)   renal impairment (failure to excrete hydrogen ions);
    d)   splanchnic or limb ischaemia (excess production of hydrogen ions);
    e)   endocrine - hyperglycaemia, thyrotoxic crisis.

●   Respiratory acidosis - CO_2 retention.

5   **What are the principles of managing acidosis post-cardiac surgery?**
●   Identify the underlying cause:

    a)   assess for clinical aetiology as described above (e.g. volume status, temperature, inotropy, urine output);
    b)   determine pH, pCO_2, base excess, lactate, anion gap, blood glucose, urinary ketones, phosphate.

●   Treat the underlying cause:

    a)   increase the respiratory rate or tidal volume (i.e. minute volume to increase CO_2 expiration) to treat respiratory acidosis;
    b)   optimise cardiac output;
    c)   reduce noradrenaline and adrenaline if possible;
    d)   restore normothermia with a warming blanket;
    e)   optimise renal function with volume, furosemide or dopamine;
    f)   consider sodium bicarbonate (50mL 8.4%) or dialysis.

6   **What are the causes of hyperkalaemia following cardiac surgery?**
●   Excess intravenous or oral potassium administration.
●   Potassium-sparing diuretics (e.g. amiloride).
●   Aldosterone antagonist (e.g. spironolactone).
●   Angiotensin-converting enzyme inhibitors (ACEIs) or angiotensin receptor blockers (ARBs).

- Reduced renal excretion of potassium with renal failure or oliguria.
- Tissue ischaemia causing increased potassium release from cells.

7 **How is hyperkalaemia treated following cardiac surgery?**
- Re-check the serum potassium level (ensure the sample is not haemolysed).
- Cardiac monitoring.
- Reduce potassium uptake:

  a) stop potassium-sparing medications (ACEI, ARB, aldosterone antagonists);
  b) stop potassium supplementation (oral and intravenous);
  c) calcium resonium® to reduce gastro-intestinal absorption of potassium.

- Increase potassium movement from plasma into the cells:

  a) insulin (give 50mL 50% dextrose and 15U insulin IV);
  b) sodium bicarbonate;
  c) aerosolized β-agonist.

- Increase potassium excretion:

  a) loop diuretic (e.g. furosemide);
  b) dialysis.

- Calcium gluconate (myocyte membrane stabiliser).

8 **What are the causes of hypokalaemia following cardiac surgery?**
- Diuresis without potassium supplementation.
- Insulin.
- Alkalosis.
- Excessive nasogastric drainage.

9 **How is hypokalaemia treated following cardiac surgery?**
- Re-check the serum potassium level.
- Cardiac monitoring.
- Increase potassium uptake:

  a) potassium-sparing medications (e.g. ACEI, ARB, aldosterone antagonists);
  b) potassium supplementation (e.g. oral and intravenous).

- Reduce potassium movement from plasma into the cells (caused by insulin and aerosolized β-agonist).
- Reduce potassium excretion caused by loop diuretics (e.g. furosemide).

10 What are the causes of hyponatraemia following cardiac surgery?

- Hypervolaemic hyponatraemia:

  a) excess 5% dextrose administered as maintenance fluid;
  b) renal failure.

- Euvolaemic hyponatraemia:

  a) syndrome of inappropriate anti-diuretic hormone (SIADH) which can be diagnosed by:
     i) urinary sodium >20mmol/L;
     ii) serum sodium <130mmol/L;
     iii) serum osmolality <270mOsm/kg;
     iv) urinary osmolality >100mOsm/L;
     v) normal serum potassium and bicarbonate.

- Hypovolaemic hyponatraemia:

  a) thiazide diuretics;
  b) angiotensin-converting enzyme inhibitors (ACEIs);
  c) angiotensin receptor blockers (ARBs);
  b) diarrhoea and vomiting.

11 How is hyponatraemia treated following cardiac surgery?

- Management depends on the underlying cause and volume status.
- Hypervolaemic hyponatraemia:

  a) fluid restriction (1-1.5L/day);
  b) replace any 5% dextrose with normal hypertonic saline;
  c) loop diuretics may be used to excrete free water.

- Euvolaemic hyponatraemia:

  a) demeclocycline which reduces the effect of ADH on the distal renal tubules;

b)   arginine vasopressin antagonist (e.g. Conivaptan), which increases free water renal excretion;

c)   sodium supplements (slow Na).

- Hypovolaemic hyponatraemia:

a)   stop ACEI, ARB and thiazide diuretics;

b)   fluid replacement with normal saline.

12 What are the causes of hypernatraemia following cardiac surgery?

- Pure water depletion - diabetes insipidus.
- Water depletion exceeding sodium depletion - diarrhoea.
- Sodium excess - excess normal saline.
- Drugs - amphotericin, phenytoin, lithium, gentamicin.

13 How is hypernatraemia treated following cardiac surgery?

- Check urine and plasma sodium and osmolality.
- Treat the underlying cause.
- 5% dextrose.
- Vasopressin (anti-diuretic hormone) for diabetes insipidus.

14 What are the common causes of hypoxia in the immediate postoperative period?

- Atelectasis caused by:

a)   general anaesthesia;

b)   cardiopulmonary bypass secondary to:
   i)   inadequate surfactant from pulmonary hypoperfusion;
   ii)   small airway closure from vasoactive mediators;
   iii) increased interstitial oedema due to increased alveolar endothelial permeability;

c)   left internal mammary artery harvesting.

- Pleural effusion.
- Bronchospasm.
- Pneumonia.
- Pneumothorax.
- Cardiogenic pulmonary oedema.
- Non-cardiogenic interstitial pulmonary oedema caused by systemic inflammatory response syndrome (SIRS) secondary to complement

activation, cytokine release, oxygen-free radicals and blood transfusion products.

- Diaphragmatic dysfunction - phrenic nerve injury, which can be caused by iced pericardial slush or direct injury.

15 What are the common causes of oliguria in the immediate postoperative period?

- Pre-renal:

    a)   hypovolaemia (intravascular volume depletion);
    b)   low cardiac output;
    c)   renal artery disease - especially following aortic dissection.

- Renal:

    a)   pre-operative renal disease - hypertensive, diabetic, contrast nephropathy;
    b)   nephrotoxic drugs - gentamicin, non-steroidal anti-inflammatory drugs;
    c)   cardiopulmonary bypass-induced nephropathy;
    d)   sepsis.

- Post-renal - rare as most patients are catheterised but may be caused by blockage or kinking of the urinary catheter.

16 How is oliguria managed?

- Ensure the urinary catheter is patent.
- Optimise myocardial function to ensure adequate renal perfusion:

    a)   preload - fluid boluses;
    b)   improve contractility with inotropes;
    c)   reduce elevated afterload;
    d)   manage any dysrhythmias;
    e)   intra-aortic balloon pump if necessary.

- Diuretics - initially with boluses followed by an infusion if unsuccessful.
- Renal-dose dopamine (1-5μg/kg/min).
- Renal dialysis for hyperkalaemia, acidosis, excessive fluid retention (e.g. pulmonary oedema).

17 What are the principles of enteral feeding in cardiac surgical patients?

- Most cardiac surgical patients require approximately 25kCal/kg/day.
- Patients in a catabolic state (such as with multi-organ failure) have increased nutritional requirements (approximately 30kCal/kg/day).
- Enteral (nasogastric) feeding should be commenced if a patient is not extubated or is not able to eat within 48 hours of surgery.
- Standard feeds provide 1-1.2kCal/mL with high-energy feeds providing 1.5-2kCal/mL.
- Patients with renal failure require low-protein feeds, except those requiring renal replacement therapy, who require high-protein feeds (as haemofiltration and haemodialysis remove protein). These patients also require high-energy (low volume) and low-electrolyte feeds.
- Enteral feeding is usually given over 16-20 hours with a 4-8-hour rest period.
- Total parenteral nutrition should be used if the patient is not absorbing or if there is any contra-indication to enteral feeding.

18 What are the principles of managing sternal wound infections post-cardiac surgery?

- Prevention:

  a) antibiotic prophylaxis - cefuroxime administered 30 minutes before incision or vancomycin if the patient is at risk of methicillin-resistant *Staphylococcus aureus* (MRSA);
  b) infection control - avoid cross-contamination between patients.

- Isolate the organism and treat with the appropriate antibiotic therapy.
- Superficial sternal wound infection can be treated with drainage but may require vacuum-assisted closure (VAC) pump insertion.
- Deep sternal wound infection and mediastinitis, however, requires:

  a) sternal debridement and VAC pump insertion or closure with a continuous irrigation system;
  b) antibiotic therapy tailored to the infecting organism;
  c) sternal reconstruction is performed once inflammatory markers have normalised and the infecting organism has been eradicated as demonstrated by negative microbiological swabs, with:
  i) sternal rewiring;
  ii) pectoral advancement flaps;
  iii) plastic surgical flap reconstruction using latissimus dorsi, pectoralis major, rectus abdominis or the omentum.

19 What are the standard anticoagulation regimes following cardiac surgery?

- According to the American Heart Association (AHA) guidelines, the following INRs (international normalized ratios) are recommended using warfarin:

   a)   coronary endarterectomy - 2.0-3.0;
   b)   atrial fibrillation - 2.0-3.0;
   c)   mechanical aortic valve - 2.0-3.0;
   d)   mechanical mitral valve - 2.5-3.5.

- For patients with bioprosthetic valves, aspirin alone can be used or 3 months of warfarin (with optimal INR 2.0-3.0) followed by aspirin alone.

20 What medications are important for secondary prevention of coronary artery disease?

- Aspirin (antiplatelet agent), which reduces the risk of subsequent coronary thrombosis.
- Statin (HMG CoA reductase inhibitor), which reduces hepatic production of cholesterol and subsequent deposition in the coronary arteries and vein grafts.
- β-blocker, which decreases left ventricular work by reducing left ventricular contractility and afterload.
- Angiotensin-converting enzyme inhibitor, which reduces left ventricular afterload and encourages left ventricular reverse remodelling.

Recommended reading

1.   Bonow RO, Carabello BA, Kanu C, de Leon AC Jr, Faxon DP, Freed MD, Gaasch WH, Lytle BW, Nishimura RA, O'Gara PT, O'Rourke RA, Otto CM, Shah PM, Shanewise JS, Smith SC Jr, Jacobs AK, Adams CD, Anderson JL, Antman EM, Faxon DP, Fuster V, Halperin JL, Hiratzka LF, Hunt SA, Lytle BW, Nishimura R, Page RL, Riegel B. ACC/AHA 2006 Guidelines for the management of patients with valvular heart disease. *Circulation* 2006; 114; e84-e231.

2.   Smith SC Jr, Allen J, Blair SN, Bonow RO, Brass LM, Fonarow GC, Grundy SM, Hiratzka L, Jones D, Krumholz HM, Mosca L, Pasternak RC, Pearson T, Pfeffer MA, Taubert KA; AHA/ACC; National Heart, Lung, and Blood Institute. AHA/ACC Guidelines for secondary prevention for patients with coronary and other atherosclerotic vascular disease: 2006 update: endorsed by the National Heart, Lung, and Blood Institute. *Circulation* 2006; 113(19): 2363-72.

Appendix I

Transoesophageal echocardiographic views

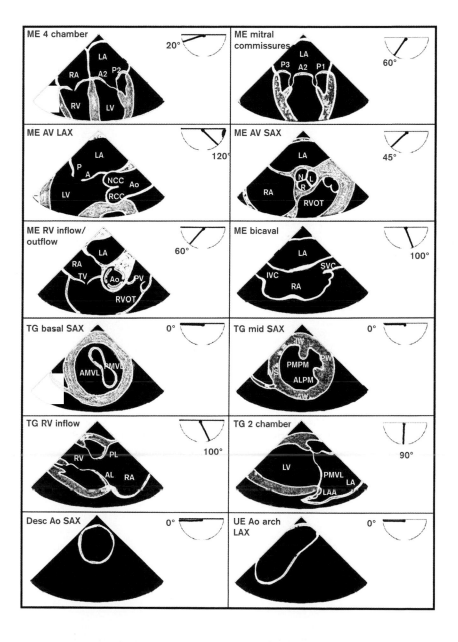

Appendix II

Transthoracic echocardiographic views

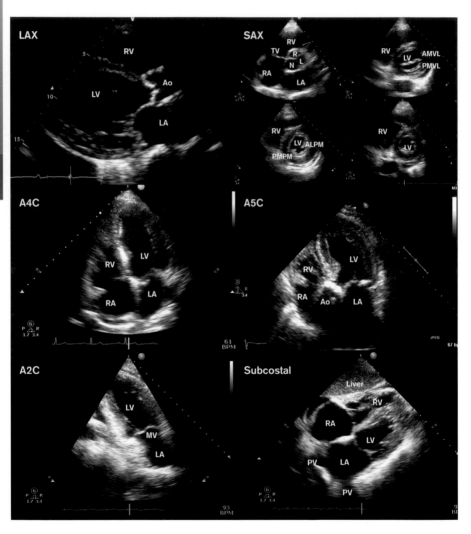

Appendix III

Normal echocardiographic values

	Diastole	Systole
Left ventricular internal diameter (cm)	3.5-5.6	2.0-4.0
Posterior wall thickness (cm)	0.6-1.2	0.9-1.8
Interventricular septum (cm)	0.6-1.2	0.9-1.8
Right ventricle (cm)	1.9-2.6	1.2-1.8

	Normal range
Left ventricular ejection fraction (%)	50-80
Fractional shortening (%)	25-45
Left ventricular mass index (g/m^2)	44-102
Right ventricular ejection fraction (%)	45-60
Aortic root (cm)	2.0-4.0
Left atrium (cm)	2.0-4.0
Left ventricular end-diastolic volume (mL)	80-140
Left ventricular end-systolic volume (mL)	25-65

Appendix IV

Standard coronary angiographic views

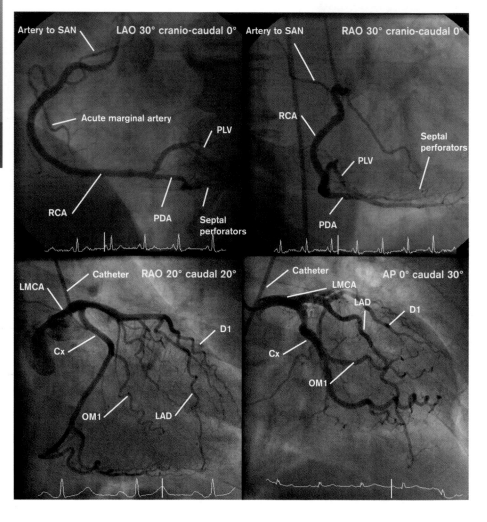

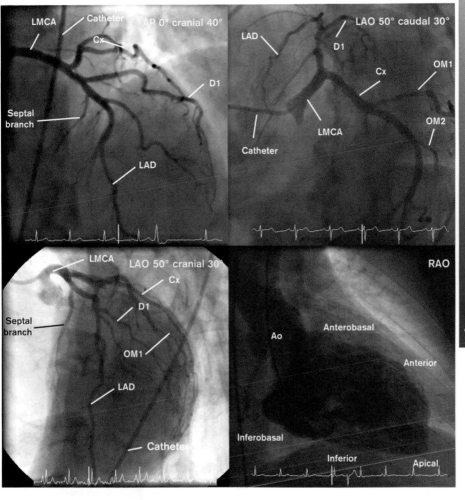

Appendix V

Normal arterial blood gas values

pH	7.35-7.45
PaO_2	10-13.3kPa; 75-100mmHg
$PaCO_2$	4.7-6.0kPa; 35-45mmHg
Bicarbonate	22-26mmol/L
Base excess	-2 to +2mmol/L
Lactate	0.5-2mmol/L
Potassium	3.5-5mmol/L
Ionised calcium	1.15-1.29mmol/L
Glucose	3.3-5.6mmol/L (fasting)

Appendix VI

Normal cardiac physiological values

	Abbreviation	Formula	Normal range
Systolic blood pressure	SBP		90-140mmHg
Diastolic blood pressure	DBP		60-90mmHg
Mean arterial blood pressure	MAP	[(SBP - DBP)/3] + DBP	70-105mmHg
Left atrial pressure	LAP		6-12mmHg
Central venous (right atrial) pressure	CVP		2-6mmHg
Arterial oxygen saturation	SaO_2		95-100%
Mixed venous saturation	SvO_2		60-80%
Pulmonary artery systolic pressure	PASP		15-30mmHg
Pulmonary artery diastolic pressure	PADP		5-15mmHg
Mean pulmonary artery pressure	MPAP	[(PASP - PADP)/3] + PADP	10-20mmHg
Pulmonary artery wedge pressure	PAWP		6-12mmHg
Systemic vascular resistance	SVR	80 x (MAP - CVP) / CO	900-1600 dyne/sec/cm^5
Systemic vascular resistance index	SVRI	SVR / BSA	1970-2390 dyne/sec/cm^5/m^2
Pulmonary vascular resistance	PVR	80 x (MPAP - PAWP) / CO	155-255 dyne/sec/cm^5
Pulmonary vascular resistance index	PVRI	PVR / BSA	255-285 dyne/sec/cm^5/m^2
Heart rate	HR		60-100 bpm
Stroke volume	SV		70-90mL (1mL/kg)
Cardiac output	CO	SV X HR	4-8L/min
Cardiac index	CI	CO / BSA	2.5-4L/min/m^2

for resistances, to convert into woods units, divide dyne/sec/cm^5 by 80

Appendix VII

AHA guidelines for quantifying the severity of valvular disease

Aortic stenosis	Mild	Moderate	Severe
Aortic valve area (cm^2)	1.5-2.5	1.0-1.5	<1.0
Mean pressure gradient (mmHg)	15-25	25-40	>40
Peak velocity (m/s)	<3.0	3.0-4.0	>4.0
Aortic regurgitation	**Mild**	**Moderate**	**Severe**
Jet width (% LVOT diameter)	<25%	25-65%	>65%
Vena contracta (cm)	<0.3	0.3-0.6	>0.6
Regurgitant volume (mL)	<30	30-60	>60
Regurgitant fraction	<30	30-50	>50
Effective regurgitant orifice area (cm^2)	<0.1	0.1-0.3	>0.3
Mitral stenosis	**Mild**	**Moderate**	**Severe**
Mitral valve area (cm^2)	>1.5	1.0-1.5	<1.0
Mean pressure gradient (mmHg)	<5	5-10	>10
Pulmonary artery systolic pressure (mmHg)	<30	30-50	>50
Mitral regurgitation	**Mild**	**Moderate**	**Severe**
Jet area (% LA area)	<20%	20-40%	>40%
Vena contracta (cm)	<0.3	0.3-0.7	>0.7
Regurgitant volume (mL)	<30	30-60	>60
Regurgitant fraction (%)	<30	30-50	>50
Effective regurgitant orifice area (cm^2)	<0.2	0.2-0.4	>0.4

Appendix VIII

EuroSCORE

Patient-related factors		Score
Age	(per 5 years or part thereof over 60 years)	1
Gender	Female	1
Chronic pulmonary disease	Long-term use of bronchodilators or steroids for lung disease	1
Extracardiac arteriopathy	Any one or more of the following: claudication, carotid occlusion or >50% stenosis, previous or planned intervention on the abdominal aorta, limb arteries or carotids	2
Neurological dysfunction	Disease severely affecting ambulation or day-to-day functioning	2
Previous cardiac surgery	Requiring opening of the pericardium	3
Serum creatinine	>200µmol/L pre-operatively	2
Active endocarditis	Patient still under antibiotic treatment for endocarditis at the time of surgery	3
Critical pre-operative state	Any one or more of the following: ventricular tachycardia or fibrillation or aborted sudden death, pre-operative cardiac massage, pre-operative ventilation before arrival in the anaesthetic room, pre-operative inotropic support, intra-aortic balloon counterpulsation or pre-operative acute renal failure (anuria or oliguria <10mL/hour)	3
Cardiac-related factors		**Score**
Unstable angina	Rest angina requiring IV nitrates until arrival in the anaesthetic room	2
LV dysfunction	Moderate LV (EF 30-50%)	1
	Poor LV (EF <30%)	3
Recent myocardial infarct	<90 days	2
Pulmonary hypertension	Systolic PA pressure >60 mmHg	2
Operation-related factors		**Score**
Emergency	Carried out on referral before the beginning of the next working day	2
Other than isolated CABG	Major cardiac procedure other than or in addition to CABG	2
Surgery on thoracic aorta	For disorder of ascending, arch or descending aorta	3
Post-infarct septal rupture		4

Index